Applied Dental Materials

Eighth Edition

J.F. McCabe
BSc, PhD, DSc
Professor of Dental Materials Science
University of Newcastle upon Tyne

A.W.G. Walls
BDS, PhD, FDSRCS
Professor of Restorative Dentistry
University of Newcastle upon Tyne

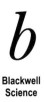

**Blackwell
Science**

© 1956, 1961, 1967, 1972, 1976, 1985, 1990, 1998 by
Blackwell Science Ltd
Editorial Offices:
Osney Mead, Oxford OX2 0EL
25 John Street, London WC1N 2BL
23 Ainslie Place, Edinburgh EH3 6AJ
350 Main Street, Malden
  MA 02148 5018, USA
54 University Street, Carlton
  Victoria 3053, Australia
10, rue Casimir Delavigne
  75006 Paris, France

Other Editorial Offices:

Blackwell Wissenschafts-Verlag GmbH
Kurfürstendamm 57
10707 Berlin, Germany

Blackwell Science KK
MG Kodenmacho Building
7–10 Kodenmacho Nihombashi
Chuo-ku, Tokyo 104, Japan

The right of the Author to be identified as the Author of
this Work has been asserted in accordance with the
Copyright, Designs and Patents Act 1988.

First published 1956
Second edtion 1961
Reprinted 1965
Third edition 1967
Fourth edition 1972
Fifth edition 1976
Sixth edition 1985
Reprinted 1987
Seventh edition 1990
Reprinted 1992, 1994, 1996, 1997
Four Dragons edition 1992
Reprinted 1994
Eighth edition 1998
Reprinted 1999

Set in 9/11 Times
by DP Photosetting, Aylesbury, Bucks
Printed and bound in the United Kingdom
at the University Press, Cambridge

The Blackwell Science logo is a
trade mark of Blackwell Science Ltd,
registered at the United Kingdom
Trade Marks Registry

DISTRIBUTORS

Marston Book Services Ltd
PO Box 269
Abingdon, Oxon OX14 4YN
(*Orders*: Tel: 01235 465500
           Fax: 01235 465555)

USA
Blackwell Science, Inc.
Commerce Place
350 Main Street
Malden, MA 02148 5018
(*Orders*: Tel: 800 759 6102
           781 388 8250
      Fax: 781 388 8255)

Canada
Login Brothers Book Company
324 Saulteaux Crescent
Winnipeg, Manitoba R3J 3T2
(*Orders*: Tel: 204 837-2987
      Fax: 204 837-3116)

Australia
Blackwell Science Pty Ltd
54 University Street
Carlton, Victoria 3053
(*Orders*: Tel: 03 9347 0300
      Fax: 03 9347 5001)

A catalogue record for this title
is available from the British Library

ISBN 0-632-04208-7

Library of Congress
Cataloging-in-Publication Data

McCabe, J.F. (John F.)
    Applied dental materials. – 8th ed./J.F. McCabe and
A.W.G. Walls.
      p.   cm.
    Includes bibliographical references and index.
    ISBN 0-632-04208-7
    1. Dental materials.   I. Walls, Angus.   II. Title.
    [DNLM: 1. Dental Materials.   WU 190 M477a 1998]
RK652.5.M38   1998
617.6′95 – dc21
DNLM/DLC
for Library of Congress   97-39634
                                                      CIP

For further information on
Blackwell Science, visit our website:
www.blackwell-science.com

Contents

Preface

As stated in the preface to the 7th edition, this textbook is written mainly with the undergraduate dental student in mind although it is hoped that many parts of the text will prove beneficial to dental technicians, dental surgery assistants and practising dentists. In order to improve the relevance of the book to the latter groups I am delighted that Professor Angus Walls has agreed to join me as a co-author in this edition. His contributions will be directed towards the clinical indications and handling of materials although it is hoped that the additional material will be closely integrated with the materials science.

As before, the layout is designed to provide a natural progression through an understanding of some simple principles of materials science by reviewing the materials primarily used in the laboratory and, finally, the products more normally used at chairside in the dental clinic.

I have been persuaded, at last, to remove the separate chapter on silicate cements since these are now only of historical influence. However, some consideration of the composition and properties of these materials is given in Chapter 20. It is important not to forget the lessons learned from our experiences with these traditional materials.

Most chapters have undergone alteration or modification compared with the previous edition – partly through the contributions of Angus Walls. In addition, full reference is now made to ISO Standards where appropriate and it is hoped that this will benefit researchers and test houses engaged in evaluating dental materials. The chapters on adhesion and ceramics have undergone major modification in order to reflect the advancements in these areas over recent years. The importance of glass ionomer cements is recognized through the introduction of a separate chapter for these materials. Additionally, the new family of products known as *resin-modified glass ionomers* have been awarded separate chapter status in recognition of their growing importance.

An attempt has been made to bring the reading list at the end of each chapter up to date and, where possible, to concentrate on review articles. At the request of many colleagues, these lists have been kept short.

Angus Walls and I hope you find the book helpful and readable.

John F. McCabe

Chapter 1
Science of Dental Materials

1.1 Introduction

The science of dental materials involves a study of the composition and properties of materials and the way in which they interact with the environment in which they are placed. The selection of materials for any given application can thus be undertaken with confidence and sound judgement.

The dentist spends much of his professional career handling materials and the success or failure of many forms of treatment depends upon the correct selection of materials possessing adequate properties, combined with careful manipulation.

It is no exaggeration to state that the dentist and dental technician have a wider variety of materials at their disposal than any other profession. Rigid polymers, elastomers, metals, alloys, ceramics, inorganic salts and composite materials are all commonly encountered. Some examples are given in Fig. 1.1 along with some of their uses in dentistry.

This classification of materials embodies an enormous variation in material properties from hard, rigid materials at one extreme to soft, flexible products at the other.

Many dental materials are fixed permanently into the patient's mouth or are removed only intermittently for cleaning. Such materials have to withstand the effects of a most hazardous environment. Temperature variations, wide variations in acidity or alkalinity and high stresses all have an effect on the durability of materials.

Normal temperature variations in the oral cavity lie between 32°C and 37°C depending on whether the mouth is open or closed. The ingestion of hot or cold food or drink however, extends this temperature range from 0°C up to 70°C. The acidity or alkalinity of fluids in the oral cavity as measured by pH varies from around pH 4 to pH 8.5, whilst the intake of acid fruit juices or alkaline medicaments can extend this range from pH 2 to pH 11.

The load on 1 mm^2 of tooth or restorative material can reach levels as high as many kilograms indicating the demanding mechanical property requirements of some materials.

Many products, for example direct filling materials, are handled entirely by the dentist and his chairside assistant and are rarely encountered by the dental technician. Other materials are generally associated with the work of the dental laboratory and in this case both technician and dentist require a thorough knowledge of the materials in order that they may communicate about selection, manipulation and any problems which arise. A third group of materials link the dental surgery and the laboratory. The most obvious example of such products is the impression materials. Whilst the latter are under the direct control of the dentist it is essential that the dental technician also has a sound knowledge of such materials.

1.2 Selection of dental materials

The process of materials selection should ideally follow a logical sequence involving (1) analysis of the problem, (2) consideration of requirements, (3) consideration of available materials and their properties, leading to (4) choice of material. Evaluation of the success or failure of a material may be used to influence future decisions on materials selection. This selection process is illustrated in Fig. 1.2. Many experienced practitioners carry out this sequence with no apparent effort since they are able to call upon a wealth of clinical experience. However, when presented with new or modified materials even the most experienced dentist should return to a more formal type of selection process based on the criteria mentioned.

Analysis: The analysis of the situation requiring selection of a material may seem obvious but it is of paramount importance in some circumstances. An incorrect decision may cause failure of the restora-

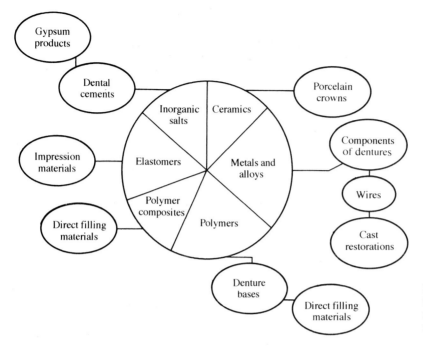

Fig. 1.1 Diagram indicating the wide variety of materials used in dentistry and some of their applications.

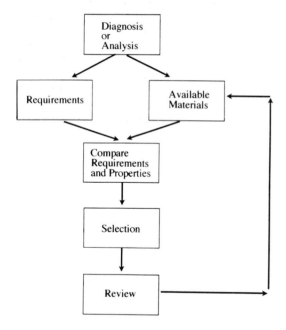

Fig. 1.2 Flow chart indicating a logical method of material selection.

tion or appliance. For example, when considering the selection of a filling material it is important to decide whether the restoration is to be placed in an area of high stress. Will it be visible when the patient smiles? Is the cavity deep or shallow? These factors and

many more must be evaluated before attempting materials selection.

Requirements: Having completed a thorough analysis of the situation it is possible to develop a list of requirements for a material to meet the needs of that situation. For the example mentioned in the previous section, it may be decided that a filling material which matches tooth colour and is able to withstand moderately high stresses without fracture is required. Some tooth cavities are caused by toothbrush/ toothpaste abrasion. In this special case the restorative material used should naturally possess adequate resistance to dentifrice abrasion. Hence, it is possible to build a profile of the ideal properties required for the application being considered.

Available materials: The consideration of available materials, their properties and how these compare with the requirements is carried out at two levels. The dentist, faced with the immediate problem of restoring the tooth of a patient in his surgery, must choose from those materials on hand at the time. Previous experience with materials in similar circumstances will be a major factor which influences selection. On a wider scale, the practitioner is able to consider the use of alternative materials or newly developed products where these appear to offer a solution to cases which have proved difficult with his existing armoury of products. It is of paramount importance that the practitioner keeps up to date with developments in materials whilst taking a conservative approach towards adopting new products for regular use in his surgery until they are properly tested.

Choice of material: Having compared the properties of the available materials with the requirement, it is possible to narrow the choice to a given generic group of products. The final choice of material brand is often a matter of personal preference on the part of the dentist. Factors such as ease of handling, availability and cost may play a part at this stage of the selection process.

1.3 Evaluation of materials

As the number of available materials increases, it becomes more and more important for the dentist to be protected from unsuitable products or materials which have not been thoroughly evaluated. It should be emphasized, however, that most manufacturers of dental materials operate an extensive quality assurance programme and materials are thoroughly tested before being released to the general practitioner.

Standard specifications: Many standard specification tests, of both national and international standards organizations, are now available which effectively maintain quality levels for some dental materials. Such specifications normally give details for the testing of certain products, the method of calculating the results of the minimum permissible result which

is acceptable. Although such specifications play a useful part they should not be seen as indicating total suitability since the tests carried out often do not cover critical aspects of the use of a material. For example, many materials fail by a fatigue mechanism in practice, but few specifications involve fatigue testing.

Laboratory evaluations: Laboratory tests, some of which are used in standard specifications, can be used to indicate the suitability of certain materials. For example, a simple solubility test can indicate the stability of a material in aqueous media – a very important property for filling materials.

It is important that methods used to evaluate materials in the laboratory give results which can be correlated with clinical experience. For example, when upper dentures fracture along the midline they do so through bending. Hence a bending or transverse strength test is far more meaningful for denture base materials than a compression test.

Clinical trials: Although laboratory tests can provide important and useful data on materials the ultimate test is the controlled clinical trial and the verdict of practitioners after a period of use in general practice. Many materials produce good results in the laboratory, only to be found lacking when subjected to clinical use. The majority of manufacturers carry out extensive clinical trials of new materials, normally in co-operation with a university or hospital department prior to releasing a product for use by general practitioners.

Chapter 2
Properties used to Characterize Materials

2.1 Introduction

Many factors must be taken into account when considering which properties are relevant to the successful performance of a material used in dentistry. The situation in which the material is to be used and the recommended technique for its manipulation define the properties which characterize the material. Laboratory tests used to evaluate materials often duplicate conditions which exist *in situ*. This is not always possible and sometimes not desirable since one aim of *in vitro* testing is to predict in a rapid laboratory test what may happen in the mouth over a number of months or years. Many tests used to evaluate dental materials involve the measurement of simple properties such as compressive strength or hardness which have been shown to correlate with clinical performance.

Many materials used in dentistry are supplied as two or more components which are mixed together and undergo a chemical reaction, during which the mechanical and physical properties may change dramatically. For example, many impression materials are supplied as fluid pastes which begin to set when mixed together. The set material may be a rigid solid or a flexible rubber depending upon the chemical nature of the product.

The acceptance of such a product by the dentist depends upon the properties of the unmixed paste, the properties during mixing and setting and the properties of the set material (Fig. 2.1). This classification of properties applies to virtually all groups of materials.

Properties of unmixed materials: Manufacturers formulate materials which give optimal performance as evaluated by their quality assurance programme and clinical trials. It is known however, that certain products deteriorate during storage and as a result may perform poorly. Such materials are said to have

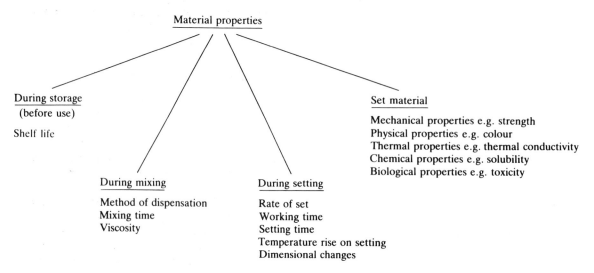

Fig. 2.1 An indication of the properties which are used to characterize dental materials.

limited *shelf life*. Some materials have an extended shelf life if refrigerated during storage. One technique commonly employed to predict stability is to carry out accelerated ageing by storing samples at elevated temperature, commonly 60°C, followed by evaluation of material properties.

Containers used for materials generally have a batch number stamped or printed onto them from which the date of manufacture can be obtained. Thus, for materials with limited shelf life it is possible to ascertain the date at which one would expect the properties to deteriorate.

Properties of materials during mixing, manipulation and setting: Properties of materials during mixing, manipulation and setting are considered together since they mainly involve a consideration of rheological properties and the way in which these change as a function of time during setting.

For materials of two or more components which set by a chemical reaction, thorough mixing is essential in order to achieve homogeneous distribution of properties throughout the material. The ease of mixing depends on factors such as the chemical affinity of the components, the viscosity, both of the components and the mixed material, the ambient temperature, the method of dispensation and the method of mixing.

Several methods of dispensation exist among materials used in dentistry. Some involve the mixing of powder and liquid components, others the mixing of two pastes, while others involve paste and liquid components. When the mixing of two pastes is required, the manufacturer often gives a good colour contrast between the two pastes. The achievement of a thorough mix of the two components can be judged by the attainment of a homogeneous colour with no streaks. When powder and liquid or paste and liquid are mixed, the achievement of a thorough mix is less certain. The components are mixed for a recommended time and/or until a recommended consistency is reached.

A growing number of materials are mixed mechanically. This method removes uncertainty and gives a more reproducible result.

The use of encapsulated materials which are mixed mechanically is becoming very popular. These offer the dual advantages of easier and more reproducible mixing coupled with pre-set proportions of components within the capsules.

Certain products have specified manipulative requirements which will be referred to later. For many applications, materials should be in a relatively fluid state at the time they are introduced into the patient's mouth but should undergo rapid setting involving a change to a more rigid or rubbery form. From the commencement of mixing, two important times can be defined which have an important bearing on the acceptability of materials. The first is the *working time*, defined as the time available for mixing and manipulating a material. For example, an impression material should be seated in the mouth before the end of the working time otherwise setting will have proceeded sufficiently for the viscosity to have increased considerably. The other time which characterizes setting is the *setting time*. This, like working time, is to some extent arbitrary since it is defined as the time taken for a material to have reached a certain level of rigidity or elasticity. It is known that many materials continue setting for a considerable time after the apparent setting and optimum properties may not be achieved until several hours later.

Properties of the set material: The properties of the unmixed material and those during mixing and setting are important and may influence the practitioner's selection. Generally, it is the properties of the set material which indicate the suitability of a product for any application. For example, in the case of a filling material, the method of dispensation, viscosity of the mixed material, working time and setting time control the ease of handling of the product, but the durability of the material in the oral environment depends on factors such as strength, solubility, abrasion resistance, etc. The properties of the set material can be conveniently divided into the following categories: mechanical properties, thermal properties, chemical properties, biological properties and miscellaneous other physical properties. Naturally, the properties relevant to any one material will depend on the application.

2.2 Mechanical properties

Most applications of materials in dentistry have a minimum mechanical property requirement. For example, certain materials should be sufficiently strong and tough to withstand biting forces without fracture. Others should be rigid enough to maintain their shape under load. Such properties of materials are generally characterized by the stress–strain relationship which is readily obtained by using a testing machine of the type shown in Fig. 2.2.

Before considering the various types of experiment which can be carried out and the relevance of the data obtained, it is necessary to define the terms stress and strain.

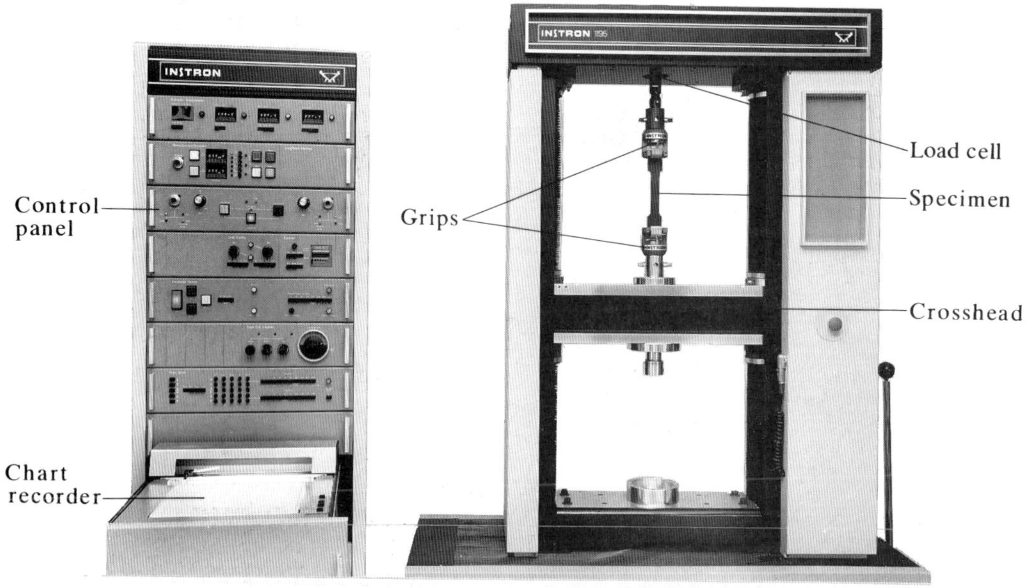

Fig. 2.2 Testing machine used for evaluating mechanical properties. Photograph shows the machine in the *tensile mode.*

Stress: When an external force is applied to a body or specimen of material under test, an internal force, equal in magnitude but opposite in direction, is set up in the body. For simple compression or tension the stress is given by the expression, Stress = F/A, where F is the applied force and A the cross-sectional area (Fig. 2.3). A stress resisting a compressive force is referred to as a compressive stress and that resisting a tensile force a tensile stress.

Tensile and compressive stresses, along with shear, are the three simple examples of stress which form the basis of all other more complex stress patterns. The unit of stress is the pascal (Pa). This is the stress resulting from a force of 1 Newton (N) acting upon one square metre of surface. Whereas the tensile stress can be visualized as a purely uni-axial stress set up within a material, the compressive stress is more complex and comprises force vectors which act to introduce elements of shear within the specimen under compression.

One test method commonly used for dental materials is the three-point bending test or transverse test (Fig. 2.4).

When an external force is applied to the midpoint of the test beam the stresses can be resolved as shown. The numerical value of stress is given by the expression

$$\text{Stress} = \frac{3FL}{2bd^2}$$

where L is the distance between the supports, b is the width of the specimen and d its depth.

When a cylinder of a brittle material is compressed across a diameter as shown in Fig. 2.5a, a tensile stress is set up in the specimen, the value of the stress being given by

$$\text{Stress} = \frac{2F}{\pi DT} \text{ at the axis of the cylinder}$$

where F is the applied force, D the diameter of the cylinder and T the length of the cylinder. This type of test is referred to as a diametral compressive tensile test and is commonly used when conventional tensile testing is difficult to carry out due to the brittle nature of the test material. For non-brittle materials the equation used to calculate stress breaks down due to the increased area of contact between the testing machine platen and the material under test (Fig. 2.5b).

Fracture stress – strength: There is a limit to the value of applied force which a body, or specimen of material, can withstand. The maximum stress is normally used to characterize the strength of a material. In a tensile test, the fracture stress is referred to as the tensile strength of a material whilst a compression test gives a value of compressive strength. The diametral compressive tensile test gives a value for tensile strength.

In the case of a bending test, fracture is normally initiated from the side of the specimen which is in

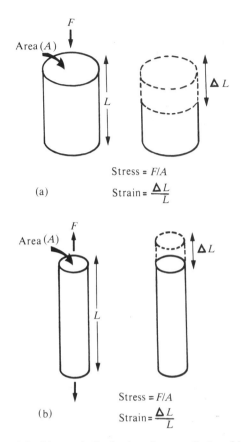

Stress = F/A

Strain = $\dfrac{\Delta L}{L}$

(a)

Stress = F/A

Strain = $\dfrac{\Delta L}{L}$

(b)

Fig. 2.3 Diagram indicating how the magnitudes of (a) compressive and (b) tensile stresses and strains are calculated.

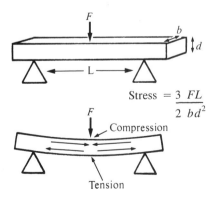

Stress $= \dfrac{3}{2}\dfrac{FL}{bd^{2}}$

Fig. 2.4 Diagrammatic representation of a 3-point bending test or transverse test. Bending of the beam introduces both tensile and compressive stresses.

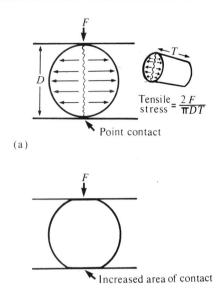

Tensile stress $= \dfrac{2F}{\pi DT}$

Point contact

(a)

Increased area of contact

(b)

Fig. 2.5 Diametral compressive test for (a) a brittle material and (b) a ductile material.

tension. The bending stress at fracture, often called the flexural stress, is closely related to the tensile strength.

For brittle materials, the flexural strength can be significantly influenced by the presence of surface defects, voids or other imperfections which may cause stress concentrations at the surface in tension. These stress concentrations may cause a material to fracture at a force lower than that which would otherwise be expected, a fact which has obvious implications for engineering design as well as dentistry.

Strain. The application of an external force to a body or test specimen results in a change in dimension of that body. For example, when a tensile force is applied the body undergoes an extension, the magnitude of which depends on the applied force and the properties of the material. The numerical value of strain is given by the expression

$$\text{Strain} = \frac{\text{Change in length}}{\text{Original length}}$$

Thus strain, which has no physical dimensions, can be seen as a measure of the fractional change in length caused by an applied force (Fig. 2.3). When strain becomes large, the dimensions of test specimens may change in a direction at 90° to that of the applied force. For example, a cylinder of material may undergo *barrelling* in addition to uni-axial compression, whilst a specimen subjected to tensile stress may become thinner in cross-section as the extension occurs. In order to monitor the way in which the stress changes with these alterations in specimen shape we need to take account of the *poissons ratio* of the material. This gives an indication of the ratio of strain occurring at 90° to the direction of the applied force to that occurring in the direction of the force.

The strain may be recoverable, that is the material will return to its original length after removal of the applied force, or the material may remain deformed, in which case the strain is non-recoverable. A third possibility is that the strain may be partially recoverable or that the recovery is time-dependent. The extent of recovery and/or rate of recovery is a function of the elastic properties of materials.

Stress–strain relationship: Stress and strain, as defined in the previous sections, are not independent and unrelated properties, but are closely related and may be seen as an example of cause and effect. The application of an external force, producing a stress within a material, results in a change in dimension or strain within the body.

The relationship between stress and strain is often used to characterize the mechanical properties of materials. Such data are generally obtained using a mechanical testing machine (Fig. 2.2) which enables strain to be measured as a function of stress and recorded automatically. Modern machines are capable of either increasing strain at a given rate and measuring the stress or increasing stress at a given rate and measuring the strain. Other applications, including fatigue testing, will be covered later.

For the simplest type of tensile or compression test, the graph displayed on the pen recorder would be as shown in Fig. 2.6.

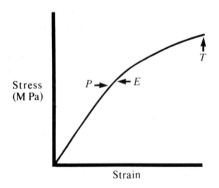

Fig. 2.6 Typical stress–strain graph obtained from a simple compressive or tensile test.

It can be seen that in this example there is a linear relationship between stress and strain up to the point *P*. Further increases in stress cause proportionally greater increases in strain until the material fractures at point *T*. The stress corresponding to point *T* is the fracture stress. In a tensile test this gives a value of *tensile strength*, whilst in a compression test a value of *compressive strength* is obtained. The value of stress which corresponds to the limit of proportionality, *P*, is referred to as the *proportional limit*.

Point *E* is the *yield stress*. This corresponds to the stress beyond which strains are not fully recovered. Hence, it is the maximum stress which a material can withstand without undergoing some permanent deformation. The *yield stress* is difficult to characterize experimentally since it requires a series of experiments in which the stress is gradually increased then released and observations on elastic recovery made.

As a consequence of these experimental difficulties the *proportional limit* is often used to give an approximation to the value of the *yield stress*. Hence, when a material is reported as having a high value of proportional limit it indicates that a sample of the material is more likely to withstand applied stress without permanent deformation.

A practical example of a situation in which a high proportional limit is required is in connectors of partial dentures. Such connectors should not undergo permanent deformation if they are to retain their shape. A material such as cobalt–chromium (Co/Cr) alloy which has a high value of proportional limit is popular for this application since it can withstand high stresses without being permanently distorted. Another way of gauging the level of stress required to produce permanent deformation is to measure the *proof stress*. This indicates the value of stress which will result in a certain degree of permanent deformation upon removal of the stress. For example, the 0.1% proof stress (commonly used for alloys) is the level of stress which would result in a 0.1% permanent deformation.

The slope of the straight-line portion of the stress–strain graph gives a measure of the *modulus of elasticity* defined as:

$$\text{Modulus of elasticity} = \frac{\text{Stress}}{\text{Strain}}$$

This has units of stress. The choice of nomenclature for this property is somewhat unfortunate since it, in fact, gives an indication of the rigidity of a material and *not* its elasticity. A steep slope, giving a high modulus value, indicates a rigid material, whilst a shallow slope, giving a low modulus value, indicates flexible material. Whereas it may be advantageous for an impression material to be flexible it is essential for a restorative material to be rigid.

The value of strain recorded between points E and T indicates the degree of permanent deformation which can be imparted to a material up to the point of fracture. For a tensile test this gives an indication of *ductility* whilst for a compressive test it indicates *malleability*. Hence, a ductile material can be bent or stretched by a considerable amount without fracture whereas a malleable material can be hammered into a thin sheet. A property often used to give an indication of ductility is the *elongation at fracture*. Alloys used to form wires must show a high degree of ductility since they are extended considerably during the production process. In addition, clasps of dentures constructed from ductile alloys can be altered by bending.

The malleability of stainless steel is utilized when forming a denture base by the swaging technique. This involves the adaptation of a sheet of stainless steel over a preformed cast.

The area beneath the stress–strain curve yields some important information about test materials (Fig. 2.7). The area beneath the curve up to the elastic limit, Fig. 2.7a, gives a value of *resilience*, the units being those of energy. Resilience may be defined as the energy absorbed by a material in undergoing elastic deformation up to the elastic limit. A high value of resilience is one parameter often used to characterize elastomers. Such materials which may, for example, be used to apply a cushioned lining to a hard denture base are able to absorb considerable amounts of energy without being permanently distorted. The energy is stored and released when the material springs back to its original shape after removal of the applied stress.

The total area under the stress–strain graph, Fig. 2.7b, gives an indication of *toughness*. This again has units of energy and may be defined as the total amount of energy which a material can absorb up to the point of fracture. A material capable of absorbing large quantities of energy is termed a *tough material*. The opposite of toughness is brittleness. This is, naturally, an important property for many dental materials. Its measurement, for example in a transverse test, depends on factors such as the speed with which the stress is increased and the presence of small imperfections in the specimen surface from which cracks can propagate.

Fracture toughness and impact strength: For brittle materials fracture may occur suddenly at a stress which is apparently well below the ideal fracture stress. This observation led to the development of theories on *fracture toughness* which takes account of the fact that small cracks can concentrate the stress at their tips. Griffith developed the theory of fracture toughness which led to the use of equations used for the calculation of stress intensification factor K. When K becomes great enough for crack propagation to occur it is termed the critical stress intensification factor K_c. This is calculated using the applied force, the specimen dimensions and the size and shape of the notch causing stress intensification. K has the units $MNm^{-1.5}$. In order to calculate K or K_c specimens of the type shown in Fig. 2.8 are most commonly used. The notch is moulded or machined into the specimen and has very well defined dimensions of notch depth and notch tip radius. This type of specimen is known as a single-edge-notched specimen (SEN). It is likely that fracture toughness is more meaningful than strength for brittle materials as the critical effect of surface defects is accounted for by the presence of a notch. The equations used to calculate fracture toughness should strictly only be applied to materials which fail by a purely brittle mechanism. When plastic deformations occur before fracture misleading results can be obtained. The speed at which testing is carried out may affect the extent to which plastic deformation may occur. It is more likely to occur when the strain is increased slowly than when the strain is increased rapidly.

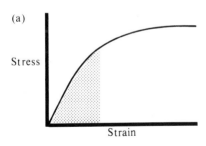

(a)

Stress

Strain

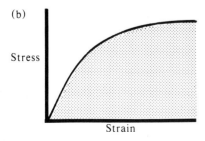

(b)

Stress

Strain

Fig. 2.7 The area under a stress–strain graph may be used to calculate either (a) resilience or (b) toughness.

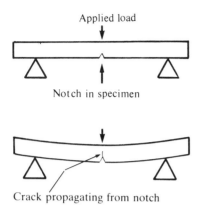

Applied load

Notch in specimen

Crack propagating from notch

Fig. 2.8 Notched specimens are often used in tests of toughness in order to overcome the effects of surface imperfections in specimens.

Hence materials are more likely to behave in a more brittle fashion when stress or strain are increased rapidly. When the stress is increased very rapidly it may be termed an *impact test* and the important practical property obtained is the *impact strength* which is normally quoted in units of energy. For this type of test the machine shown in Fig. 2.2 is often not capable of increasing stress rapidly enough and a swinging pendulum impact testing device is commonly used (Fig. 2.9). This type of instrument is known as a Charpy Impact tester. The position reached by the pendulum after fracturing the specimen gives a measure of the energy absorbed by the specimen during fracture. The absorbed energy can be resolved into several components which include friction and air resistance in the equipment. These minor components can be calculated by doing a *dummy run* with no specimens. The major components of energy are used in initiating and propagating cracks in the material. The relative magnitudes of these two components can be investigated by testing specimens with and without preformed cracks or notches. When the presence of a small notch or crack in the surface of a material has a marked effect on impact strength the material is said to be *notch sensitive*. Specimens of the type shown in Fig. 2.8 are often used in impact testing. Impact strength is not a fundamental material property (as is modulus of elasticity, for example) and it is not possible to fully account for differences in specimen size and shape. Values of impact strength measured in this way may only be considered of limited use in making direct comparisons with other materials of the same specimen size tested on the same instrument. For this reason the method is of limited

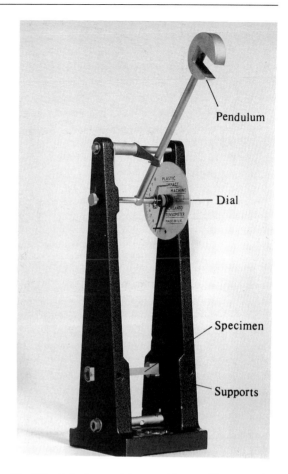

Pendulum

Dial

Specimen

Supports

Fig. 2.9 Swinging pendulum machine used for measuring impact strength.

scientific use, but is widely used in industry for quality control and development. Impact strength is an important property for acrylic denture base materials which have a tendency to fracture if accidentally dropped onto a hard surface.

Figure 2.10 gives examples of various types of stress–strain graphs which may be encountered, along with an explanation of the way in which the graphs can be used to characterize materials.

Fatigue properties: Many materials which are used as restoratives or dental prostheses are subjected to intermittent stresses over a long period of time – possibly many years. Although the stresses encountered may be far too small to cause fracture of a material when measured in a direct tensile, compressive or transverse test it is possible that, over a period of time, failure may occur by a fatigue process. This involves the formation of a microcrack,

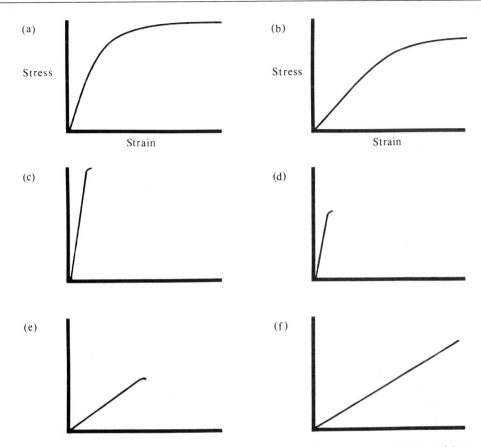

Fig. 2.10 Six different types of stress–strain graphs. These may be used to characterize materials as follows: (a) rigid, strong, tough, ductile; (b) flexible, tough; (c) rigid, strong, brittle; (d) rigid, weak, brittle; (e) flexible, weak, brittle; (f) flexible, resilient.

possibly caused by stress concentration at a surface fault or due to the shape of the restoration or prosthesis. This crack slowly propagates until fracture occurs. Final fracture often occurs at quite a low level of stress, a fact which often surprises patients who claim that their denture fractured when biting on soft food.

Fatigue properties may be studied in one of two ways. Firstly, it is possible to apply a cyclic stress at a given magnitude and frequency and to observe the number of cycles required for failure. The result is often referred to as the *fatigue life* of a material. Another approach is to select a given number of stress cycles, say 10 000, and determine the value of the cyclic stress which is required to cause fracture within this number of cycles. The result in this case is referred to as the *fatigue limit*. Both methods play an important part in materials evaluation. The most rigorous approach is to test many specimens at different cyclic stress levels and to determine the

number of cycles to failure in each case. The result is then given in the form of a graph as shown in Fig. 2.11. As the applied cyclic stress increases, the number of cycles to failure decreases.

One of the most important factors involved in such tests is the quality of the specimen used in the test since faults introduced during preparation can drastically reduce both fatigue life and fatigue limit.

Fatigue failure has often received only scant consideration in the past as a possible mode of failure for dental materials. It is now recognized that stress concentrations within materials can occur to an extent where cracks can propagate to cause failure within the normal lifetime of the material. Where fatigue cracks occur near the surface of a material and result in material loss from the surface they can be considered to contribute towards the overall wear observed for the material. Thus it is often not possible to separate the fracture and wear characteristics of materials.

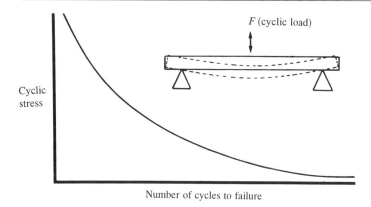

Cyclic stress

Number of cycles to failure

Fig. 2.11 Fatigue testing. Results are often given as a graph of cyclic stress versus number of cycles to failure. At smaller stress levels a greater number of cycles are required to cause fracture.

Abrasion resistance: The oral cavity is a relatively harsh environment in which to place either a restoration or prosthesis. *Wear* can occur by one or more of a number of mechanisms, some of which may be considered to be of mechanical origin and others chemical. Wear caused by indenting and scratching of the surface by abrasive toothpastes or food is termed *abrasive wear* and the hardness of a material is often used to give an approximate indication of the resistance to this type of abrasion.

Wear due to intermittent stresses caused by, for example, tooth-restorative contacts where the degree of scratching may be minimal is termed *fatigue wear* and the fatigue life and fatigue limit mentioned in the previous section are thought to give a guide to the fatigue wear resistance.

In practice the position is not as clear cut as it would seem from the previous two paragraphs since most wear processes occur by a combination of two or more mechanisms. Consequently, laboratory experiments devised to measure wear rates of dental materials often produce unconvincing or even misleading results.

Chemical factors may play an important role in many wear mechanisms. For example, water absorption may cause structural changes within a material which accelerate the rate of degradation by abrasive wear or fatigue. Likewise, solvents may cause surface softening which accelerates wear.

A process closely related to wear is erosion. This is the loss of surface material caused by impinging particles (such as sand or raindrops). The term erosion has been used in dentistry to imply the loss of material through a chemical effect such as acid attack.

The most important comparative information about the abrasion resistance values of different materials comes from well-controlled clinical trials.

Hardness: The hardness of a material gives an indi-

cation of the resistance to penetration when indented by a hard asperity. The value of hardness, often referred to as the hardness number, depends on the method used for its evaluation. Generally, low values of hardness number indicate a soft material and vice versa.

Common methods used for hardness evaluation include Vickers, Knoop, Brinell and Rockwell. Vickers and Knoop both involve the use of diamond pyramid indentors. In the case of Vickers hardness, the diamond pyramid has a square base, whilst for Knoop hardness, one axis of the diamond pyramid is much larger than the other. The Brinell hardness test involves the use of a steel ball indentor producing an indentation of circular cross-section. Figure 2.12 shows the types of indentation produced in test specimens. The hardness is a function of the diameter of the circle for Brinell hardness and the distance across the diagonal axes for Vickers and Knoop hardness. Allowance is naturally made for the magnitude of the applied loads.

Measurements are normally made using a microscope since the indentations are often too small to be

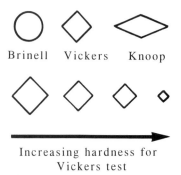

Brinell   Vickers   Knoop

Increasing hardness for Vickers test

Fig. 2.12 Shapes of indentations produced by three types of hardness test. A decrease in the size of the indentation indicates a harder material.

seen with the naked eye. In the case of Rockwell hardness, a direct measurement of the depth of penetration of a conical diamond indentor is made. Table 2.1 shows Vickers hardness numbers for some common dental materials.

Table 2.1 Vickers hardness numbers of some selected dental materials.

Material	VHN
Enamel	350
Dentine	60
Acrylic resin	20
Dental amalgam	100
Porcelain	450
Co/Cr alloys	420

It is worth giving some consideration to what is actually being measured during a hardness test. For those methods involving the measurement of an indentation with a microscope after the indenting force has been removed, the hardness value is related to the degree of permanent deformation produced in the surface of the test material by the indentor under a given load. The pyramidal designs of indentors used in Vickers and Knoop tests dictate that when they come into contact with the surface of a test material the initial contact stress is very high. As the indentor penetrates further the applied load is spread over a greater area and the stress is reduced. The indentor comes to rest when the applied stress is equivalent to the elastic limit of the test material and the hardness measurement gives an indication of yield stress. Any other deformation of the material is likely to be elastic in nature and will not be recorded as part of the material hardness measurement since elastic recovery may occur before the measurement is made with the microscope. Occasionally it is possible to observe the size of the indentation shrinking as elastic recovery occurs. When this happens it is important to allow the size of the indentation to stabilize before measurements are made. Methods which involve the direct measurement of depth of indentation may produce results which are difficult to analyse unless the elastic and plastic parts of the deformation can be separated.

Hardness is often used to give an indication of the ability to resist scratching. Hence, acrylic materials are easily scratched because they are relatively soft whereas Co/Cr alloys are unlikely to become scratched because they are relatively hard. As a corollary to this, harder materials are more difficult to polish by mechanical means.

Hardness is also used to give an indication of the abrasion resistance of a material, particularly where the wear process is thought to include scratching as in abrasive wear.

Elasticity and viscoelasticity: The property of yield stress has previously been used to define the elastic range of a material. The yield stress is the value of stress beyond which the material becomes permanently distorted, that is, the strain is not completely recovered after the applied load is removed.

Although yield stress is an important property it does not, on its own, fully characterize the elastic properties of a material. Elastic properties are often defined in terms of the ability of a material to undergo *elastic recovery*. When a material undergoes full elastic recovery immediately after removal of an applied load it is *elastic*. If the recovery takes place slowly, or if a degree of *permanent deformation* remains, the material is said to be *viscoelastic*.

Models involving the use of springs and dashpots can be used to explain the elastic and viscoelastic behaviour of materials (Fig. 2.13). When a spring, which represents an elastic material, is fixed at one end and a load applied at the other it becomes instantaneously extended. When the load is removed it immediately recovers its original length (Fig. 2.14a). This behaviour is analogous to that of a perfectly elastic material. The two things that characterize the material are firstly the perfect recovery after removal of the force and secondly the lack of any time dependency of either the deformation under load or the recovery after removal of the applied force. The extent of deformation under load is characterized by the modulus of elasticity of the material (analogous to the spring constant of the spring).

When a load is applied to a dashpot, which represents a viscous material, it opens slowly, strain being a function of the *time* for which the load is applied (Fig. 2.14b). When the load is removed the dashpot remains open and no recovery occurs. This is in distinct contrast to the behaviour of an elastic material. The time-dependent opening of the dashpot is akin to the way in which the flow of a viscous or plastic material is controlled by its viscosity.

For the material behaving as a spring and dashpot in series (Maxwell model), application of a load causes the spring to be extended instantaneously followed by slow opening of the dashpot (Fig. 2.14c). On removal of the load the spring recovers but the dashpot remains permanently distorted. The magnitude of the distortion depends on the *applied load* and the *time* for which the load is applied.

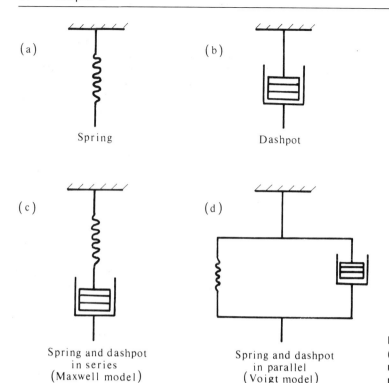

(a)

Spring

(b)

Dashpot

(c)

Spring and dashpot
in series
(Maxwell model)

(d)

Spring and dashpot
in parallel
(Voigt model)

Fig. 2.13 Models used to represent (a) elastic materials, (b) plastic materials and (c) and (d) viscoelastic materials.

For the material behaving as a spring and dashpot in parallel (Voigt model), application of load causes slow opening of the spring under the damping effect of the dashpot (Fig. 2.14d). Following removal of the load the dashpot and spring slowly recover to their original state under the elastic influence of the spring and the damping influence of the dashpot. The time taken to recover is a function of the *applied load* and the *time* of application of the load. For materials which exhibit either Voigt or Maxwell type behaviour, the deformation under load is described by a value of modulus of elasticity, viscosity and time.

Many viscoelastic materials used in dentistry behave like a combination of the Voigt and Maxwell models (Fig. 2.15). Such materials show an instantaneous increase in strain due to the spring (A) followed by a gradual increase in strain as the dashpot (B) and spring/dashpot (C/D) system open. On removal of the load the spring (A) recovers instantaneously followed by gradual recovery of the spring/dashpot (C/D). Some permanent distortion remains as a consequence of the dashpot (B). Again, the magnitude of the permanent deformation is a function of the *applied load* and the *time* of application.

This type of behaviour has important practical significance for many dental materials and particularly for *elastic* impression materials. All such materials are viscoelastic to some extent and may become distorted when being removed over undercuts. The permanent deformation depends on the applied load, which in this case is a function of the force required to remove the impression from the mouth, and the time for which that force is applied. The magnitude of the force is dictated by the modulus of elasticity of the material, its thickness and the severity of the undercuts.

Creep and *stress relaxation* are two other phenomena which can be explained using the viscoelasticity models.

Creep involves a gradual increase in strain under the influence of a constant applied load similar to that which takes place in the Maxwell model (Fig. 2.13c). The phenomenon of *creep* can only be distinguished from that of *flow* by the extent of the deformation and the rate at which it occurs. The term *creep* implies a relatively small deformation produced by a relatively large stress over a long period of time whereas *flow* implies a greater deformation produced more rapidly with a smaller applied stress.

Stress relaxation involves the application of a constant strain. Under such conditions the stress decreases as a function of time for Maxwell-type viscoelastic materials. Although stress relaxation experiments can be used to classify materials, creep tests have more practical significance for dental materials. Such tests are relatively simple to carry out. A constant load is applied to a test specimen in either compression or tension. The strain or creep is measured as a function of time. Dynamic creep tests are also carried out in which the load is applied at regular intervals and the change in the value of strain measured as a function of the number of loading cycles.

Values of creep obtained by such techniques are particularly important for dental amalgam. It is thought that creep is a precursor to fracture at the edge of the filling and hence failure for such materials.

Stress relaxation is a measure of decreasing stress at constant strain. It is not of direct relevance for most dental applications.

2.3 Rheological properties

Rheology is the study of the flow or deformation of materials. The term can be applied to both solids and liquids and in the case of solids or elastomers involves the use of elasticity and viscoelasticity theory mentioned in Section 2.2. A study of the rheological properties of liquids and pastes normally involves the measurement of viscosity and the determination of the way in which this varies with factors such as rate of shear and time.

By definition viscosity (η) is given by the equation

$$\eta = \frac{\text{Shear stress } (\sigma)}{\text{Shear rate } (E)}$$

The phenomena of *shear stress* and *shear rate* can be visualized by considering the extrusion of a fluid material from a syringe (Fig. 2.16). When the material is extruded at a constant rate the shear stress is related to the pressure required to depress the barrel of the syringe, whereas the shear rate is a function of the flow rate. Thus, a material of low viscosity requires only a low pressure to produce a high flow rate, whereas a more viscous material may require a high pressure to produce a relatively small rate of flow.

Further characterization of the rheological properties of materials is obtained by reference to the equation

$$\text{Shear stress} = K (\text{Shear rate})^n$$

where K and n are constants. The constant n is referred to as the *flow index*. For the simplest case,

where n = 1, the shear stress is directly proportional to shear rate and the viscosity of the material is constant and independent of shear rate. Materials which behave in this way are referred to as *Newtonian fluids*.

When the flow index value is less than unity an increase in shear rate produces a less than proportionate increase in shear stress. Thus the viscosity is effectively decreased with increasing shear rate (shear thinning). Such materials are referred to as being *pseudoplastic*. When the flow index value is greater than unity an increase in shear rate produces a more proportionate increase in shear stress, thus effectively increasing viscosity (shear thickening). Such materials are said to be *dilatant*.

Figure 2.16 illustrates the result which may be obtained for Newtonian, pseudoplastic and dilatant materials when viscosity is measured as a function of shear rate. For dental materials, Newtonian and pseudoplastic behaviour are commonly encountered, whereas dilatancy is rare. The rheological properties are important for many different materials since they often control the ease of use.

Some materials exhibit so-called Bingham characteristics. Here, a finite stress, referred to as the yield stress of the substance, is required in order to cause the material to flow. Once the yield stress is exceeded the material may behave as a Newtonian, pseudoplastic or dilatant fluid. In Fig. 2.17 curve A represents the behaviour of a normal Newtonian fluid, curve B the behaviour of a normal pseudoplastic fluid, curve C the behaviour of a material with a yield stress (value E) followed by Newtonian behaviour and curve D the behaviour of a material with a yield stress followed by pseudoplastic behaviour.

Viscosity values of materials are temperature-dependent, an increase in temperature generally causing a significant reduction in viscosity.

Time-dependence of viscosity (working times and setting times): Many materials used in dentistry involve the mixing of two components, thus initiating a chemical reaction which causes the material to change from a fluid to a rigid solid or elastomer. The initial viscosity of the mixed material often governs its ease of handling. The rate at which the viscosity increases as a function of time is of equal importance. Manipulation becomes impossible when viscosity has increased beyond a certain point. The time taken to reach that point is the *working time* of the material.

Figure 2.18 shows a typical plot of viscosity against time for a material setting by a chemical reaction

(a)

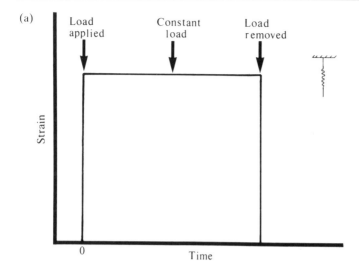

(b)

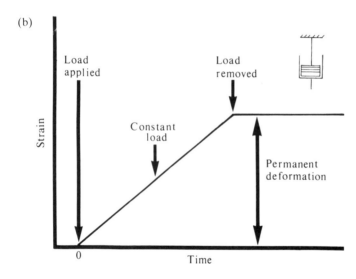

Fig. 2.14 Strain versus time graphs obtained for various types of model materials: (a) elastic material, (b) plastic material, (c) viscoelastic material (Maxwell type), (d) viscoelastic material (Voight type).

(curve A). The material may become unmanageable when it reaches a viscosity value of V_1, thus the material has a working time of T_1. Curve B is the plot of a material for which the viscosity does not begin to increase until the time T_2 and the viscosity has not reached V_1 until the time T_3. Thus the working time for this material is considerably longer than that for material A. The shape of curve B suggests that the chemical reaction involved in setting has an induction period, probably produced by chemical retarders which manufacturers sometimes use to extend working times.

The other important time used to define setting characteristics is the *setting time*. This is related to the time taken for the material to reach its final set

state or to develop properties which are considered adequate for that application. Methods used for measuring setting characteristics vary from one type of material to another. Many types of rheometer, both simple and complex, are capable of monitoring changes in viscosity as a function of time. Unfortunately, few instruments are able to monitor both the subtle changes occurring during the early stages of setting whilst the material is still relatively fluid and the changes occurring later when the material is highly viscous and rigid. Hence, two separate instruments are sometimes required to fully characterize setting. One convenient and commonly used method is resistance to penetration. Thus a material may be considered set when it is able to resist

(c)

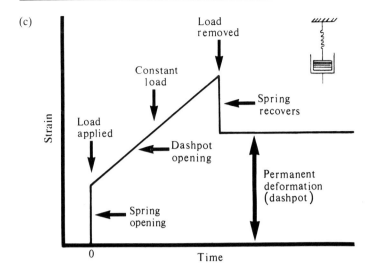

(d)

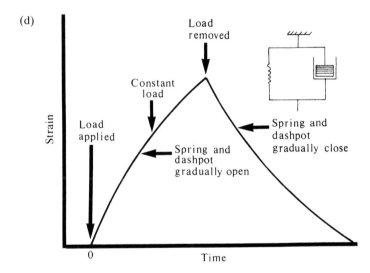

Fig. 2.14   (continued)

penetration by a probe of known weight and tip diameter (Fig. 2.19). It can be seen that in Fig. 2.19a the material is readily penetrated by the probe indicating that it has not set, whilst in Fig. 2.19b the probe is supported by the material, indicating that it is now set. As with most other methods of setting-time evaluation, this one is to some extent arbitrary in that the value obtained depends on the weight and tip diameter of the probe. Further consideration of the arrangement illustrated in Fig. 2.19 suggests that the setting time determined by this method is the time required to produce a particular value of yield stress within the setting material. For this test to be meaningful the critical yield stress which corresponds to the applied load and probe tip diameter

should have some practical significance related to the intended use of the material. Some products develop elastic properties during setting. These working times and setting times can be determined through measurement of the initial onset of elastic behaviour and the attainment of the final, optimum elastic state.

2.4 Thermal properties

Wide temperature fluctuations occur in the oral cavity due to the ingestion of hot or cold food and drink. In addition, more localized temperature increases may occur due to the highly exothermic nature of the setting reaction for some dental

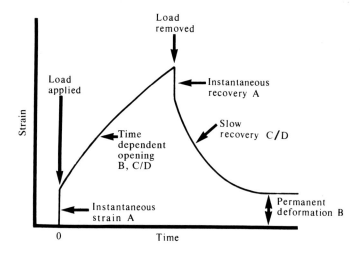

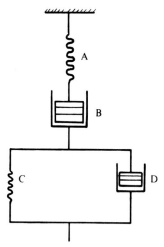

Fig. 2.15 Universal model which can be used to explain the viscoelastic properties of most materials.

materials. The dental pulp is very sensitive to temperature change and in the healthy tooth is surrounded by dentine and enamel, which are relatively good thermal insulators. It is important that materials which are used to restore teeth should not only offer a similar degree of insulation but also should not undergo a large temperature rise when setting *in situ*.

Another consequence of thermal change is dimensional change. Materials generally expand when heated and contract when cooled. These dimensional changes may cause serious problems for filling materials, particularly in the region of the tooth/restorative interface.

Thermal conductivity: Thermal conductivity is defined as the rate of heat flow per unit temperature gradient. Thus, good conductors have high values of conductivity. Table 2.2 gives values of thermal con-

Table 2.2 Thermal conductivity values of some selected dental materials.

Material	Thermal conductivity (W m^{-1} $^\circ$C^{-1})
Enamel	0.92
Dentine	0.63
Acrylic resin	0.21
Dental amalgam	23.02
Zinc phosphate cement	1.17
Zinc oxide/eugenol cement	0.46
Silicate materials	0.75
Porcelain	1.05
Gold	291.70

ductivity for some dental materials along with those for enamel and dentine. It is clear that heat is conducted through metals and alloys more readily than through polymers such as acrylic resin. The relatively

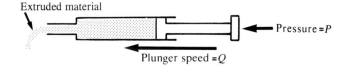

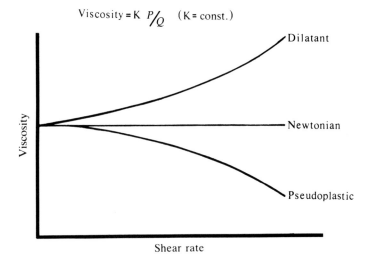

Fig. 2.16 The rheological properties of fluids and pastes can be represented by the extrusion of materials from a syringe.

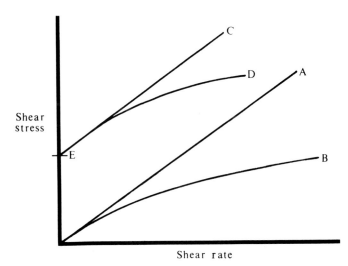

Fig. 2.17 Shear stress–shear rate plots of four materials. Two (A and B) have no yield stress whilst the other two (C and D) exhibit a yield stress of value E.

high value of conductivity for dental amalgam indicates that this material could not provide satisfactory insulation of the pulp. For this reason it is normal practice to use a cavity base of a cement such as zinc phosphate which has a lower thermal conductivity value.

Thermal conductivity is an equilibrium property and since most thermal stimuli encountered in the mouth are transitory in nature the value of *thermal diffusivity* may be of more practical use in predicting materials behaviour.

Thermal diffusivity: Thermal diffusivity (D) is defined by the equation

$$D = \frac{K}{Cp \times \rho}$$

where K is the thermal conductivity, Cp is the heat capacity and ρ the density. This property gives a better indication of the way in which a material responds to transient thermal stimuli. Thus, if a cold drink is taken and the cooling effect on any tooth or restoration surface is maintained for only a second or

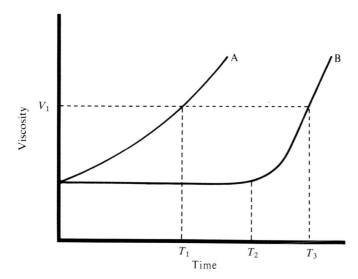

Fig. 2.18 Viscosity increasing with time for two materials during setting. Material B has an induction period during which the viscosity is unchanged.

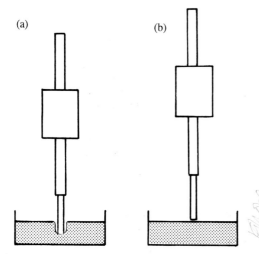

Fig. 2.19 Assessment of setting time by determination of resistance to penetration. (a) Material is unset. (b) Material is set.

two, the diffusivity allows calculation of the temperature change in the pulp. This should, naturally, be as small as possible. The diffusivity value recognizes that when transient thermal stimuli are applied a certain amount of heat will be absorbed in raising the temperature of the material itself. This will effectively reduce the quantity of heat available to be transported through the material.

Measurements of thermal diffusivity are often made by embedding a thermocouple in a specimen of material and plunging the specimen into a hot or cold liquid (Fig. 2.20a). If the temperature recorded by the thermocouple rapidly reaches that of the liquid, this indicates a high value of diffusivity. A slow response, on the other hand, indicates a lower value of diffusivity (Fig. 2.20b). In many circumstances a low value of diffusivity is preferred. However, there are occasions on which a high value is beneficial. For example, a denture base material, ideally, should have a high value of thermal diffusivity in order that the patient retains a satisfactory response to hot and cold stimuli in the mouth.

Exothermic reactions: Many dental materials involve the mixing of two or more components followed by setting. The setting process often occurs *in situ* and very often the chemical reaction occurring during setting is exothermic in nature. For industrial production processes, exothermic reactions must be closely controlled in order to avoid explosions. For dental materials this is not a problem due to the relatively small sample sizes used. However, the heat liberated and the associated rise in temperature may cause clinical problems.

Table 2.3 gives typical values of temperature rise recorded for small samples of some dental materials.

Table 2.3 Temperature rise during setting of some selected materials (100 mg sample).

Material	Temperature rise (°C)
Zinc oxide/eugenol cement	0.2
Zinc phosphate cement	1.9
Acrylic resin	9.6
Composite resin	4.0
Glass ionomer cement	1.0

(a)

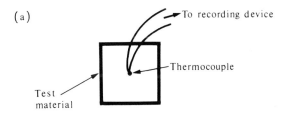

To recording device

Thermocouple

Test
material

(b)

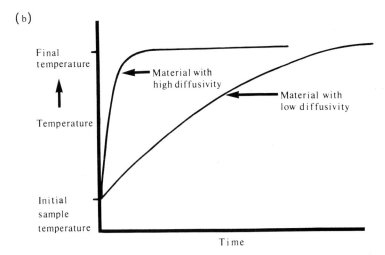

Final
temperature

↑

Temperature

Material with
high diffusivity

Material with
low diffusivity

Initial
sample
temperature

Time

Fig. 2.20 (a) Measuring thermal diffusivity by embedding a thermocouple in a sample of the material. The sample is plunged into a hot or cold fluid and (b) temperature change plotted against time.

Naturally, the temperature rise increases with an increasing amount of material. Hence, due regard must be paid to the possible effect that such materials may have on the dental pulp when used as restoratives, particularly when a large bulk of material is used.

Following the course of an exothermic chemical reaction using a calorimeter is an accurate way of evaluating the setting characteristics of some dental materials. Consideration of the temperature against time curve which results from such experiments may produce a convenient method for measuring working times and setting times. The temperature rise occurring during setting has become even more significant with the growing number of light-activated materials used in dentistry. For these products setting often occurs very rapidly, leading to a more marked rise in temperature. In addition, the light sources used to activate setting produce heat. Hence, the combined effect of the setting reaction and the heating effect of the light can cause short-lived temperature rises in excess of 20°C for even small quantities of some resin-based materials.

Coefficient of thermal expansion: The linear coefficient of thermal expansion is defined as the fractional increase in length of a body for each degree centigrade increase in temperature. Thus,

$$\alpha = \frac{\triangle L / L_0}{\triangle T} \; {}^{\circ}\mathrm{C}^{-1}$$

where the coefficient α is defined in terms of the change in length $\triangle L$, the original length L_0 and the temperature change $\triangle T$.

Because the values of α are often very small numbers (typically $0.000\,025\,{}^{\circ}\mathrm{C}^{-1}$ for amalgam) they are often quoted as parts per million (ppm). For example, the value for a typical amalgam specimen would be quoted as 25 ppm ${}^{\circ}\mathrm{C}^{-1}$. (Values for some common materials are given in Table 2.4.)

This property is particularly important for filling materials. When the patient takes a cold drink, both the filling material and tooth substance contract, the amount of contraction depending on the value of α for each. If the value of α for the material is significantly greater than that for tooth substance a small gap will develop down which fluids containing bacteria can penetrate, as illustrated in Fig. 2.21. The magnitude of the gap, shown as x in the diagram, is minimized for both hot and cold stimuli if the values of α for tooth substance and filling are matched. Hence, it can be seen from Table 2.4 that certain

Table 2.4 Coefficient of thermal expansion values of some selected materials.

Material	Coefficient of thermal expansion (ppm $°C^{-1}$)
Enamel	11.4
Dentine	8.0
Acrylic resin	90
Porcelain	4
Amalgam	25
Composite resins	25–60
Silicate cements	10

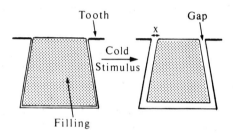

Fig. 2.21 Diagram illustrating the production of a marginal gap due to thermal contraction.

materials, for example silicate cements, perform very well in this respect, whilst others, such as acrylic resin, perform badly.

(In practice, however, the situation is not so clear cut. Coefficient of thermal expansion is an equilibrium property and the expansion or contraction due to transient stimuli is a function of both coefficient of thermal expansion and thermal diffusivity.) For filling materials, the most ideal combination of properties would be a low value of diffusivity combined with a coefficient of thermal expansion value similar to that for tooth substance.

2.5 Adhesion

Adhesion may be defined simply as an interaction between two materials at an interface where they are in contact. The nature of the interaction is such that their separation is prevented. The property of adhesion is recognized as being of major importance for filling materials, luting materials and fissure sealants. In each case the aim is to produce a tight seal between tooth substance and material with minimal destruction of tooth tissue.

Materials which are capable of bonding two surfaces together are called *adhesives* whilst the material to which the adhesive is applied is termed the *adherend*. In dentistry, an adhesive may, typically, be required to bond dentine and gold or, if the adhesive also acts as a filling material, may simply be required to attach to one surface, for example enamel or dentine. The latter is an ideal situation in which the restorative material possesses inherent adhesive characteristics which enable it to bond to dentine. This ideal is not always possible to achieve and dental adhesives are commonly used to form a thin layer between tooth substance and a restorative material.

Bonding may be achieved by one of two mechanisms – *mechanical attachment* or *chemical adhesion*.

In *mechanical attachment* the adhesive simply engages in undercuts in the adherend surface as shown in Fig. 2.22. When the surface irregularities responsible for bonding have dimensions of only a few micrometres the process is known as *micromechanical attachment*. This should be distinguished from *macromechanical attachment* which forms the basis of retention for many filling materials, using undercut cavities. In the case of *chemical adhesion* the adhesive has a chemical affinity for the adherend surface. If the attraction is caused by Van der Waals forces or hydrogen bonds, the resultant bond may be relatively weak. On the other hand, the formation of ionic or covalent links may result in a stronger bond.

Whichever mechanism of bonding is utilized the

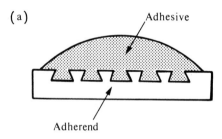

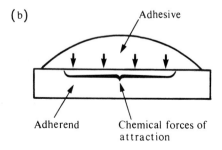

Fig. 2.22 Diagram illustrating the difference between (a) micromechanical attachment and (b) chemical adhesion.

adhesive must be capable of *wetting* the adherend surface. In the case of mechanical attachment the adhesive must flow readily across the adherend surface and enter into all the surface undercuts in order to form the bond. For chemical adhesion the adhesive must *wet* the adherend surface in order that intimate contact between the adhesive and adherend may result in the formation of specific links which cause bonding.

The ability of an adhesive to wet an adherend surface is evaluated by measuring the *contact angle* which is formed when a drop of adhesive is applied to the surface. Figure 2.23 shows that for good wetting, a low contact angle, ideally approaching $0°$, is required. High contact angles indicate poor wetting and globule formation, and would probably result in poor adhesion.

The surface tension of the adhesive is the property which maintains it in the form of a droplet and acts to prevent wetting. There must be sufficient energy liberated through the forces of attraction between the adhesive and adherend in order to break down the surface tension of the adhesive and enable the materials to come into intimate contact. This affinity which is a prerequisite to adhesion has posed dental researchers with a great dilemma since the majority of resins used in dental fillings are relatively hydrophobic whilst dentine and enamel are relatively moist. This implies that there will be little natural affinity between the two materials which the dentist is trying to join together. The development of *primers* has helped to solve the problem. These materials change the nature of the adherend surface

and improve affinity for resins used in restorative materials.

Adhesive forces are maximized if the adhesive and adherend are in intimate contact over a large surface area. This generally requires that adhesives should be applied to the adherend in the form of a low viscosity fluid or paste. Figure 2.24a illustrates the situation which arises if two solid surfaces are placed in contact. The rigid nature of the materials dictates that unless the two surfaces are perfectly flat (very difficult to achieve), they are in contact over only a very small proportion of their surface and the actual area of contact is only a fraction of the apparent area of contact. Hence, even if interactions between the two surfaces are favourable the adhesive strength is unlikely to be great enough to maintain the adhesive and adherend in contact in the presence of even a small displacing force. If the adhesive is fluid but does not adequately wet the adherend surface the situation may not be much better, as illustrated in Fig. 2.24b. The ideal situation of a fluid adhesive which fully wets the adherend surface is illustrated in Fig. 2.24c. Here the two interacting materials take full advantage of the adhesive forces set up over the whole surface. In this case the actual area of contact is greater than the apparent area.

The way in which the preceding argument relates to certain dental adhesives is illustrated in Fig. 2.25. Figure 2.25a represents a cross-section through acid-etched enamel. Figure 2.25b illustrates the situation which may exist when a resin is applied. Close adaptation and penetration of the resin into the enamel surface has not occurred due to poor wetting

(a)

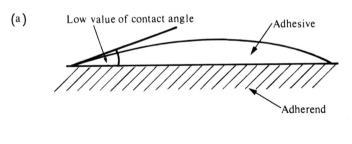

(b)

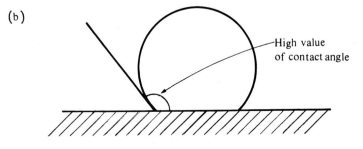

Fig. 2.23 Diagram showing (a) good wetting of an adherend surface and (b) poor wetting and globule formation.

(a)

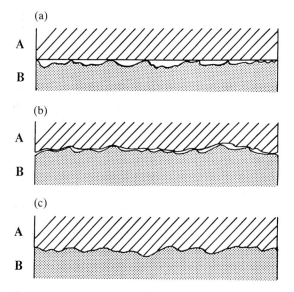

(b)

(c)

Fig. 2.24 Diagram illustrating adhesive (A) and adherend (B) surfaces in contact. (a) Two rigid surfaces make contact over a relatively small area. (b) The adhesive is fluid but does not wet the adherend surface. (c) The adhesive is fluid and wets the adherend surface.

and/or the viscosity of the resin being too great. In Fig. 2.25c a resin of low viscosity and good wetting characteristics ensures good adaptation to and penetration of the etched enamel surface, probably resulting in good bonding characteristics.

2.6 Miscellaneous physical properties

Properties of materials which may influence their acceptability but which do not fall into any of the other categories are (1) dimensional changes during and after setting, (2) density, and (3) appearance.

Dimensional changes: Dimensional accuracy is an important requirement of many dental materials. The success of many restorative procedures depends on dimensional changes which occur during impression recording, casting of alloys or setting of direct restorative materials.

The manipulation of many materials involves the mixing of two or more components followed by a chemical reaction which brings about setting. Chemical reactions are invariably accompanied by dimensional changes. In the case of polymerization reactions, a contraction normally occurs whereas other types of reaction may result in an expansion.

Where several stages are involved in the production of a restoration or appliance it is possible that

(a)

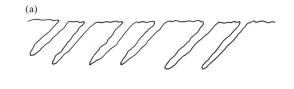

(b)

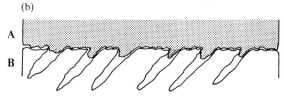

(c)

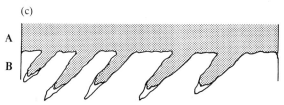

Fig. 2.25 Diagram illustrating application of a resin adhesive (A) to an etched-enamel surface (B). (a) View of section through etched enamel. (b) The adhesive is too viscous or does not wet the enamel surface. (c) Good penetration of etched-enamel by resin resulting from good wetting characteristics and relatively fluid resin.

dimensional changes occur at each stage. In such a case it is possible that an expansion at one stage can be used to partly counteract a contraction which occurs at another stage. For example, when constructing a cast metal restoration the setting expansion of the investment material partially compensates for the casting shrinkage of the alloy.

Dimensional changes may continue to occur in materials long after the apparent setting. There are many possible causes. Firstly, the changes may be due to continued slow setting or release of stresses set up during setting. Alternatively, they may be due to water absorption by, or loss of constituents from, the material. The degree to which the dimensions of a material alter after setting is said to be a measure of its *dimensional stability*.

Density: Density is a fundamental property which affects design aspects of dental appliances. If, for example, one were choosing an alloy with which to construct components of an upper denture, it would be necessary to consider density. A bulky design in a heavy alloy would result in large displacing forces making retention difficult. In order to reduce such destabilizing forces one may choose to use a lower density alloy and to keep the alloy bulk to a minimum. These considerations become even more significant when other design parameters are taken into account. For example, if a rectangular cross-section beam is subjected to three-point bending, the force to cause a given deflection at the centre of the beam depends upon the square of the thickness. Hence, if a rigid (high modulus of elasticity), low density material is used equal performance can be achieved with a considerable saving in weight.

Appearance: One of the most demanding requirements of dental restorative materials is that they should match the natural hard and soft tissues in appearance. Colour may be described quantitatively in terms of a three-dimensional colour chart such as that shown in Fig. 2.26. The three independent parameters represented in the diagram are as follows.

(1) The dominant wavelength or *hue*, represented by the position of the circumference.
(2) The colour intensity or *chroma*, represented by the radial distance from the centre of the circle.
(3) The *brightness* as represented by the position in the vertical column.

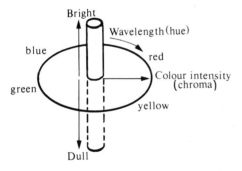

Fig. 2.26 Three-dimensional representation of colour, including wavelength of light, intensity and brightness.

The *hue* and *chroma* are inherent properties of materials whereas the *brightness* may be affected by factors such as surface finish.

In many materials (e.g. resin-based products) the initial hue and chroma are controlled by the manufacturer through the incorporation of pigments and the use of fillers having varying translucency/opacity. The passage of light through a material having a composite structure is influenced by the degree to which the filler and matrix phases have a matched refractive index.

Changes in hue and chroma which occur over time can be due to either changes in the bulk of the material, i.e. through molecular transformations or reactions of one or more of the material components, or through the absorption of stains onto the surface of the material. To distinguish these two processes the terms intrinsic and extrinsic staining are often used. The latter is normally related to the surface roughness of the material.

2.7 Chemical properties

One of the main factors which determines the durability of a material used in the mouth is its chemical stability. Materials should not dissolve, erode or corrode, nor should they leach important or toxic constituents into the oral fluids.

Solubility and erosion: The solubility of a material is simply a measurement of the extent to which it will dissolve in a given fluid, for example, water or saliva. Erosion, on the other hand, is a process which combines the chemical process of dissolution with a mild mechanical action. Hence it is possible to envisage a situation in which the surface layer of a material becomes weakened and undermined by dissolution and then becomes totally detached by mild abrasion.

There is occasionally some confusion over the term erosion. This is because in materials science the term is normally used to imply damage produced by the impingement of particles on an object. In dentistry the term has gained widespread use to describe the destruction of natural hard tissues by acids (either occurring naturally or present in food/drinks). This usage has been widened to include the degradation of restorative materials by a combination of chemical and mild mechanical action.

These properties are particularly important for all restorative materials since a high solubility or poor resistance to erosion will severely limit the effective lifetime of the restoration.

When assessing the solubility or erosion rate of materials it is important to consider the vast range of conditions which may exist in the mouth. The pH of oral fluids may vary from pH 4 to pH 8.5, representing a range from mildly acidic to mildly alkaline. Highly acidic soft drinks and the use of chalk-containing toothpastes extend this range from a lower end of pH 2 up to pH 12. It is possible for a material to be stable at near neutral pH values but to erode rapidly at extremes of either acidity or alkalinity. This partially explains why certain materials perform adequately with some patients but not with others.

Standard tests of solubility often involve the storage of disc specimens of materials in water for a period of time, the result being quoted as the percentage weight loss of the disc. Such methods, however, often give misleading results because they do not represent what occurs in the mouth. New methods of testing which have been incorporated in some ISO standards involve dripping or spraying sets of aqueous acidic solutions onto the surfaces of test specimens. This involves the use of a more aggressive fluid (typically pH 4) and the mildly abrasive effect of the impinging liquid droplets. The most appropriate method for measuring material loss is to estimate volume loss as this can be correlated with material loss from restorations as judged clinically. Judging material loss by weight change is less satisfactory as even though material is lost from the surface the weight of a specimen may increase if water absorption is great enough.

Leaching of constituents: Many materials, when placed in an aqueous environment, absorb water by a diffusion process. Constituents of the material may be lost into the oral fluids by a diffusion process commonly referred to as leaching. This may have serious consequences if it results in a change of material properties or if the leached material is toxic or irritant.

Some soft acrylic polymers used for cushioning the fitting surfaces of dentures rely on the presence of relatively large quantities of plasticizer in the acrylic resin for their softness. The slow leaching of plasticizer causes the resin to become hard and therefore ineffective as a cushion.

Occasionally leaching is used to the benefit of the patient. For example, in some cements containing calcium hydroxide, slow leaching causes an alkaline environment in the base of deep cavities. This has the dual benefit of being antibacterial and of encouraging secondary dentine formation.

Some restorations leach fluoride which is thought to have a beneficial effect on the surrounding dental hard tissues. It is important that this process does not have a deleterious effect on the properties of the material (e.g. cement). Much depends on the mechanism of leaching. If this occurs by ion exchange there is a good chance that fluoride ions will be replaced by another anion (e.g. hydroxyl) and the integrity of the material is maintained. If the leaching occurs by *washout*, however, the process is likely to be accompanied by gradual degradation.

Corrosion: Corrosion is a term which specifically characterizes the chemical reactivity of metals and alloys. The major requirement of any such material used in the mouth is that it should have good corrosion resistance.

Metals and alloys are good electrical conductors and many corrosion processes involve the setting up of an electrolytic cell as a first stage in the process.

The tendency of a metal to corrode can be predicted from its electrode potential. It can be seen from Fig. 2.27 that materials with large negative electrode potential values are more reactive whilst those with large positive values are far less reactive and are often referred to as *noble* metals. The electrode potential is a measure of the extent to which the reaction

$$M \rightarrow M^+ + \text{electron}$$

will occur.

In an electrolytic cell involving two metals, material is lost from the metal with the most negative electrode potential. Thus, when zinc and copper come into contact in the presence of a suitable electrolyte (Fig. 2.28), material loss occurs from the zinc by the reaction:

$$Zn \rightarrow Zn^{2+} + 2 \text{ electrons}$$

Hydrogen is liberated at the copper by the reaction:

$$2H^+ + 2 \text{ electrons} \rightarrow H_2$$

In this simple type of electrolytic cell the zinc is referred to as the *anode*. This is the electrode at which positive ions are formed and therefore the electrode at which corrosion occurs. The copper is referred to as the *cathode*. The more negative a value of electrode potential which a metal possesses the more likely it is to form the anode in an electrolytic cell.

If a voltmeter is placed between the anode and cathode an electrical potential difference can be measured, thus illustrating the flow of electrons within the electrolytic cell.

The conditions under which an electrolytic cell may be set up in the mouth involve the presence of two or more metals of different electrode potential and a suitable electrolyte. Saliva and tissue fluids are good electrolytes. The two metals may be derived from restorations constructed from different metals or alloys, or from areas of different composition within one restoration, for example amalgam, as illustrated in Fig. 2.29.

Generally, the more homogeneous the distribution of metal atoms within an alloy the less tendency there is for corrosion to occur. Consequently, many manufacturers of alloys carry out homogenization heat treatments to help to eliminate the possibility of electrolytic corrosion.

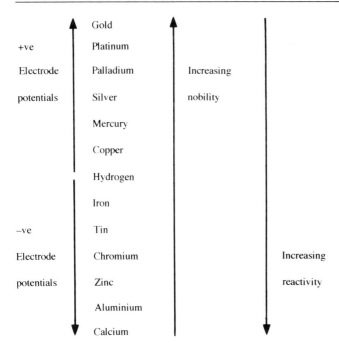

+ve
Electrode
potentials

−ve
Electrode
potentials

Gold
Platinum
Palladium
Silver
Mercury
Copper
Hydrogen
Iron
Tin
Chromium
Zinc
Aluminium
Calcium

Increasing
nobility

Increasing
reactivity

Fig. 2.27 Ranking orders of electrode potentials and reactivities for various metals.

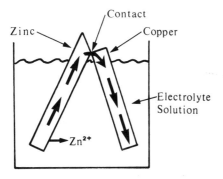

Fig. 2.28 Electrolytic cell involving two dissimilar metals in contact and an electrolyte. Corrosion of the most electronegative metal occurs. Arrows represent flow of electrons.

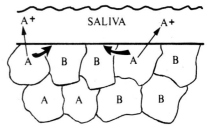

Fig. 2.29 An electrolytic cell involving different phases within one alloy. Saliva acts as the electrolyte. Phase A is more electronegative than phase B. Arrows represent flow of electrons.

It can be seen from Fig. 2.27 that chromium has a negative value of electrode potential and is at the reactive end of the series of metals shown. It is therefore surprising to learn that chromium is included as a component of many alloys in order to improve corrosion resistance. This apparent contradiction can be explained by the *passivating effect*. Although chromium is electrochemically active it reacts readily forming a layer of chromic oxide which protects the metal or alloy from further decomposition.

Other factors which can affect the corrosion of metals and alloys are stress and surface roughness.

Stress in metal components of appliances produced, for example, by excessive or continued bending can accelerate the rate of corrosion and may lead to failure by *stress corrosion cracking*. Pits in rough surfaces can lead to the setting up of small corrosion cells in which the material at the bottom of the pit acts as the anode and that at the surface acts as the cathode. The mechanism of this type of corrosion, sometimes referred to as *concentration cell corrosion*, is complicated but is caused by the fact that pits tend to become filled with debris which reduces the oxygen concentration in the base of the pit compared with the surface. In order to reduce corrosion by this mechanism, metals and alloys used in the mouth should be polished to remove surface irregularities.

An appreciation of the principles of electrolytic corrosion should help the dentist to design the arrangement of restorations and appliances in such a manner that dissimilar materials are not allowed to come into close contact. The consequences of corrosion can be varied and include: pain due to the flow of galvanic current, metallic taste due to the release of ions, deterioration in appearance and mechanical properties and, most seriously, an increased body burden of metallic ions. There is increasing concern over the effects of increasing the body's burden of heavy metals such as mercury and nickel.

2.8 Biological properties

It is a primary requirement of any dental material that it should be harmless to the patient and to those involved in its manufacture and handling. Whilst the manufacture of materials may involve the use of relatively toxic raw materials, close control of production processes reduces or eliminates the risk to personnel.

Ideally, a material placed into a patient's mouth should be non-toxic, non-irritant, have no carcinogenic or allergic potential and, if used as a filling material, should be harmless to the pulp.

Biological evaluation of dental materials is carried out on three levels. At the first level, simple screening tests can be used to evaluate acute systemic toxicity, irritational potential and carcinogenic potential. The second level of testing involves limited usage tests in experimental animals. For example, when evaluating filling materials it is common to place restorations in the teeth of monkeys or ferrets. If the tests carried out at the first and second levels produce satisfactory results then it is possible to consider moving to the third level of testing – the controlled clinical trial involving volunteer human subjects. Hence, every effort is made to ensure the safety of new products.

The effect of materials on the dentists, surgery assistants and technicians involved in their handling is an important consideration. Materials are normally in their most reactive and potentially harmful state during mixing and manipulation. In addition, dental personnel may be exposed to materials over a long period of time. For example, mercury is known to have certain toxic effects and the most potent mechanism for incorporation of mercury into the body is by inhaling mercury vapour. A patient may spend only a few minutes each year in a mercury-contaminated dental surgery and is thus subjected to only minimal exposure. The dentist and his assistant, on the other hand, may spend all of their working lives in such an environment. The need for adequate mercury hygiene is therefore apparent.

Many materials are used in the mouth despite the fact that for some patients they may have the potential to cause problems. Studies of biocompatability suggest that the term can only be used relatively and a product which is perfectly tolerated by one patient may cause problems of irritancy with another. Each material/patient combination must in some ways be the subject of a risk/benefit analysis. Potentially toxic materials are used when the risk only applies to a very small number of people and/or when there is no viable alternative material.

Materials used for certain applications have specific biological requirements which will be discussed in the relevant chapters dealing with those groups of products.

2.9 Suggested further reading

Ashby, M.F. & Jones, D.R.H. (1980) *Engineering Materials 1. An Introduction to their Properties and Applications.* Pergamon Press, Oxford.

Ashby, M.F. & Jones, D.R.H. (1986) *Engineering Materials 2. An Introduction to Microstructures, Processing and Design.* Pergamon Press, Oxford.

Cottrell, A. (1975) *An Introduction to Metallurgy.* Arnold, London.

Gordon, J.E. (1976) *The New Science of Strong Materials.* Penguin Books, Harmondsworth.

Kinloch, A.J. (1987) *Adhesion and Adhesives.* Chapman & Hall, London.

Chapter 3
Gypsum Products for Dental Casts

3.1 Introduction

Gypsum is a naturally occurring, white powdery mineral with the chemical name calcium sulphate dihydrate ($CaSO_4 \cdot 2H_2O$). Gypsum products used in dentistry are based on calcium sulphate hemihydrate ($CaSO_4)_2 \cdot H_2O$. Their main uses are for casts or models, dies and investments, the latter being considered in Chapter 5.

Many dental restorations and appliances are constructed outside the patient's mouth using models and dies which should be accurate replicas of the patient's hard and soft tissues.

The term *model* is normally used when referring to a replica of several teeth and their associated soft tissues or, alternatively, to an edentulous arch. The term *die* is normally used when referring to a replica of a single tooth.

The morphology of the hard and soft tissues is recorded in an impression and models and dies are prepared using materials which are initially fluid and can be poured into the impression, then harden to form a rigid replica.

Many materials have been used for producing models and dies but the most popular are the materials based on gypsum products.

The current ISO Standard for Dental Gypsum Products identifies five types of material as follows:

Type 1   Dental plaster, impression
Type 2   Dental plaster, model
Type 3   Dental stone, die, model
Type 4   Dental stone, die, high strength, low expansion
Type 5   Dental stone, die, high strength, high expansion

The Type 1 material will be discussed in Chapter 17 (Non-elastic Impression Materials).

3.2 Requirements of dental cast materials

The main requirements of model and die materials are dimensional accuracy and adequate mechanical properties. The accuracy of fit of any restoration or appliance constructed outside the mouth depends *inter alia* on the dimensional accuracy of the replica on which it is constructed. Thus, the dimensional changes which occur during and after the setting of these model materials should, ideally, be minimal in order to produce an accurate model or die. The final fit of the appliance may depend upon a balancing of small expansions or contractions which occur at different stages in its construction and it would be unwise to consider, in isolation, dimensional changes occurring with the model and die materials.

Although small dimensional changes during setting can often be tolerated and even compensated for, changes occurring during storage are a more serious problem. Hence, the dimensional stability after setting should be as good as possible.

The material should, ideally, be fluid at the time it is poured into the impression so that fine detail can be recorded. A low contact angle between the model and impression materials would help to minimize the presence of surface voids on the set model by encouraging surface wetting.

The set material should be sufficiently strong to resist accidental fracture and hard enough to resist abrasion during the carving of a wax pattern.

The material should be compatible with all the other materials with which it comes into contact. For example, the set model should easily be removed from the impression without damage to its surface and fracture of teeth. It should give a good colour contrast with the various waxes which are often used to produce wax patterns.

3.3 Composition

Gypsum products used in dentistry are formed by driving off part of the water of crystallization from gypsum to form calcium sulphate hemihydrate.

$$\begin{array}{lcl}
\text{Gypsum} & \rightarrow & \text{Gypsum product} + \text{water} \\
2CASO_4 \cdot 2H_2O & \rightarrow & (CaSO_4)_2 \cdot H_2O + 3H_2O \\
\text{Calcium sulphate} & & \text{Calcium sulphate} \\
\text{dihydrate} & & \text{hemihydrate}
\end{array}$$

Applications of gypsum products in dentistry involve the reverse of the above reaction. The hemihydrate is mixed with water and reacts to form the dihydrate.

$$(CaSO_4)_2 \cdot H_2O + 3H_2O \rightarrow 2CaSO_4 \cdot 2H_2O$$

The various types of gypsum product used in dentistry are chemically identical, in that they consist of calcium sulphate hemihydrate, but they may differ in physical form depending upon the method used for their manufacture.

Dental plaster (plaster of Paris): Dental plaster is produced by a process known as calcination. Gypsum is heated to a temperature of about 120°C in order to drive off part of the water of crystallization. This produces irregular, porous particles which are sometimes referred to as β-hemihydrate particles (Fig. 3.1a). Overheating the gypsum may cause further loss of water to form calcium sulphate anhydrite ($CaSO_4$), whilst underheating produces a significant concentration of residual dihydrate. The presence of both components has a marked influence upon the setting characteristics of the resultant plaster.

Dental stone: Dental stones may be produced by one of two methods. If gypsum is heated to about 125°C under steam pressure in an autoclave a more regular and less porous hemihydrate is formed (Fig. 3.1b). This is sometimes referred to as an α-hemihydrate.

Alternatively, gypsum may be boiled in a solution of a salt such as $CaCl_2$. This gives a material similar to that produced by autoclaving but with even less porosity. Manufacturers normally add small quantities of a dye to dental stones in order that they may be differentiated from dental plaster, which is white.

3.4 Manipulation and setting characteristics

Plaster and stone powders are mixed with water to produce a workable mix. Hydration of the hemihydrate then occurs producing the gypsum model or die.

Table 3.1 gives an indication of the water/powder (W/P) ratio used for each material along with the theoretical ratio required to satisfy the chemical reaction which occurs. Although a ratio of only 0.186 is required to satisfy the reaction, such a mix would

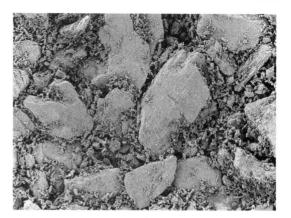

Fig. 3.1(a) Particles of calcium sulphate β-hemihydrate (dental plaster) ($\times$ 235).

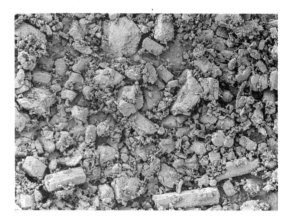

Fig. 3.1(b) Particles of calcium sulphate α-hemihydrate (dental stone) ($\times$ 235).

Table 3.1 Water/powder ratios for gypsum model and die materials.

	Water (ml)	Powder (g)	W/P ratio (ml/g)
Plaster	50–60	100	0.55
Stone	20–35	100	0.30
Theoretical ratio	18.6*	100	0.186

* Sometimes referred to as gauging water.

be too dry and unworkable. In the case of the more dense material, dental stone, a ratio of about 0.3 is required to produce a workable mix, whereas for the more porous plaster a higher W/P ratio of 0.55 is required. The excess water is absorbed by the porosities of the plaster particles. Considerable quantities of air may be incorporated during mixing and this may lead to porosity within the set material. Air porosity may be reduced either by vibrating the mix of plaster or stone in order to bring air bubbles to the surface or by mixing the material mechanically under vacuum, or both.

For hand mixing a clean, scratch free rubber or plastic bowl having a top diameter of about 130 mm is normally recommended. The presence of gypsum residues in the mixing bowl can noticeably alter the working and setting characteristics of a fresh mix and so the need for cleanliness is emphasized. A stiff spatula with a round-edged blade of around 20–25 mm width and 100 mm length is used. The requisite amount of water is added to a moist bowl and the powder added slowly to the water over about 10 seconds. The mix is allowed to soak for about another 20 seconds and then mixing/spatulation carried out for around 60 seconds using a circular stirring motion. After the material has been mixed and used, the mixing bowl should be thoroughly cleaned before the next mix is performed.

The fluidity of dental gypsum products is normally measured by one of two methods outlined in the ISO Standard. For types 1 and 2 materials a *slump* test is recommended. Here, a known volume of mixed material is allowed to *slump* onto a glass plate at a time indicated by the manufacturer as the pouring time (2–3 minutes for most materials). The fluidity is defined as the average of the major and minor diameters of the slumped material.

The fluidity of types 3, 4 and 5 materials is determined using a core penetration test. The depth of penetration of a core falling under a load for 15 seconds into a known quantity of material is measured 3 minutes after starting to mix powder and water.

The setting process begins rapidly after mixing the powder and water. The first stage in the process is that the water becomes saturated with hemihydrate, which has a solubility of around 0.8% at room temperature. The dissolved hemihydrate is then rapidly converted to dihydrate which has a much lower solubility of around 0.2%. Since the solubility limit of the dihydrate is immediately exceeded it begins to crystallize out of solution. The process continues until most of the hemihydrate is converted to dihydrate.

The crystals of dihydrate are spherulitic in nature and grow from specific sites called nuclei of crystallization. These may be small particles of impurity, such as unconverted gypsum crystals, within the hemihydrate powder. If a thin mix of material is used, containing more water than that indicated in Table 3.1, the formation of the supersaturated solution of dihydrate which is a precursor to crystallization is delayed and the centres of nucleation are more widely dispersed by the dilution effect. The set plaster is therefore less dense with greater spaces between crystals leading to a significant reduction in strength.

The material should be used as soon as possible after mixing since its viscosity increases to the stage where the material is unworkable within a few minutes. Two stages can be identified during setting. The first is the time at which the material develops the properties of a weak solid and will not flow readily. At this time, often referred to as the initial setting time, it is possible to carve away excess material with a knife. The materials continue to develop strength for some time after initial setting and eventually reach a stage when the models or dies are strong and hard enough to be worked upon. The time taken to reach this stage is referred to as the final setting time, although this term is misleading since it implies that the material has reached its ultimate strength. This may not be reached until several hours after mixing.

The setting characteristics of gypsum products can be affected not only by the presence of unconverted dihydrate but also by the presence of anhydrite, the age of the material and the storage conditions experienced by the material prior to use. Small quantities of unconverted dihydrate act as centres of nucleation as mentioned earlier. Anhydrite reacts very rapidly with water producing a marked acceleration in setting. Freshly produced plaster may contain significant quantities of anhydrite (Section 3.3) and this may accelerate setting to the extent that manipulation becomes difficult. To overcome this problem plaster is often allowed to mature before use, the anhydrite absorbs moisture and is converted to the less reactive hemihydrate. If the plaster is allowed to mature for too long in a humid environment the hemihydrate crystals become coated with a layer of dihydrate and the reactivity is markedly reduced.

The setting characteristics of gypsum products have traditionally been measured in terms of their ability to resist penetration by needles, such as those shown in Fig. 3.2. The heavier needle has a smaller tip diameter than the lighter one and hence applies a considerably greater pressure to the surface of the material under test. The initial setting time is defined as the time taken for the material to develop sufficient strength such that it is able to support the lighter of the needles. The time at which the material is able to support the heavier needle has doubtful practical significance since it indicates a time some-

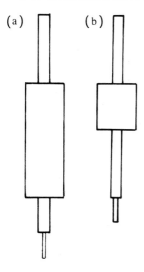

Fig. 3.2 Indentors used to assess setting characteristics of gypsum products. Sometimes referred to as Gilmore needles. Ability to support needle (b) indicates the initial set. Ability to support needle (a) indicates final set.

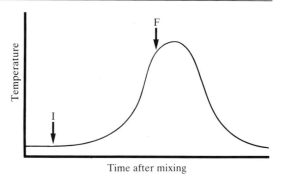

Fig. 3.3 Temperature–time profile for a gypsum material during setting. Points I and F correspond to the initial set and final set points indicated by indentors (Fig. 3.2).

where between the initial and final setting times and is not indicative of the fact that the model or die is hard enough to be used.

The ISO specification for dental gypsum products requires the use of a Vicat needle for judging setting time. This system has a built-in dial gauge allowing depth of penetration to be measured. Also the load can be varied in order to satisfy the requirements of several standard tests. The setting material is indented by a needle of 1 mm diameter under a load of 300 g. The setting time in this test is defined rather arbitrarily as the time when the needle is no longer able to penetrate to a depth of 2 mm into the material. The setting time measured using this method is normally less than 30 minutes, however a longer time is required before the material has matured sufficiently to allow any further work to be performed on the cast without damaging the surface.

The setting reaction is exothermic, the maximum temperature being reached during the stage when final hardening occurs (Fig. 3.3). It is interesting to note that the temperature rise is still negligible at the time of the initial set. The magnitude of the temperature rise depends on the bulk of material used and can be as great as 30°C at the centre of a mass of setting material. This temperature may be maintained for several minutes due to the thermal insulating characteristics of the materials. This marked rise in temperature can be used to good effect when flasking dentures since it softens the wax of the trial denture and enables it to be easily removed from the mould.

Another physical change which accompanies setting is a small expansion caused by the outward thrust of growing crystals as shown in Fig. 3.4. The maximum rate of expansion occurs at the time when the temperature is increasing most rapidly. The

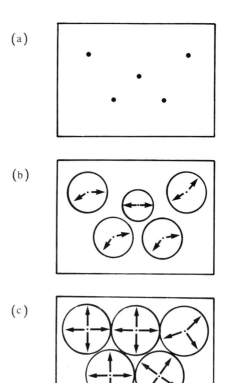

Fig. 3.4 Diagram showing growth of spherulitic gypsum crystals, indicating (a) the nuclei from which crystals grow, (b) spherulitic growth and (c) the outward thrust as spherulites make contact.

expansion is, in fact, only apparent since the set material contains a considerable volume of porosity. If the material is placed in water at the initial set stage, considerably more expansion occurs during setting. This increased expansion is called *hygroscopic expansion* and is sometimes used to increase the setting expansion of gypsum-bonded investment materials (Chapter 5).

The setting expansion is measured using a special trough with a moveable end-plate which pushes against an extensometer. Mixed material is poured into the trough and as it solidifies and expands the extensometer is displaced, giving a value of linear expansion. The maximum expansion values are as great as 0.15% for type 1 and 4 materials and 0.30% for type 2 and 5 materials. Type 3 materials have a maximum expansion of 0.20%. Some individual products have much lower values of expansion (see Table 3.2).

Control of setting time: Factors which control the setting times of gypsum products can be divided into those controlled by manufacturers and those controlled by the operator.

The manufacturer can control the concentration of nucleating agents in the hemihydrate powder. A higher concentration of nucleating agent, produced by ageing or from unconverted calcium sulphate dihydrate, results in more rapid crystallization. Also, the manufacturers may add chemical accelerators or retarders to dental stones. Potassium sulphate is a commonly used accelerator which is thought to act by increasing the solubility of the hemihydrate. Borax is the most widely used retarder, although the mechanism by which it works is not clear.

Factors under the control of the operator are temperature, W/P ratio and mixing time. Surprisingly, temperature variation has little effect on the setting times of gypsum products. This is due to the fact that the setting involves a dissolution of one sparingly soluble salt followed by crystallization of another. Increasing the temperature accelerates the solution process but retards the crystallization. Thus the two effects tend to cancel out. Increasing the W/P ratio retards setting by decreasing the concentration of crystallization nuclei. Increasing mixing time has the opposite effect. This accelerates setting by breaking up dihydrate crystals during the early stages of setting, thus producing more nuclei on which crystallization can be initiated. These effects are shown in Fig. 3.5.

Control of setting expansion: In order to produce an accurate model or die it is necessary to maintain the setting expansion at as low a value as possible. Accelerators or retarders which are added by manufacturers to dental stones in order to control the setting time also have the effect of reducing the setting expansion and are sometimes referred to as *antiexpansion agents*. The final values of expansion observed for typical materials are given in Table 3.2. The very low value of expansion for some stones may be considered negligible in terms of its effect on the accuracy of restorations or appliances which are to be constructed.

Alterations in W/P ratio and mixing time have only a minimal effect on setting expansion.

3.5 Properties of the set material

The strength of gypsum depends, primarily, on the porosity of the set material and the time for which the material is allowed to dry out after setting.

The porosity, and hence the strength, is proportional to the W/P ratio as shown in Fig. 3.6.

Since stone is always mixed at a lower W/P ratio than plaster it is less porous and consequently much stronger and harder.

Although a gypsum model or die may appear completely set within a relatively short period its strength increases significantly if it is allowed to stand for a few hours. The increase in strength is a

Table 3.2 Properties of dental gypsum products (typical values).

Property	Type 1	Type 2	Type 3	Type 4	Type 5
Initial setting time (min)	–	5–10	5–20	5–20	5–20
Setting time (min)	4	20	20	20	20
Setting expansion (%)	0–0.15	0–0.30	0–0.20	0–0.15	0.16–0.3
Compressive strength 1 h (MPa)	6	12	25	40	40
Compressive strength 24 h (MPa)	–	24	70	75	75
Flexural strength 24 h (MPa)	1	1	15	20	20
Detail reproduction (μm)	75	75	50	50	50

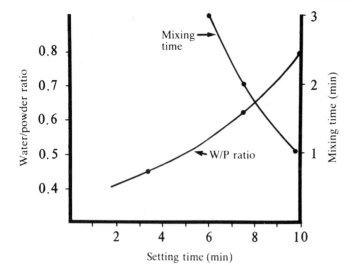

Fig. 3.5 The effect of water/powder ratio and mixing time on setting time for a typical dental plaster.

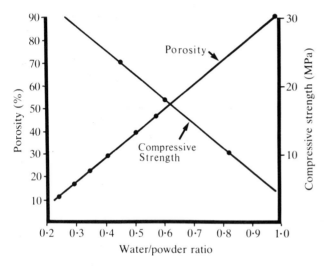

Fig. 3.6 The effect of water/powder ratio on the porosity and compressive strength of gypsum products.

function of the loss of excess water by evaporation. It is thought that evaporation of water causes a precipitation of any dissolved dihydrate and that this effectively cements together the crystals of gypsum formed during setting.

Despite precautions which may be taken to ensure optimum mechanical properties, gypsum is a very brittle material. The very low value of flexural strength of plaster shown in Table 3.2 is indicative of how fragile this material is. Stone is less fragile but must be treated with care if fracture is to be avoided. It is relatively rigid but has a poor impact strength and is likely to fracture if dropped. Attempts to improve the mechanical properties have involved the impregnation by a polymer such as acrylic resin and the use of wetting agents which enable the materials to be used at a lower W/P ratio.

The dimensional stability of gypsum is good. Following setting, further changes in dimensions are immeasurable and the materials are sufficiently rigid to resist deformations when work is being carried out upon them.

The ability of dental gypsum products to reproduce surface details of hard or soft tissues either directly or from impressions is central to their suitability as model and die materials. This ability is judged by measuring the extent to which accurately machined lines in a block of stainless steel can be reproduced in a sample of the material. Types 1 and 2 materials can reproduce a groove 75 µm wide whilst types 3, 4 and 5 are able to reproduce grooves of only 50 µm width. Hence, types 3, 4, and 5 stones are capable of recording greater fine detail than type 2 (plaster) material.

Set plaster is slightly soluble in water. Solubility increases with the temperature of the water and if hot water is poured over the surface of a plaster cast, as happens during the boiling out of a denture mould, a portion of the surface layer becomes dissolved leaving the surface roughened. Frequent washing of the surface with hot water should therefore be avoided.

Table 3.2 gives comparative values of properties for the different types of dental gypsum products.

3.6 Applications

When strength, hardness and accuracy are required dental stones are normally used in preference to dental plaster. The stone materials are less likely to be damaged during the laying down and carving of a wax pattern and give optimal dimensional accuracy. Thus, these materials are used when any work is to be carried out on the model or die as would be the case when constructing a denture on a model or a cast alloy crown on a die.

When mechanical properties and accuracy are not of primary importance the cheaper dental plaster is used. Thus, plaster is often used for mounting stone models onto articulators and sometimes for preparing study models.

3.7 Advantages and disadvantages

Gypsum model and die materials have the advantages of being inexpensive and easy to use. The accuracy and dimensional stability are good and they are able to reproduce fine detail from the impression, providing precautions are taken to prevent blow holes.

The mechanical properties are not ideal and the brittle nature of gypsum occasionally leads to fracture – particularly through the teeth, which form the weakest part of any model.

Problems occasionally arise when gypsum model and die materials are used in conjunction with alginate impression. The surface of the model may remain relatively soft due to an apparent retarding effect which hydrocolloids have on the setting of gypsum products. It is not certain whether the retarding effect is due to borax in the hydrocolloid or to the absorption of hydrocolloid onto the gypsum crystals which act as nuclei of crystallization. Despite these observations it cannot be said that gypsum products are incompatible with alginate impression materials since problems arise very infrequently.

Alternative materials for the production of models and dies exist but are hardly ever used. These include various resins, cements and dental amalgam. The alternatives may be stronger but are generally less stable, difficult to use and more expensive. The surface of a gypsum die can be hardened by electroplating the impression prior to constructing the die. The thin layer of metal, copper for impression compound and silver for some elastomers, is transferred to the surface of the die on separation from the impression.

Another treatment which has been suggested for improving the durability of gypsum is to partly saturate the set material in a polymerizable monomer such as methylmethacrylate or styrene. Polymerization of the monomer produces a polymer phase which occupies many of the porosities in the set gypsum and increases its strength and toughness. Despite these apparent advantages these techniques are rarely used in practice.

3.8 Suggested further reading

Combe, E.C. & Smith, D.C. (1964) Some properties of gypsum plasters. *Br. Dent. J.* **117**, 237.

Earnshaw, R. & Marks, B.I. (1964) The measurement of the setting time of gypsum products. *Aust. Dent. J.* **9**, 17.

Fairhurst, C.W. (1960) Compressive properties of dental gypsum. *J. Dent. Res.* **39**, 812.

Chapter 4
Waxes

4.1 Introduction

The waxes used in dentistry normally consist of two or more components which may be natural or synthetic waxes, resins, oils, fats and pigments. Blending is carried out to produce a material with the required properties for a specific application.

Waxes are thermoplastic materials which are normally solids at room temperature but melt, without decomposition, to form mobile liquids. They are, essentially, soft substances with poor mechanical properties and their primary uses in dentistry are to form *patterns* of appliances prior to casting.

Following the production of a stone model or die (Chapter 3), the next stage in the formation of many dental appliances, dentures or restorations is the production of a wax pattern of the appliance on the model. The wax pattern defines the shape and size of the resulting appliance and is eventually replaced by either a polymer or an alloy using the *lost-wax technique*. Methods which involve the production of a model followed by the laying down of a wax pattern are known as *indirect techniques*. Some dental restorations, such as inlays, may be produced by a *direct wax pattern* technique in which the inlay wax is adapted and shaped in the prepared cavity in the mouth. Waxes used in the production of patterns by either the direct or indirect technique must have very precisely controlled properties in order that well-fitting restorations or appliances may be constructed. Other waxes used in dentistry have less rigorous property requirements. One such material is used by manufacturers for attaching denture teeth to display sheets (*carding wax*). Another product is used for boxing in impressions prior to making a gypsum model (*boxing-in wax*). A third material is used for temporarily joining two components of an appliance, for example, during soldering (*sticky wax*).

An important group of waxes used in dentistry are the impression waxes. These are discussed in Section 17.4.

4.2 Requirements of wax-pattern materials

The major requirements of waxes used to construct wax patterns by either the direct or indirect technique are as follows.

(1) The wax pattern must conform to the exact size, shape and contour of the appliance which is to be constructed.
(2) No dimensional change should take place in the wax pattern once it has been formed.
(3) After formation of the casting mould, it should be possible to remove the wax by boiling out or burning without leaving a residue.

The ability to record detail depends on the flow of the material at the moulding temperature, which is just above mouth temperature for direct techniques and just above room temperature for indirect techniques. Accuracy and dimensional stability depend on dimensional changes which occur during solidification and cooling of the wax. Distortions may also occur if thermal stresses are introduced.

4.3 Composition of waxes

Dental waxes are composed of mixtures of thermoplastic materials which can be softened by heating then hardened by cooling. The major components may be of mineral, animal or vegetable origin.

Mineral: Paraffin wax and the closely related microcrystalline wax are both obtained from petroleum residues following distillation. They are both hydrocarbons, paraffin wax being a simple straight-chain hydrocarbon whilst the microcrystalline material has a branched structure.

Paraffin waxes soften in the temperature range 37–55°C and melt in the range 48–70°C. They are brittle at room temperature. Microcrystalline waxes melt in the range 65–90°C and when added to paraffin waxes they raise its melting point. At the same

36

time they lower the softening temperature and render the material less brittle than paraffin wax alone.

Animal: Beeswax, derived from honeycombs, consists of a partially crystalline natural polyester and is often blended with paraffin wax in order to modify the properties of the latter. The effect of adding beeswax to paraffin wax is to render the material less brittle and to reduce the extent to which it will flow under stress at temperatures just below the melting point.

Vegetable: Carnauba wax and candelilla wax are derived from trees and plants. They are blended with paraffin wax in order to control the softening temperature and modify properties.

4.4 Properties of dental waxes

Waxes are generally characterized by their thermal properties such as *melting point* and *solid–solid transition temperature* which is closely related to the *softening temperature* observed in practice. The *coefficient of thermal expansion* is a major factor affecting accuracy. *Dimensional stability* is primarily a function of the magnitude of the stresses which become incorporated during thermal contraction after moulding. Important mechanical properties are *brittleness* and the degree of *flow* which a material will undergo in its working temperature range.

Thermal properties: All the waxes used in dentistry have a predominantly crystalline structure and are characterized by a well-defined melting point. On heating, a second endothermic peak exists at a temperature somewhat lower than the melting point. This peak is indicative of a solid–solid transition involving a change in the crystal structure of the wax. The change in crystal structure is accompanied by a change in mechanical properties and the wax is converted from a relatively brittle solid to a much softer, mouldable material. For this reason, the solid–solid transition temperature is sometimes referred to as the *softening temperature*. For many applications of waxes the softening temperature should be just above mouth temperature. This is in order that the material may be introduced into the mouth in a mouldable state but will become relatively rigid at mouth temperature. The manufacturers can control the melting point and softening temperature by blending mixtures of various mineral, animal and vegetable components.

Waxes are very poor thermal conductors and must be maintained above the solid–solid transition temperature for long enough to allow thorough softening to occur throughout the material before moulding is attempted.

Following moulding, the waxes are allowed to cool, During this cooling period they may undergo potentially significant contraction due to the high values of coefficient of expansion exhibited by these products.

The thermal contraction may not be fully exhibited immediately after cooling. The low thermal conductivity values of the materials result in solidification of the surface layers of the wax well before the bulk becomes rigid. This reduces the magnitude of the thermal contraction and produces significant internal stresses. Dimensional changes may occur due to relief of the stresses. This is more likely to occur at elevated temperatures. Greater stresses may be incorporated if the wax is not properly softened before moulding.

Methods for softening wax prior to moulding include a water bath, an infra-red lamp and a bunsen burner. In order to achieve even heating with the latter it is important that the wax should be held in the warm rising air above the flame and not in the flame itself. If the surface becomes shiny it indicates that the wax is becoming too hot and the outer layers are beginning to melt.

Heating in warm water causes more regular softening although this method has been frowned upon since it was thought that some constituents may be leached out and small quantities of water may become incorporated causing an alteration in properties. These problems are probably overstated since most waxes contain few leachable components.

The method of softening used in standardization testing of waxes involves the use of a 250 W infra-red lamp. When using this method, the distance of the wax from the lamp must be carefully controlled in order to cause softening but not melting.

The ideal method for softening wax is to use a wax *annealer*. This is a thermostatically controlled oven which keeps the wax at a constant temperature, just above the softening point, ready for use. The annealer is most useful for inlay waxes.

Mechanical properties: A major factor which determines the mouldability and stability of a wax is its *flow* value. This property is related to *creep* which is discussed on p. 14. Creep and flow are both measured by applying a load to a cylindrical specimen and measuring the extent to which the specimen becomes compressed after a given time. Materials should, ideally, exhibit considerable flow at the moulding temperature but should show little or no flow at mouth temperature or room temperature so that they are not easily distorted. The determination of flow is made on cylindrical specimens 10 mm diameter by 6 mm. They are loaded across their flat faces using a 2 kg weight for the specified time (10 minutes). The flow is recorded as the percentage change in the height of the cylinder. The nature of the materials dictates that very precise temperature control be maintained ($\pm 0.1°$C) during these tests. Flow values for some typical materials are given in Table 4.1.

Brittleness is another important property which the manufacturers can, to some extent, control. For some waxes, for example denture waxes, toughness is required since the wax denture base may have to be removed from a slightly undercut cast many times without fracturing. In other cases, such as inlay waxes, brittleness is preferred in order that the wax will fracture rather than distort on removal from an undercut cavity. This will indicate to the dental surgeon that a modification to the cavity shape is required.

4.5 Applications

Apart from their uses as impression materials, the major applications of waxes in dentistry are as modelling waxes and inlay waxes, collectively termed pattern waxes.

Denture modelling waxes: The manufacture of dentures involves several stages with wax being used in at least two of these.

Following the production of a stone model from an impression, a wax *rim* is constructed, either directly on the model, or on a denture base which has been adapted to the model. The rim is inserted into the patient's mouth at the 'registration' stage in order to record a satisfactory occlusal relationship. The next stage is to mount artificial teeth on the wax rim and to check the suitability of the wax denture at the 'try in' stage.

Waxes used for this purpose should have a softening temperature well above mouth temperature so that they are not distorted at either the registration or try in stages. They should be tough in order to reduce the chances of fracture during removal from the stone model. Three types of material are available, designated as follows:

Type 1   soft wax
Type 2   hard wax
Type 3   extra hard

These products differ primarily in regard to their softening temperature. Only the type 3 material can be considered relatively stable at mouth temperature. Type 1 material is designed to be hard at room temperature but soft at mouth temperature and is used only for building contours and veneers in the laboratory. The type 2 material is suitable for pattern production in temperate climates. Type 3 material is designed primarily for use in warmer climates.

Modelling waxes consist mainly of mixtures of paraffin wax and beeswax and have melting points in the range 49–58°C. They are generally supplied in sheet form, the sheets being produced either by rolling or by cutting from a block. Rolled sheets often change shape on softening due to the relief of stresses which are introduced during rolling. Some denture modelling waxes are referred to as *toughened* by their manufacturers. This probably reflects attempts to control the rolling procedure to optimize crystal alignments which may influence mechanical properties. Sheets of toughened modelling wax can typically be bent without fracturing.

Softening of the sheets is normally carried out under controlled conditions using a water bath. This enables the thickness of the sheet (typically 1–2 mm)

Table 4.1 Flow values of some dental waxes.

Material	Flow value % at specified temperature				
	23°C	30°C	37°C	40°C	45°C
Casting wax					
Type 1	—	1.0 max	—	50 min	70–90
Type 2	—	—	1.0 max	20 max	70–90
Modelling wax					
Type 1	1.0 max	—	5–90	—	—
Type 2	0.6 max	—	10 max	—	50–90
Type 3	0.2 max	—	1.2 max	—	5–50

to be maintained which is important since the thickness of the wax will control the thickness of the denture base.

Although the softening temperatures of modelling waxes are above mouth temperature, even type 2 and 3 materials will slightly soften and distort if left in the mouth for more than a few minutes. This should be taken into account during registration and try in.

Modelling waxes are tough enough to resist fracture when withdrawn from shallow undercuts. An important requirement of denture modelling waxes is that they can easily be trimmed with a sharp instrument without tearing, chipping or flaking. These characteristics are determined at room temperature since they dictate the ease with which trimming can be performed in the laboratory situation.

Waxes tend to have high values of coefficient of thermal expansion, which coupled with the manner in which the materials are used (softening with heat and cooling) suggests that a significant dimensional change can occur. An upper limit of 0.8% expansion on heating from 25°C to 40°C is allowed in the ISO specification. When the wax denture is invested, prior to formation of an acrylic denture base, the wax can be removed from the mould by melting in boiling water, leaving no detectable residue.

Some metal components of partial dentures are formed in wax on the model. Small sheets of casting wax are used, which have been rolled to a precise thickness, according to the metal gauge required. In manipulating this wax it is important that the thickness is maintained. It is usual to soften it in hot water and adapt it into position with a soft material such as cotton wool or rubber. Pre-formed polymeric components can be used as an alternative to waxes for modelling the metal components of partial dentures.

Temporary denture bases constructed from wax and used during denture construction are prone to distortions unless great care is taken. For this reason alternative materials/techniques are sometimes used.

Shellac, a wax-like resin which is more stable at mouth temperature, has been used for construction of the temporary denture base. The wax rim is then built on top of this more stable base. Shellac is a natural beetle exudate which has a considerably higher softening temperature than ordinary modelling wax. Care must be taken to ensure thorough softening prior to moulding, otherwise considerable stresses are introduced which eventually lead to distortion.

Another widely used approach to denture construction is to use either a temporary or permanent acrylic base-plate on which to construct the wax rim. The advantages and disadvantages of the various approaches are beyond the scope of this book and are covered adequately in other excellent texts.

Inlay waxes: Wax patterns for inlays or cast posts can be produced either by a direct or indirect technique as mentioned previously. The use of direct wax patterns is normally reserved only for the most simple designs of cast posts/cores on anterior teeth. These patterns can be removed from the prepared tooth or root with a minimum of distortion. Inlay casting waxes are currently classified as follows:

Type 1   soft
Type 2   hard

This has caused some confusion because in the past the opposite classification was used. The type 1 materials are designed for use in the indirect technique, being suitable for making patterns outside the mouth for the production of inlays, crowns and cast pontics. The type 2 materials are suitable for use in the direct technique (and may also be suitable for indirect use) for the production of inlays and crowns. The difference between the two types of wax is characterized by their flow behaviour as shown in Table 4.1. Both types are commonly produced in the form of cones and sticks.

For direct wax patterns the softened wax is forced into the tooth cavity and held under pressure until it cools. The wax should soften just above mouth temperature and should not be raised to a higher temperature than necessary, in order to reduce the magnitude of thermal contraction and internal stresses. In addition, the softening temperature must be tolerated without pain by the patient. The thermal contraction occurring on removal of the direct pattern material from the mouth is of the order of 0.1–0.5%. This would seem sufficient to cause problems of fit with the final cast restoration although serious problems are rarely encountered in practice, possibly because of the relatively simple nature of the restorations produced by the direct technique. Dimensional changes caused by stress relief are minimized by investing the pattern as soon as possible.

The material should be hard at mouth temperature and when removed from the cavity should fracture rather than flow if the cavity has unwanted undercuts. This enables the undercuts to be located and removed.

The wax should ideally have a good colour contrast with enamel and be easy to carve without flaking so that the exposed surfaces of wax can be easily contoured to shape and the margins readily observed. When a direct pattern for a two-surface restoration is removed there is a need to increase the bulk of material in the contact area between teeth to ensure that the correct pattern of tooth to tooth contact is recreated. This can be achieved either by using a very low fusing point wax and adding to the pattern or by soldering additional precious metal to the casting. Direct patterns for post cores are built up using a different approach. The post channel is usually prepared using a proprietary system and a pre-formed pattern for the post is installed into the canal. The core is then built up in wax by melting the wax on an instrument and carrying the molten wax into the tooth.

The required properties are produced by using a blend of several types of wax including paraffin wax, carnauba, candelilla and beeswax with small quantities of other resins.

The procedure for indirect patterns is similar to that described for direct patterns except that the softened wax is forced into a cavity on the gypsum die. Since this procedure is carried out at room temperature rather than mouth temperature, inlay waxes for indirect patterns may soften at a somewhat lower temperature than direct pattern waxes, although the softening temperature should not be so low that the wax will flow at room temperature (Table 4.1). The value of thermal contraction for the indirect technique is much lower as a result of the lower softening temperature. This may be considered a distinct advantage of the indirect technique. However, it should be appreciated that the die has been produced in an impression which was itself recorded at mouth temperature and then cooled to room temperature – thus undergoing a thermal contraction which may approach the value of a direct wax pattern material. The normal method of softening for inlay casting waxes is using dry heat. When using a flame, care should be taken not to overheat the wax whilst at the same time thorough softening throughout the whole bulk of material occurs. When material in stick form is used it is gently rotated above the flame until it becomes shiny. It is then removed and then replaced and the process repeated until it is warmed throughout. At this stage the softened material can be kneaded before pressing into the prepared cavity.

Inlay waxes are also used widely in the dental laboratory to prepare casting patterns for metallic restorations, either crowns or bridges. The first layer of wax is applied to a die either by adapting a softened thin sheet of wax or using a hot dipping technique. The wax pattern is then developed using a wax-additive technique in which molten wax is applied to the die of the tooth to rebuild gradually the form of the tooth. Pre-formed resin components are available to facilitate the manufacture of patterns for bridge pontics.

4.6 Suggested further reading

Craig, R.G., Eick, J.D. & Peyton, F.A. (1965) The properties of natural waxes used in dentistry. *J. Dent. Res.* **44**, 1308.

Warth, A.H. (1956) *The Chemistry and Technology of Waxes.* Von Nostrand Reinhold, New York.

Chapter 5
Investments and Refractory Dies

5.1 Introduction

Following the production of a wax pattern by either the direct or indirect method (Chapter 4), the next stage in many dental procedures involves the *investment* of the pattern to form a mould. A sprue is attached to the pattern and the assemblage is located in a casting ring (Fig. 5.1). Investment material is poured around the wax pattern whilst still in a fluid state. When the investment sets hard, the wax and sprue former are removed by softening and/or burning out to leave a mould which can be filled with an alloy or ceramic using a casting technique.

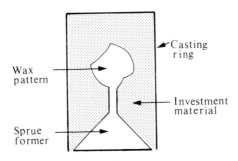

Fig. 5.1 Diagram illustrating how an investment mould is constructed from a wax pattern.

In the case of acrylic denture production the base-plate wax is invested in a two-part split mould using dental plaster or stone as the investment. Following removal of the wax the resulting mould is filled with acrylic resin.

The investment mould used for casting alloys and some castable ceramics needs to be constructed from a material which retains its integrity at the casting temperature. Unmodified dental plasters or stones are not suitable for this purpose.

A group of materials which are closely related to the investment materials are the refractory die materials. These products are used for making dies on which ceramic restorations (e.g. porcelain crowns) are constructed. As for the investments used in casting, a prerequisite of the refractory die materials is an ability to retain their structural integrity at the temperatures used to *fire* ceramics.

Phosphate-bonded die materials are most commonly used for the construction of refractory dies and since these are similar to phosphate bonded investments they will be covered in that section.

5.2 Requirements of investments for alloy casting procedures

The investment material forms the mould into which an alloy will be cast and it therefore follows that the accuracy of the casting can be no better than the accuracy of the mould.

The investment should be capable of reproducing the shape, size and detail recorded in the wax pattern. Since casting is carried out at very high temperatures, often in excess of 1000°C, the investment mould should be capable of maintaining its shape and integrity at these elevated temperatures. In addition, the investment should have a sufficiently high value of compressive strength at the casting temperature so that it can withstand the stresses set up when the molten metal enters the mould.

Alloy castings undergo considerable contraction when cooling from the casting temperature to room temperature. Such contraction may result in a casting with a very poor fit, for example a simple class I inlay would be loose fitting, whereas a crown would be too small and short at the margin. One function of the investment mould is to compensate for this casting shrinkage. This is generally achieved by a combination of setting expansion during the hardening of the investment mould and thermal expansion during the heating of the mould to the casting temperature.

The main factors involved in the selection of investment material are the casting temperature to be used and the type of alloy to be cast. Some gold alloys are cast at relatively low casting temperatures of around 900°C whilst some chromium alloys require casting temperatures of around 1450°C.

The investment which is best able to retain its integrity at the casting temperature and able· to provide the necessary compensation for casting shrinkage is chosen.

5.3 Available materials

Investment materials consist of a mixture of a refractory material, normally silica, which is capable of withstanding very high temperatures without degradation, and a binder which binds the refractory particles together. The nature of the binder characterizes the material.

There are three main groups of investment material in common use. They are referred to as *gypsum-bonded, silica-bonded* or *phosphate-bonded.*

Gypsum-bonded materials

These materials are supplied as powders which are mixed with water and are composed of a mixture of silica (SiO_2) and calcium sulphate hemihydrate (gypsum product) together with other minor components including powdered graphite or powdered copper and various modifiers to control setting time.

Silica is a refractory material which adequately withstands the temperatures used during casting. It is available in three allotropic forms – quartz, cristobalite and tridymite – which are all chemically identical but differ slightly in crystalline form. Quartz and cristobalite are used extensively in investments. In addition to imparting the necessary refractory properties to the investment, the silica is responsible for producing much of the expansion which is necessary to compensate for the casting shrinkage of the alloy. The expansion is accomplished by a combination of simple thermal expansion coupled with a crystalline *inversion* which

results in a significant expansion. Quartz undergoes *inversion* at a temperature of 575°C from the so-called 'low' form or α-quartz to the so-called 'high' form or β-quartz. For cristobalite, conversion from the low to the high form occurs at a lower temperature of around 210°C. The expansion is probably due to a straightening of chemical bonds to form a less dense crystal structure as illustrated in Fig. 5.2. The change is reversible and both quartz and cristobalite revert back to the low form on cooling. The overall thermal expansion and *inversion* expansion of materials containing cristobalite is greater than those containing quartz as illustrated in Fig. 5.3.

The calcium sulphate hemihydrate is an essential component since it reacts with water to form calcium sulphate dihydrate (gypsum) which effectively binds together the refractory silica. The chemistry of setting and important properties of gypsum products are dealt with in Chapter 3. The setting expansion of the calcium sulphate dihydrate, when mixed with water, is used to partially compensate for the shrinkage of the alloy which occurs on casting. Further compensation can be achieved by employing the hygroscopic setting expansion which occurs if the investment mould is placed into water at the initial set stage. The latter method is known as the *water immersion* hygroscopic expansion technique and can result in an expansion of five times the normal setting expansion. Another method is the *water added* technique in which a measured volume of water is placed on the upper surface of the investment material within the casting ring. This produces a more readily controlled expansion. Hygroscopic expansion is further encouraged by lining the casting ring with a layer of damp asbestos which is able to feed water to a large surface area of the investment mould. The latter technique is routinely employed even when no attempt is made to maximize hygroscopic expansion by immersing in water or adding water.

The mechanism of hygroscopic expansion is not

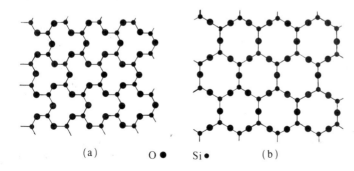

(a)   O ●   Si ●   (b)

Fig. 5.2 Bond straightening during 'inversion' of quartz at 575°C. (a) More dense structure existing below 575°C. (b) Less dense structure existing above 575°C.

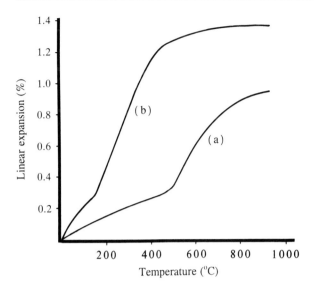

Fig. 5.3 Linear expansion versus temperature curves for two types of investment. (a) Containing quartz. (b) Containing crystobalite.

fully understood. However, it may be envisaged that water is attracted between crystals by capillary action and that the extra separation of particles causes an expansion. The magnitude of the hygroscopic setting expansion which occurs with gypsum-bonded investments is greater than that which occurs with gypsum model and die materials.

Gypsum alone is not satisfactory as an investment for alloy casting since it contracts on heating as water is lost and fractures before reaching the casting temperature. The magnitude of the contraction, which occurs rapidly above 320°C, is significantly reduced in investment materials by the incorporation of sodium chloride and boric acid.

Three types of gypsum bonded investments can be identified as follows:

Type 1   thermal expansion type; for casting inlays and crowns.

Type 2   hygroscopic expansion type; for casting inlays and crowns.

Type 3   for casting complete and partial dentures.

The ISO Standard for gypsum bonded investments allows individual products to be described by more than one of the above. Hence, materials may be both type 1 and type 3 but must satisfy the most stringent of the requirements outlined in the two standards. Interestingly, the ISO Standard describes all of these materials as 'Dental gypsum-bonded casting investments for gold alloys', implying that they are suitable only for a limited range of alloys. This is confirmed by a consideration of their properties (Section 5.4).

Silica-bonded materials

These materials consist of powdered quartz or cristobalite which is bonded together with silica gel. On heating, the silica gel turns into silica so that the completed mould is a tightly packed mass of silica particles.

The binder solution is generally prepared by mixing ethyl silicate or one of its oligomers with a mixture of dilute hydrochloric acid and industrial spirit. The industrial spirit improves the mixing of ethyl silicate and water which are otherwise immiscible. A slow hydrolysis of ethyl silicate occurs producing a sol of silicic acid with the liberation of ethyl alcohol as a byproduct,

$$(C_2H_5O)_4Si + 4H_2O \rightarrow Si(OH)_4 + 4C_2H_5OH$$

The silicic acid sol forms silica gel on mixing with quartz or cristobalite powder under alkaline conditions. The necessary pH is achieved by the presence of magnesium oxide in the powder.

Stock solutions of the hydrolysed ethyl silicate binder are normally made and stored in dark bottles. The solution gels slowly on standing and its viscosity may increase noticeably after three or four weeks. When this happens it is necessary to make up a fresh solution.

Simultaneous hydrolysis and gelation can be promoted by amines such as piperidine. Unfortunately, such a procedure is accompanied by an unacceptable shrinkage which is a result, mainly, of the hydrolysis reaction.

In order that the material should have sufficient strength at the casting temperature it is necessary to incorporate as much powder as possible into the binder solution. This process is aided by a gradation of particle sizes such that small grains fill in the spaces between the larger grains. A very thick, almost dry mix of investment is used and it is vibrated in order to encourage close packing and produce as strong an investment as possible.

A small shrinkage occurs during the early stages of the heating of the investment prior to casting. This is due to loss of water and alcohol from the gel. The contraction is followed by a more substantial thermal expansion and inversion expansion of the silica similar to that for gypsum-bonded investments.

Ethyl-silicate bonded investments do not expand on setting in the same way that gypsum-bonded and phosphate-bonded materials do. The total linear expansion is therefore identical with the linear thermal expansion.

Phosphate-bonded materials

These materials consist of a powder containing silica, magnesium oxide and ammonium phosphate. On mixing with water or a colloidal silica solution, a reaction between the phosphate and oxide occurs to form magnesium ammonium phosphate.

$$NH_4 \cdot H_2PO_4 + MgO + 5H_2O \rightarrow Mg \cdot NH_4 \cdot PO_4 \cdot 6H_2O$$

This binds the silica together to form the set investment mould. The formation of the magnesium ammonium phosphate involves a hydration reaction followed by crystallization similar to that for the formation of gypsum. As in the case of gypsum, a small expansion results from the outward thrust of growing crystals. The material is also able to undergo hygroscopic expansion if placed in contact with moisture during setting. Moisture adversely affects the unmixed material and the container should always be kept closed when not in use.

The use of colloidal solution of silica instead of water for mixing with the powder has the dual effect of increasing the setting expansion and strengthening the set material.

On heating the investment prior to casting, mould enlargement occurs by both thermal expansion and inversion of the silica. Thermal expansion is greater for the colloidal silica-mixed materials than for the water-mixed materials. At a temperature of about 300°C ammonia and water are liberated by the reaction:

$$2(Mg \cdot NH_4 \cdot PO_4 \cdot 6H_2O) \rightarrow Mg_2 \cdot P_2O_7 + 2NH_3 + 13 H_2O$$

At a higher temperature some of the remaining phosphate reacts with silica forming complex silico-phosphates. These cause a significant increase in the strength of the material at the casting temperature.

Two types of phosphate-bonded investment can be identified as follows:

Type 1:   for inlays, crowns and other fixed restorations.

Type 2:   for partial dentures and other cast, removable restorations.

5.4 Properties of investment materials

Thermal stability: One of the primary requirements of an investment is that it should retain its integrity at the casting temperature and have sufficient strength to withstand the stresses set up when the molten alloy enters the investment mould.

Gypsum-bonded investments decompose above 1200°C by interaction of silica with calcium sulphate to liberate sulphur trioxide gas.

$$CaSO_4 + SiO_2 \rightarrow CaSiO_3 + SO_3$$

This not only causes severe weakening of the investment but would lead to the incorporation of porosity into the castings. Thus, gypsum-bonded materials are generally restricted to use with those alloys which are cast well below 1200°C. This includes the majority of the gold alloys and some of the lower melting, base metal alloys. The majority of base alloys, however, have higher casting temperatures and require the use of a silica-bonded or phosphate-bonded material.

Another reaction which may take place on heating gypsum-bonded investments is that between calcium sulphate and carbon:

$$CaSO_4 + 4C \rightarrow CaS + 4CO$$

The carbon may be derived from the residue left after burning out of the wax pattern or may be present as graphite in the investment. Further reaction can occur liberating sulphur dioxide:

$$3CaSO_4 + CaS \rightarrow 4CaO + 4SO_2$$

These reactions occur above 700°C and their effects can be minimized by 'heat soaking' the investment mould at the casting temperature to allow the reaction to be completed before casting commences.

The presence of an oxalate in some investments reduces the effects of gypsum decomposition products by liberating carbon dioxide at elevated temperatures.

Phosphate- and silica-bonded materials have sufficient strength at the high temperatures used for casting base metal alloys. The strength of the phosphate-bonded materials is aided by the formation of silicophosphates on heating.

The cohesive strength of the phosphate investments is such that they do not have to be contained in a metal casting ring. The material is generally allowed to set inside a plastic ring which is removed before heating.

Although it is the strength of the investment material at the casting temperature which is most critical this is difficult to measure (for obvious reasons). The normal method used for evaluating strength is therefore to measure compressive strength at room temperature 2 hours after starting to mix the material. Values specified in the various ISO Standards for investments are given in Table 5.1.

Table 5.1 Compressive strength values for investment and refractory die materials.

Material	Compressive strength (MPa) at 2 h (minimum values allowed in ISO Standards)
Gypsum-bonded investment	1.5
Silica-bonded investment	1.5
Phosphate-bonded investment – type 1	2.5
Phosphate-bonded investment – type 2	3.0
Phosphate-bonded refractory die	13.0

The higher strengths of the phosphate-bonded materials mean that these products are becoming widely used for casting all types of alloys (precious, semi-precious and base-metal). The wax burn-out temperature is varied to suit the type of alloy being cast. Typical wax burn-out temperatures are as follows:

gold alloys	700–750°C
palladium-silver alloys	730–815°C
base-metal alloys	815–900°C

This temperature is normally held for 30 minutes for small moulds and 1 hour for larger moulds before the metal is cast. Burn-out times need to be extended when resin-based pattern materials are used.

Porosity: The gypsum-bonded and phosphate-bonded materials are sufficiently porous to allow escape of air and other gases from the mould during casting. The silica-bonded materials, on the other hand, are so closely packed that they are virtually porosity-free and there is a danger of 'back pressure' building up which will cause the mould to be incompletely filled or the castings to be porous. These problems can be overcome by making vents in the investment which prevent the pressure from increasing.

Compensating expansion: The accuracy of fit of a casting depends primarily on the ability of the investment material to compensate for the shrinkage of the alloy which occurs on casting. The magnitude of the shrinkage varies widely but is of the order of 1.4% for most gold alloys, 2.0% for Ni/Cr alloys and 2.3% for Co/Cr alloys.

The compensating expansion is achieved by a combination of setting expansion, thermal expansion and the expansion which occurs when silica undergoes *inversion* at elevated temperatures.

Hygroscopic expansion can be used to supplement the setting expansion of gypsum-bonded materials. This is also possible for phosphate-bonded materials but is rarely used in practice for these products.

The setting expansion of a typical gypsum-bonded material is of the order of 0.3% which may be increased to around 1.3% by hygroscopic expansion.

The degree of thermal expansion depends on the nature of the silica refractory used in the investment and the temperature to which the mould is heated. Investments containing cristobalite undergo greater thermal expansion than those containing quartz, as shown in Fig. 5.3 for a gypsum-bonded material. If hygroscopic expansion has been used to achieve expansion it is likely that the magnitude of the thermal expansion required will be relatively small. When thermal expansion is used as the primary means of achieving compensation a cristobalite-containing investment mould heated to around 700°C is required.

Silica-bonded investments undergo a slight contraction during setting and the early stages of heating. This is due to the nature of the setting reaction and the subsequent loss of water and alcohol from the material. Continued heating causes considerable expansion due to the close-packed nature of the silica particles. A maximum linear expansion of approximately 1.6% is reached at a temperature of about 600°C.

For phosphate-bonded materials a combined setting expansion and thermal expansion of around 2.0% is normal, provided the special silica liquid is used with the investment. Many manufacturers of phosphate-bonded investments supply instructions which enable the expansion to be varied so that the casting shrinkage of the alloy can be compensated more precisely. This variation is achieved by diluting the *special liquid* with water. Table 5.2 gives an example of how this works out in practice. Hence, by selecting the most appropriate liquid dilution the investment can be made to compensate casting shrinkages for both base-metal alloys and gold alloys.

Table 5.2 Effect of special liquid dilution on the expansion of phosphate-bonded investment at 700–900°C.

Special liquid: water	Expansion (%)
Neat liquid	1.9–2.1
3:1	1.7–1.9
1:1	1.5–1.7
1:3	1.3–1.5

The expansion reaches a maximum at 700°C and remains the same to 1000°C. The lowest permissible burn-out temperature for any particular alloy normally gives the best results so it is essential to follow the directions given for any particular alloy.

Consideration of the relatively large casting shrinkages which can occur with some base-metal alloys in comparison with the compensating expansions possible with the investments may suggest that ideal compensation is not always possible.

It should be remembered, however, that further compensation may take place during other stages in the production of the casting. A small contraction of the impression, for example, may give the required compensation.

5.5 Applications

Table 5.3 gives the primary applications of the three main groups of investment materials.

Of the three main types of investment material, the phosphate-bonded products are becoming the most widely used. Silica-bonded materials are rarely used nowadays due to the fact that they are less

Table 5.3 Applications of the various types of investment material.

Investment	Primary use
Dental plaster or stone	Mould for acrylic dentures
Gypsum-bonded materials	Mould for gold casting alloys
Silica-bonded materials	Mould for base metal casting alloys (rarely used)
Phosphate-bonded materials	Mould for base metal and gold casting alloys; mould for cast ceramics and glasses
	Refractory die for ceramic build-up

convenient to use than the other products and that the ethanol produced in the liquid can spontaneously ignite or explode at elevated temperatures. Some laboratories regularly use phosphate-bonded materials even for gold castings. This practice allows the laboratory to stock only one type of investment, which is suitable for all cases.

The phosphate-bonded refractory die materials are used in a different way to the investments. A duplicating impression of the working die is made usually using a proprietary material. The mixed material is poured into this impression and allowed to set. It is then removed from the impression and consolidated by *firing* at about 1000°C. The surface is then coated with a thin layer of glaze and the die refired at a slightly lower temperature (e.g. 970°C). The surface glaze helps to prevent moisture from the porcelain from being soaked up into the porous die material.

5.6 Suggested further reading

Earnshaw, R. (1960) Investments for casting cobalt–chromium alloys, parts I and II. *Br. Dent. J.* **108**, 389 and 429.

Jones, D.W. (1967) Thermal behaviour of silica and its application to dental investments. *Br. Dent. J.* **122**, 489.

Chapter 6
Metals and Alloys

6.1 Introduction

Metals and alloys have many uses in dentistry. Steel alloys are commonly used for the construction of instruments and of wires for orthodontics. Gold alloys and alloys containing chromium are used for making crowns, inlays and denture bases whilst dental amalgam, an alloy containing mercury, is the most widely used dental filling material.

With the exception of mercury, metals are generally hard and lustrous at ambient temperatures, and have crystalline structures in which the atoms are closely packed together. Metals are opaque and are good conductors of both heat and electricity.

The shaping of metals and alloys for dental use can be accomplished by one of three methods, namely, casting, cold working or amalgamation. Casting involves heating the material until it becomes molten, when it can be forced into an investment mould which has been prepared from a wax pattern. Cold working involves mechanical shaping of the metal at relatively low temperatures, taking advantage of the high values of ductility and malleability possessed by many metals. Some alloys can be mixed with mercury to form a plastic mass which gradually hardens by a chemical reaction followed by crystallization. The material is shaped by packing it into a tooth cavity whilst still in the plastic state. This specific technique of shaping by amalgamation is dealt with in detail in the chapter devoted to dental amalgam (Chapter 21).

6.2 Structure and properties of metals

Crystal structure

Metals usually have crystalline structures in the solid state. When a molten metal or alloy is cooled, the solidification process is one of crystallization and is initiated at specific sites called nuclei. The nuclei are generally formed from impurities within the molten mass of metal (Fig. 6.1a). Crystals grow as dendrites, which can be described as three-dimensional, branched network structures emanating from the central nucleus (Fig. 6.1b). Crystal growth continues until all the material has solidified and all the dendritic crystals are in contact (Fig. 6.1c). Each crystal is known as a *grain* and the area between two grains in contact is the *grain boundary*.

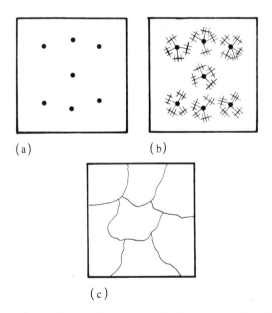

Fig. 6.1 Diagram illustrating crystallization of a metal (a) from nuclei, (b) through dendritic growth, (c) to form grains.

After crystallization, the grains have approximately the same dimensions in each direction, measured from the central nucleus. They are not perfectly spherical or cubic however, nor do they conform to any other geometric shape. They are said to have an *equiaxed* grain structure. A change from an equiaxed structure to one in which the grains have a more elongated, fibrous structure can cause important changes in mechanical properties.

The atoms within each grain are arranged in a regular three-dimensional lattice. There are several possible arrangements such as cubic, body-centred cubic and face-centred cubic as shown in Fig. 6.2. The arrangement adopted by any one crystal depends on specific factors such as atomic radius and charge distributions on the atoms. Although there is a tendency towards a perfect crystal structure, occasional defects occur, as illustrated, two-dimensionally, in Fig. 6.3. Such defects are normally referred to as *dislocations* and their occurrence has an effect on the *ductility* of the metal or alloy. When the material is placed under a sufficiently high stress the dislocation is able to move through the lattice until it reaches a grain boundary. The plane along which the dislocation moves is called a *slip plane* and the stress required to initiate movement is the yield stress.

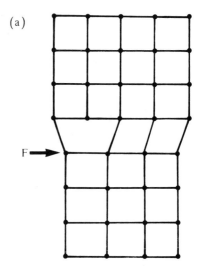

(a)

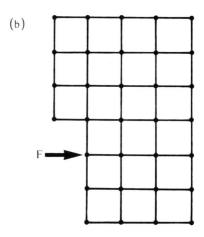

(b)

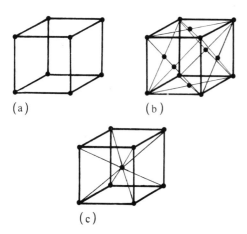

Fig. 6.2 Some possible arrangements of atoms in metals and alloys: (a) cubic structure; (b) face-centred cubic; (c) body-centred cubic.

Fig. 6.3 (a) Simplified, diagrammatic indication of an imperfection in a crystal structure. (b) Under the influence of sufficient force atoms may move to establish a more perfect arrangement.

In practical terms, the application of a stress greater than the yield stress causes the material to be permanently deformed as a result of movement of dislocations. Depending upon the circumstances, this can be a disadvantage or, alternatively, may be used to advantage, as in the formation of wires.

Grain boundaries form a natural barrier to the movement of dislocations. The concentration of grain boundaries increases as the grain size decreases. Metals with finer grain structure are generally harder and have higher values of yield stress than those with coarser grain structure. Hence it can be seen that material properties can

be controlled to some extent by controlling the grain size.

As stated in Chapter 2, the yield stress is not easily determined experimentally. The proportional limit is therefore often used as an indication of yield stress. Alternatively the *proof stress* is used. The proof stress is the stress required to produce a certain level of permanent strain. For example the 0.2% proof stress indicates the stress required to produce a strain of 0.002.

A fine grain structure can be achieved by rapid cooling of the molten metal or alloy following casting. This process, often referred to as *quenching*, ensures that many nuclei of crystallization are formed, resulting in a large number of relatively small grains as shown in Fig. 6.4a. Slow cooling causes relatively few nuclei to be formed which results in a larger grain size as shown in Fig. 6.4b. Some metals and alloys are said to have a *refined grain structure*. This is normally a fine grain structure which is achieved by *seeding* the molten material with an additive metal which forms nuclei for crystallization.

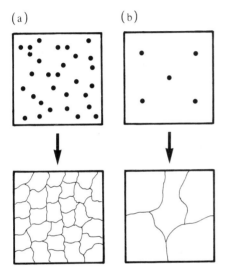

Fig. 6.4 Control of metallic grain size by controlling the rate of cooling from the melt. (a) Rapid cooling – more nuclei, smaller grains. (b) Slow cooling – fewer nuclei, larger grains.

Cold working

In the previous section it was mentioned that permanent deformation takes place on the application of a sufficiently high force, due to the movement of dislocations along slip planes. For an applied tensile force the maximum degree of extension is a measure of the *ductility* of the metal or alloy. For an applied compressive force the maximum degree of compression is a measure of *malleability*. These changes occur when the stress is greater than the yield stress and at relatively low temperatures. Such *cold working* not only produces a change in microstructure, with dislocations becoming concentrated at grain boundaries, but also a change in grain shape. The grains are no longer equiaxed but take up a more *fibrous* structure (Fig. 6.5a). The properties of the material are altered, becoming harder and stronger with a higher value of yield stress. The ductility or

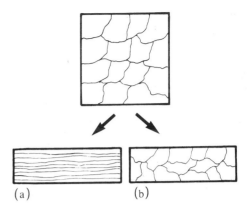

Fig. 6.5 Mechanical work carried out on a sample of metal or alloy. (a) Below the recrystallization temperature – produces a fibrous grain structure. (b) Above the recrystallization temperature – retains an equiaxed grain structure.

malleability is decreased because the potential for further cold working is reduced. Cold working is sometimes referred to as *work hardening* due to the effect on mechanical properties. When mechanical work is carried out on a metal or alloy at a more elevated temperature it is possible for the metal object to change shape without any alteration in grain shape or mechanical properties (Fig. 6.5b). The temperature below which work hardening is possible is termed the *recrystallization temperature*. Examples of cold working in dentistry include the following.

(1) The formation of wires, in which an alloy is forced through a series of circular dies of gradually decreasing diameter. The resulting fibrous grain structure is responsible for the special *springy* properties possessed by most wires.
(2) The bending of wires or clasps during the construction and alteration of appliances.
(3) The swaging of stainless steel denture bases.

Since metals and alloys have finite values of ductility or malleability there is a limit to the amount of cold working which can be carried out. Attempts to carry out further cold working beyond this limit may result in fracture. This limitation should be remembered when carrying out alterations to clasps constructed from low-ductility alloys.

If a cold-worked metal or alloy with a fibrous grain structure is heated to above its recrystallization temperature it gradually reverts to an equiaxed form and becomes softer with a lower value of yield stress but a higher ductility. Hence, recrystallization can be used as a softening heat treatment. In many applications of wrought alloys however, it is something which must be avoided because of the adverse effect on mechanical properties. If the material is maintained above the recrystallization temperature for sufficient time, diffusion of atoms across grain boundaries may occur, leading to *grain growth*. The effect of grain size on mechanical properties has already been discussed and it is clear that grain growth should be avoided if the properties are not to be adversely affected.

Cold working may cause the formation of internal stresses within a metal object. If these stresses are gradually relieved they may cause distortion which could lead to loss of fit of, for example, an orthodontic appliance. For certain metals and alloys the internal stresses can be wholly or partly eliminated by using a low temperature heat treatment referred to as *stress relief annealing*. This heat treatment is carried out well below the recrystallization temperature and has no deleterious effect on mechanical properties since the fibrous grain structure is maintained.

6.3 Structure and properties of alloys

An alloy is a mixture of two or more metals. Mixtures of two metals are termed binary alloys, mixtures of three metals ternary alloys etc. The term *alloy system* refers to all possible compositions of an alloy. For example the silver–copper system refers to all alloys with compositions ranging between 100% silver and 100% copper.

In the molten state metals usually show mutual solubility, one within another. When the molten mixture is cooled to below the melting point one of four things can occur.

(1) The component metals may remain soluble in each other forming a *solid solution*. The solid solution may take one of three forms. It may be a *random solid solution* in which the component metal atoms occupy random sites in a common crystal lattice. Another possibility is the formation of an *ordered solid solution* in which component metal atoms occupy specific sites within a common crystal lattice. The third type of solid solution is the *interstitial solid solution* in which, for binary alloys, the primary lattice sites are occupied by one metal atom and the atoms of the second component do not occupy lattice sites but lie within the interstices of the lattice. This is normally found where the atomic radius of one component is much smaller than that of the other. Solid solutions are generally harder, stronger and have higher values of elastic limit than the pure metals from which they are derived. This explains why pure metals are rarely used. The hardening effect, known as *solution hardening*, is thought to be due to the fact that atoms of different atomic radii within the same lattice form a mechanical resistance to the movement of dislocations along slip planes.

(2) The component metals may be completely insoluble in the solid state. Examination of a binary alloy of two metals, A and B, showing this behaviour reveals the presence of some areas containing pure metal A and others containing pure metal B. This type of alloy is susceptible to electrolytic corrosion, as described in Section 2.7, particularly if the component metals have widely differing electrochemical potentials. Complete insolubility of two metals is rarely encountered in practice.

(3) The two metals may be partially soluble in the solid state. For metals A and B two distinct phases exist within the solid state. One phase consists of a solid solution of metal B in metal A, whilst the other phase consists of a solid solution of A in B. There is a limit to the solubility of the two metals one within the other in each of the two types of grain. The solubility is temperature dependent and normally decreases markedly as the temperature is reduced from the melting point down to room temperature. These *partially soluble solid solutions* are far more commonly encountered than the completely insoluble material covered in the previous paragraph.

(4) If the two metals show a particular affinity for one another they may form intermetallic compounds with precise chemical formulation (e.g. Ag_3Sn). Since intermetallic compounds have specific valence requirements there are fewer crystal imperfections and the potential for movement along slip planes is reduced. Such materials therefore tend to be relatively hard and brittle with low ductility.

Most alloys have properties which are specific to the particular system being considered. The general principles discussed for metals in the previous section, however, also hold true for most alloy systems. Hence, the grain size of alloys can be controlled by the rate of cooling from the melt. Alloys can be work hardened and they undergo recrystallization and grain growth under the correct conditions.

6.4 Cooling curves

Metals and alloys are sometimes characterized using cooling curves. The material is heated till molten then allowed to cool and a plot of temperature against time is recorded, as shown in Fig. 6.6. For a pure metal (Fig. 6.6a) the cooling curve displays a distinct plateau region at the melting point (Tm) indicating that temperature remains constant over a period of time during crystallization. With few exceptions, the cooling curves for alloys show no such plateau region (Fig. 6.6b). Crystallization begins at temperature T_1, and is complete at temperature T_2. Hence crystallization takes place over a range of temperatures.

(a)

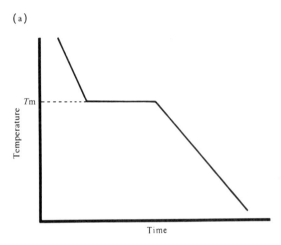

(b)

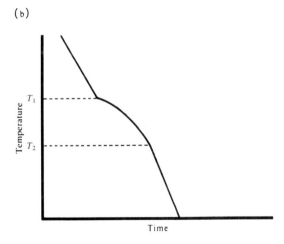

Fig. 6.6 Cooling curves for (a) a pure metal, showing solidification at a fixed temperature and (b) an alloy showing solidification over a range of temperatures.

For a binary solid solution alloy of two metals, A and B, in which the melting point of metal A is greater than that of metal B, the first material to crystallize, at just below temperature T_1, will be rich in the higher melting point metal A, whilst the last

material to crystallize, at a temperature just above T_2, is rich in the lower melting point metal B. Each alloy grain can be envisaged as having a concentration gradient of metals; the higher melting metal being concentrated close to the nucleus and the lower melting metal close to the grain boundaries.

The material is said to have a *cored* structure. Such *coring* may influence corrosion resistance since electrolytic cells may be set up on the surface of the alloy between areas of different alloy composition.

If a series of cooling curves for alloys of different composition within a given alloy system are available a *phase diagram* can be constructed from which many important predictions regarding coring and other structural variations can be made.

6.5 Phase diagrams

The temperature range over which an alloy crystallizes can readily be obtained from the cooling curve, as illustrated in Fig. 6.6b. If the temperatures T_1 and T_2 are obtained over a range of compositions for an alloy system and their values plotted against percentage composition, a useful graph emerges. This is illustrated in Fig. 6.7 for a hypothetical solid solution alloy of metals A and B. The melting points of the pure metals are indicated by the temperatures TmA and TmB. The upper and lower temperature limits of the crystallization range, T_1 and T_2, are shown for four alloys ranging in composition from 80% A/20% B to 20% A/80% B.

The phase diagram is completed by joining together all the T_1 points and all the T_2 points, together with the melting points of the pure metals, TmA and TmB. At temperatures in the region above the top line, known as the *liquidus line*, the alloy is totally liquid. At temperatures in the region below the bottom line, known as the *solidus line*, the alloy is totally solid. At temperatures in the region between the solidus and liquidus lines the alloy consists of a mixture of solid and liquid. The composition of the solid and liquid phases at any temperature between T_1 and T_2 can be predicted with the aid of the phase diagram.

Solid solution phase diagrams

Figure 6.7 shows how the phase diagram for a binary solid solution alloy is constructed. The diagram is redrawn in Fig. 6.8 in order to illustrate how it may be used to predict some of the characteristics of the alloy. Consider, for example, an alloy of composition X (approximately 60% A and 40% B). This alloy may be rendered completely molten by

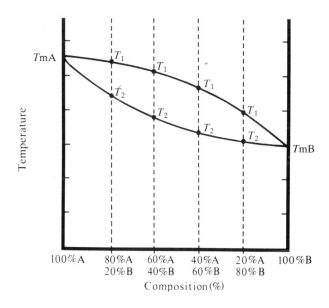

Fig. 6.7 Phase diagram of a solid solution alloy constructed from a series of cooling curves (Fig. 6.6). The temperatures T_1 and T_2 are obtained from experiments using alloys of varying composition.

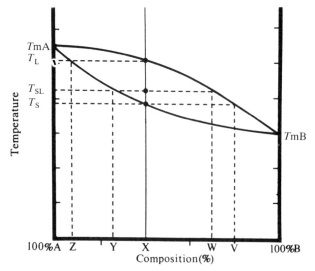

Fig. 6.8 Diagram illustrating how a solid solution phase diagram can be used to predict or explain certain alloy characteristics.

heating it to a temperature above T_1 which represents the liquidus temperature for that particular composition. If the alloy is cooled from above T_L it remains molten until the temperature T_L is reached, when the first solid begins to form. The composition of the first solid to form is given by drawing a horizontal line or *tie line* to intersect the solidus. In this case, drawing such a tie line reveals that the first solid to form has composition Z (approximately 90% A/10% B). As the alloy is cooled further, more crystallization occurs and between temperatures T_L and T_S a mixture of solid and liquid exists. Selecting one temperature, T_{SL}, within this region, the composition of both solid

and liquid can be predicted, by noting where the tie line intersects both solidus and liquidus. Thus, at temperature T_{SL} the composition of the solid is Y (approximately 80% A/20% B) and the composition of the remaining liquid is W (approximately 75% B/25% A). On further cooling, the alloy becomes completely solid at temperature T_S. The last liquid to crystallize has the composition V (approximately 80% B/20% A). This confirms the previous observation that for solid solution alloys a cored structure exists in which the first material to crystallize is rich in the metal with the higher melting point (A), whilst the last material to solidify is rich in the other metal (B). In the case of the alloy described, the variation in composition within the solidified alloy grains ranges from 90% A/10% B near the nuclei to 80% B/20% A at the grain boundaries. An indication of the degree of coring is given by the separation of the solidus and liquidus lines on the phase diagram. The potential for coring is greater when there is wide separation of solidus and liquidus lines as shown in Fig. 6.9.

The previous discussion describes what happens when a solid solution alloy is cooled rapidly, as occurs for example, during casting. With slow cooling the crystallization process is accompanied by diffusion and a random distribution of atoms results, with no coring. Rapid cooling quickly denies the alloy the energy and mobility required for diffusion of atoms to occur and the cored structure is 'locked in' at low temperatures. Reducing the cooling rate as a means of eliminating coring would be self-defeating since it would produce an alloy with large grain size which, of course, would have inferior mechanical properties.

The coring may markedly reduce the corrosion resistance of some alloys, a heat treatment is sometimes used to eliminate the cored structure. Such a heat treatment is termed a *homogenization* heat treatment. This involves heating the alloy to a temperature just below the solidus temperature for a few minutes to allow diffusion of atoms and the establishment of an homogeneous structure. The alloy is then normally quenched in order to prevent grain

(a)

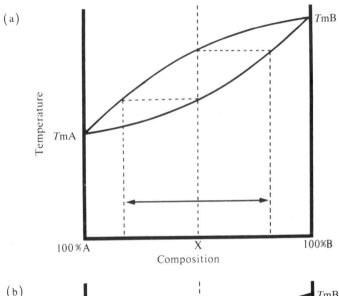

(b)

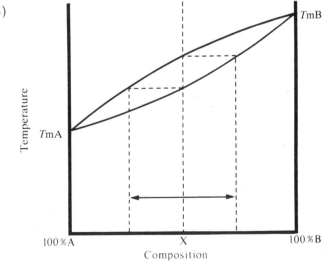

Fig. 6.9 Diagram to show how the extent of coring depends on the separation of solidus and liquidus line. (a) Solidus and liquidus widely separated. Extensive coring as illustrated by arrows. (b) Solidus and liquidus closer together resulting in less extensive coring.

growth from occurring. An example of a solid solution alloy is the gold–silver system.

Eutectic phase diagrams

It has already been pointed out that some metals are completely insoluble in the solid phase and an alloy of such metals consists of a mixture of grains of the pure metal components. Phase diagrams may be constructed by exactly the same technique as that described for solid solutions – by constructing cooling curves and noting the temperatures at which crystallization commences and is complete. Such a phase diagram for a hypothetical alloy of two metals, A and B, is shown in Fig. 6.10. The liquidus line is given by joining points A, C and E, whilst the solidus is given by A B C D E. The temperatures TmA and TmB are again the melting points of the pure metals A and B. In the two triangular regions between the solidus and liquidus lines a mixture of solid and liquid exists. The solid is always one of the pure metals. To the right of point C it is always pure B and to the left of point C it is always pure A. The alloy with composition corresponding to point C is called the *eutectic alloy* and is of particular interest since it crystallizes at a given temperature and not over a range of temperatures. In this respect, the eutectic alloy behaves in a similar fashion to a pure metal. Alloys with composition close to the eutectic composition have narrow melting ranges and melting points considerably lower than those of the component pure metals. For these reasons they are often used as solders.

The eutectic phase diagram can be used to predict composition changes during crystallization in just the same way as the solid solution diagram was used. For the most simple case of the eutectic alloy, it solidifies at temperature T_E to give a mixture of metals A and B. Figure 6.11 illustrates what happens during crystallization for an alloy, X, not having the eutectic composition. On cooling, crystallization begins at temperature T_L. The intersection of the horizontal tie line with the solidus indicates that the first material to crystallize is pure metal A. At temperature T_1 the alloy lies in the region between solidus and liquidus lines, indicating that a mixture of solid and liquid exists. The compositions of solid and liquid are given by the points of intersection of the tie line with the solidus and liquidus lines. Thus it can be seen that at T_1 the solid formed is still pure metal A whilst the remaining liquid has composition Y. On cooling further to temperature T_2, the solid is still pure metal A but the remaining liquid has composition Z, very close to the eutectic composition (E). Finally, on reaching temperature T_E the eutectic mixture of metals remaining in the liquid phase crystallize out.

Hence, a simplified explanation of what happens during cooling is that one of the pure metals crystallizes until the remaining mixture of molten metals has a composition equivalent to the eutectic. At this stage the remaining metals crystallize together.

The solidified alloy consists of a mixture of insoluble metals which often has inferior corrosion resistance due to the potential for the establishment of electrolytic cells on the surface of the alloy.

The situation of complete solid insolubility as described above is rarely met in practice. Much more common is the case of limited solubility. Where the solubility of one metal in the other in the solid state is

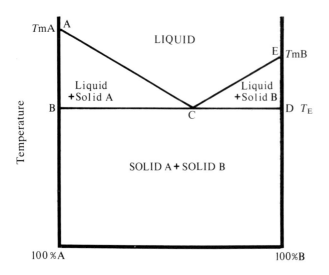

Fig. 6.10 Phase diagram of an alloy of two metals (A and B) which are completely insoluble in the solid phase. The alloy with compositions equivalent to point C is termed a eutectic alloy. The type of phase diagram is sometimes called a eutectic phase diagram.

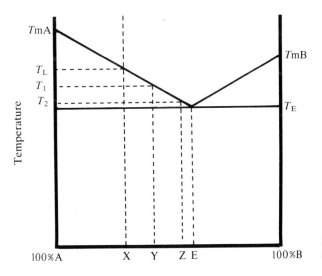

Fig. 6.11 Diagram illustrating how a eutectic phase diagram can be utilized.

low, the behaviour of the alloy is similar to that of a eutectic alloy except that instead of grains of pure metals being produced we get grains of two dilute solid solutions.

Other alloy systems

The preceding discussion of alloy cooling curves and the formation of phase diagrams for solid solutions and eutectics illustrates how important information on alloy systems can be gathered and utilized. Every alloy system has its own distinctive phase diagram which can be used to characterize that system. The principles behind the use of such diagrams are the same as those described here.

In the following chapters, specific alloy systems used in dentistry are discussed and some of their properties are illustrated with the aid of phase diagrams where necessary. In some cases, structural transitions of alloys occur, not during crystallization, but within the solid phase. Such solid–solid transitions complicate phase diagrams by adding more lines but do not alter the way in which the diagrams are used.

6.6 Suggested further reading

Cottrell, A. (1975) *An Introduction to Metallurgy*. Edward Arnold, London.

Chapter 7
Gold and Alloys of Noble Metals

7.1 Introduction

In the 'as cast' condition, pure gold is too soft to maintain its shape under the forces of mastication. Its strength and hardness can be greatly improved by either cold working or alloying.

Gold is very malleable and ductile and can be readily cold worked. This characteristic is utilized in the restoration of teeth using pure gold fillings. Alloys of gold are commonly used for cast restorations. The use of wrought gold wires is dealt with in a separate chapter dealing with wrought alloys.

7.2 Pure gold fillings (cohesive gold)

When two pieces of pure gold are pressed together, metallic bonds are formed at their point of contact and the gold is welded together, without the application of heat. This property of *cold welding* is utilized when building up a pure gold filling. The surfaces of the two pieces of gold must be perfectly clean to allow intimate contact and the applied force must be great enough to encourage the formation of bonds.

Cohesive gold is normally used in the form of a very thin gold sheet or 'foil', approximately 0.001 mm thick. On condensation into the prepared cavity, each layer of foil becomes welded to the material already condensed. It is normal practice to heat the gold foil to about 250°C in an electric furnace or a gas flame before use to remove any adsorbed grease or gases which would prevent efficient welding. The tooth to be filled must be isolated from the saliva using rubber dam and thoroughly dried to avoid contamination during condensation.

Condensation or 'plugging' of the gold may be carried out by hand, with an automatic mallet, or by the application of a mechanical vibrator. The use of an automatic mallet involves the application of a relatively large force at infrequent intervals, whereas a pneumatic or electrically driven condenser delivers much lighter, but more frequent blows. Care must be taken not to overheat the filling during the finishing procedures where the occlusal contour of the tooth is 'carved' using rotary finishing instruments then polished. Marked heating can cause damage to the pulp. The tooth and its supporting structures must withstand the fairly harsh treatment they receive during condensation without becoming damaged. Fortunately, both the dentine and periodontal membrane are fairly resilient.

The mechanical properties of the pure gold filling depend on the amount of cold working carried out on the material. The degree of work hardening depends on the pressure applied during condensation and the length of time for which the material is condensed. Practical limitations of time and the pressure which can be tolerated by the patient restrict the hardness of the pure gold filling to values similar to those for the softer (type I) casting gold alloys. Sandwich foils of gold and platinum are also available which produce a condensed restoration with better physical characteristics. These can be used to produce small class II restorations using a similar approach.

The advantages of the gold foil filling are that it is perfectly corrosion resistant and does not rely on a relatively soluble cement lute for retention. In cavities where the filling is surrounded by tooth substance, or where there is little or no opposing force, the mechanical properties are adequate and the pure gold filling offers a very durable restoration. In high load bearing areas, certain properties of pure gold such as rigidity and elastic limit are insufficient to resist distortion. Apart from this, the high cost of these restorations in terms of material used and the time taken to produce the restoration precludes their use in all but a minimal number of cases.

7.3 Traditional casting gold alloys

An indication of the composition of the traditional casting gold alloys is given in Table 7.1. The

Table 7.1 Typical compositions of casting gold alloys.

Type	Au (%)	Ag (%)	Cu (%)	Pt/Pd (%)	Zn (%)
1 (soft)	85	11	3	—	1
2 (medium)	75	12	10	2	1
3 (hard)	70	14	10	5	1
4 (extra hard)	65	9	15	10	1

descriptions of those alloys has changed over the years and the wording used in current ISO Standards is now:

Type 1   low strength – for castings subject to very slight stress, e.g. inlays.

Type 2   medium strength – for castings subject to moderate stress, e.g., inlays and onlays.

Type 3   high strength – for castings subject to high stress, e.g. onlays, thin cast backings, pontics, full crowns and saddles.

Type 4   extra high strength – for castings subject to very high stress and thin in cross section, e.g. saddles, bars, clasps, crowns, bridges and partial denture frameworks.

Standards for 'dental gold casting alloys' require a noble metal content of at least 75%. It can be seen that the gold content or *nobility* decreases on going from the type 1 (soft) alloy to the type 4 (extra hard) alloy. Nobility of gold alloys is often indicated by either a *carat* value or a *fineness* value. The carat value indicates the number of parts by weight of gold in 24 parts of alloy. Thus, a type 2 alloy containing 75% gold has a carat value of 18. The fineness value indicates the number of parts by weight of gold in 1000 parts of alloy. The type 2 alloy would have a fineness value of 750.

The increase in hardness observed when nobility decreases is primarily due to the *solution hardening* effect of the alloying metals which all form solid solutions with gold.; The types 3 and 4 alloys can be further hardened by heat treatments.

The presence of significant quantities of platinum and palladium, as in the type 4 alloys, not only causes considerable solution hardening but also leads to a widening of the separation between the solidus and

liquidus lines of the solid solution phase diagram. The results of this is an increase in *coring* as explained on p. 51. The cored structure can be removed by carrying out a *homogenization* heat treatment. Platinum and palladium also significantly increase the melting point and recrystallization temperature of gold alloys, a fact which can be used to advantage when selecting alloys for components which may require soldering.

Zinc, which is present to a concentration of about 1% in most alloys, acts as a *scavenger* during casting. It is the most chemically reactive of all the metals used and becomes preferentially oxidized at the high temperatures of casting. The resulting zinc oxide slag can be removed from the molten alloy. It is normal to re-use any excess alloy which is left after a casting has been produced (e.g. the alloy from the sprue). Care should be taken when doing this to ensure that sufficient zinc remains to have an effective scavenging action. When all the zinc has been oxidized the other metals of the alloy, particularly copper, become prone to attack. In order to minimize the chances of this occurring it is good practice to always include some fresh alloy in each alloy melt prepared for casting.

Table 7.2 gives an indication of the comparative properties of the four types of casting gold alloys. Moving through the series from type 1 to type 4, there is an increase in hardness, strength and proportional limit. The corrosion resistance decreases as the gold content is reduced, although for practical purposes all of the alloys may be considered adequate from this point of view. Ductility and malleability also decrease when the gold content is reduced. Table 7.3 gives more detailed information regarding the properties of the alloys. Table 7.4 gives

Table 7.2 Comparative properties of casting gold alloys.

Type	Hardness	Proportional limit	Strength	Ductility	Corrosion resistance
1					
2	⏐	⏐	⏐	⏐	⏐
3	Increases	Increases	Increases	Decreases	Decreases
4	↓	↓	↓	↓	↓

Table 7.3 Properties of casting gold alloys.

Property	1	2	3	4	4 (hardened)
Hardness (VHN)	50–90	90–120	120–160	150–230	250–300
Modulus of elasticity (GPa)	80	80	85	95	100
Tensile strength (MPa)	250	340	360	500	750
Proportional limit (MPa)	120	200	290	350	500
Elongation at break (%)	35	25	20	15	8
Melting range (°C)	950–1100	920–980	900–1000	870–950	870–950

the ISO specification limits which apply to the materials.

The variation in alloy properties with composition is reflected in the applications for which the materials are chosen. The relatively soft, type 1 alloys are used for inlays which are well supported by tooth substance and which do not have to resist large masticatory forces. The high values of ductility of these alloys enables them to be burnished – a process which improves the marginal fit of the inlay and increases surface hardness. The need to improve the fit of inlays by burnishing has decreased with improvements in casting accuracy.

The type 2 alloys are the most widely used alloys for inlays. They have superior mechanical properties when compared with the type 1 materials, though at the expense of a slight decrease in ductility.

The type 3 (hard) alloys are used where there is less support from tooth substance and when opposing stresses are likely to be relatively high. Examples of the use of these materials include the production of crowns and inlays for high stress areas such as class II cavities in molars. Type 3 alloys with a high copper content (>8%) can be heat treated in air at 400°C for 10 minutes to produce a stable copper oxide layer on their surface. Chemically active adhesive luting resins can then be used to bond such structures to tooth tissue rather than relying upon mechanical retention form and a conventional luting cement for retention. The high platinum and/or palladium content of the type 3 alloys, leading to a higher melting point, is beneficial when constructing components for bridges which are joined by soldering.

Type 4 alloys are used in high stress areas and for constructing components of partial dentures and for this reason are normally referred to as *partial denture casting alloys*. Partial dentures normally have clasps or other devices for retaining the denture. These must be flexible enough to engage undercuts in standing teeth but have sufficiently high values of proportional limit such that they do not become distorted. The type 4 gold alloys possess this useful combination of properties. In addition, the alloys have sufficient ductility in the softened state to allow slight adjustments to be made. Attempts to carry out adjustments on a heat hardened alloy may lead to fracture due to the decrease in ductility which accompanies hardening.

The connectors of partial dentures, be they bars or plates, should be rigid and resist distortion. Whereas the proportional limit of type 4 gold alloys is sufficiently high to resist distortion, the connectors must be constructed in fairly thick section in order to produce sufficient rigidity due to the relatively low value of modulus of elasticity of these alloys. Some base metal denture casting alloys have higher values of modulus and from this point of view are more satisfactory for producing connectors (see Table 8.1).

7.4 Hardening heat treatments (theoretical considerations)

The type 3 (hard) and type 4 (extra hard) casting gold alloys can be further hardened by heat treatments. Hardening heat treatments are hardly ever performed for type 3 materials but are occasionally used for type 4 materials which are to be used in very high stress bearing situations. The hardening process can be explained by consideration of the phase diagrams for the silver–copper and gold–copper systems. Hardening heat treatments are not beneficial for the types 1 and 2 alloys because they contain insufficient quantities of copper and silver.

Silver–copper system

The silver–copper system is a good example of an alloy in which the component metals are only partially soluble in the solid state. The solidified alloy consists of a mixture of two solid solutions, one in which small quantities of copper are dissolved in silver (called the α solid solution) and one in which small quantities of silver are dissolved in copper (the β solid solution.

The phase diagram for the silver–copper system is shown in Fig. 7.1. In some respects it resembles the eutectic phase diagram given in Fig. 6.10. The solidus is defined by the line A B E C D, whilst the liquidus is given by A E D. The compositional limits of the α and β solid solutions are denoted by the areas marked α and β on the phase diagram. The lines B F and C G are termed *solvus lines* and indicate the decreasing solubility of copper in silver and silver in copper as the temperature decreases. Thus the solubility of copper in silver is around 9% at 780°C (the eutectic temperature) but only around 2% at 400°C. This relationship between solubility and temperature is normal for any system of limited solubility.

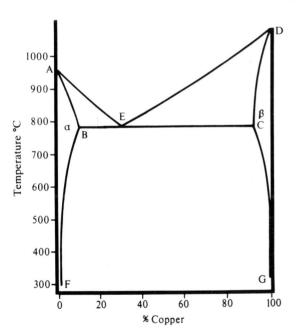

Fig. 7.1 Phase diagram of the silver–copper system.

When an alloy of the eutectic composition (72% Ag/28% Cu) is cooled from the molten state it undergoes solidification at a constant temperature, equivalent to point E on the phase diagram. The solid formed is a mixture of α and β solid solutions in which the α has composition equivalent to point B (approximately 9% Cu/91% Ag) and the β has a composition equivalent to point C (approximately 8% Ag/92% Cu). An alloy with slightly more copper than the eutectic composition (a hypereutectic alloy) solidifies to give the eutectic mixture plus additional

β solid solution. An alloy with slightly more silver (a hypoeutectic alloy than the eutectic composition solidifies to give the eutectic mixture and additional α solid solution. Using tie lines it can be shown that during crystallization the excess solid solution crystallizes first and that the eutectic mixture is always the last to crystallize.

If the alloy has either less than 9% or greater than 92% copper then the solid formed is either α *or* β solid solution – no eutectic mixture is formed.

When casting, generally alloys are cooled rapidly to encourage the formation of a fine grain structure. At low temperatures the alloys become rigid and atomic diffusions become difficult if not impossible. The structure of the alloy which was formed during crystallization becomes 'frozen' into the alloy at room temperature. Despite the fact that the solubilities of silver in copper and copper in silver are negligible at room temperature, there exist, within the eutectic mixture, α and β solid solutions in which 9% copper remains dissolved in silver and 8% silver remains dissolved in copper. If diffusion were possible, there would be a tendency for copper to precipitate from the α solid solution and silver to precipitate from the β solid solution.

It is possible to heat the alloy to a temperature at which the solubility is exceeded but at which atomic diffusions are possible. In the temperature range 300–600°C slow diffusion of copper atoms can occur. Given sufficient time in this temperature range copper would begin to precipitate from the α solid solution. Well before any precipitated phase can be observed however, a significant hardening of the alloy takes place, presumably because the diffusing atoms have effectively prevented movement of slip planes. This forms the basis of the *precipitation hardening* procedure used for type 3 and type 4 casting gold alloys.

The same process may occur to a lesser extent and at a much slower rate at room temperature. Hardening which occurs in this way is referred to as *age hardening*.

Gold–copper system

Gold and copper form a continuous series of solid solutions over the whole range of compositions. The solid solutions are random-substitutional solid solutions with face-centred cubic lattices (Fig. 7.2).

The phase diagram for the gold–copper system is shown in Fig. 7.3. It can be seen that the solidus and liquidus are close together and almost coincide at point M. Two other areas on the phase diagram, at compositions between 40% gold and 90% gold,

Disordered

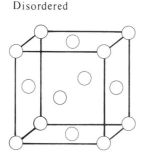

Fig. 7.2 Disordered, face-centred cubic, gold–copper alloy. Circles represent either gold or copper.

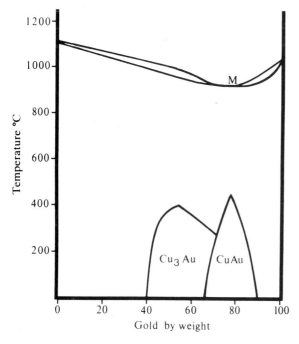

Fig. 7.3 Simplified phase diagram of the gold–copper system.

indicate regions in which the alloys are capable of undergoing a solid–solid transition to form an ordered rather than disordered lattice. The ordered lattice, in which gold and copper take up specific lattice sites, is often referred to as a superlattice.

Formation of the superlattice requires that an atomic rearrangement must take place by diffusion of atoms. This cannot occur at normal temperatures since there is insufficient energy in the system to allow diffusion to occur. Consider, for example, an alloy containing 75% gold which lies within one of the areas of interest. If this alloy is heated to a temperature in the region 200–400°C, sufficient

energy is imparted to the system to allow atomic diffusions to occur, atoms take up their preferred sites and the superlattice is formed. In this case the superlattice has the formula CuAu and the superlattice has an ordered tetragonal structure as shown in Fig. 7.4. In alloys containing 40–60% gold an ordered superlattice, based on the formula Cu_3Au, is formed. The change in size and shape of the gold–copper lattice sets up a resistance to the movement of slip planes within the multi-component casting gold alloy which results in a significant increase in hardness and strength and a reduction in ductility. Heat treatments which are used to carry out this hardening procedure are termed *order hardening* heat treatments.

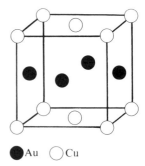

● Au   ○ Cu

Fig. 7.4 Ordered, tetragonal structure of a heat-treated gold–copper alloy containing 75% gold.

7.5 Heat treatments (practical considerations)

On melting the alloy prior to casting, any metallographic structure which it possessed as an ingot is lost and a new crystal structure is created as the metal 'freezes' inside the mould.

It is important to quench the gold alloy castings before they cool to the range of temperatures within which heat hardening takes place. An alloy which is allowed to cool slowly to room temperature will undergo both precipitation and order hardening prematurely. Before any alteration in shape of such a casting is attempted, it must be softened by cooling rapidly from above 600°C. Normal casting procedure is to leave the mould until the gold, visible in the sprues of the casting, is no longer at red heat. This indicates that the internal metal temperature is about 600°C. The mould is then plunged into cold water in order to chill the metal quickly and cause disintegration of the mould. Rapid cooling also helps to ensure a fine grain structure.

The casting is then cleaned and when platinum or

palladium are present a homogenization heat treatment may be carried out to remove coring. This involves heating to 700°C for 10 minutes, then quenching. The casting is then polished and its fit in the mouth is checked. Any minor adjustments, such as bending of clasps, etc., are made at this stage whilst the alloy is still in the softened state. If adjustments are made, a low temperature *stress relief anneal* should be carried out.

The hardening heat treatment may then be carried out with type 3 and type 4 alloys by heating the casting to above 450°C and allowing it to cool slowly until its temperature has dropped to about 200°C, then quenching. This takes about 20 minutes for an average-sized casting. The precise details of the heat treatment vary from one alloy to another and the manufacturer's instructions should be followed. The procedures are designed such that hardening by both precipitation and ordering can occur. In practice, hardening heat treatments are hardly ever performed on type 3 alloys and only infrequently for type 4 materials, indicating that the properties of the as-cast material are adequate for most purposes.

Following hardening the casting is repolished and, in the case of a denture, the teeth are added in order to complete the job.

Ideally, all hardening and softening heat treatments should be carried out in a pyrometrically controlled furnace. The castings should be supported by sand or another refractory material in order to prevent 'sag' at elevated temperatures.

7.6 Low gold-content alloys

Large increases in the price of gold have led to the development and increased use of alloys with lower gold content than those described previously. Some alloys contain as little as 10% gold but more normally a gold content of around 45–50% is used. They have a high palladium content which imparts a characteristic 'whitish' colour to the alloys.

The increased popularity and use of these 'low gold' alloys has led to the development of an ISO Standard for dental casting alloys with a noble metal content of 25% up to but not including 75%. There are four types of alloy equivalent to those previously described for the high gold materials. The mechanical properties for both high gold and low gold alloys are characterized in the standards using measurements of proof stress and elongation at break (a measure of ductility). The specification limits are shown in Table 7.4, where it can be seen that the requirements for the two groups of alloys are identical.

Table 7.4 Specification limits for both traditional dental casting gold alloys and dental casting alloys with noble metal content of 25% up to but not including 75%.

Type	0.2% Proof stress (MPa)	Elongation (%)
1	80–180	18 minimum
2	180–240	12 minimum
3	240 minimum	12 minimum
4	300 minimum	10 minimum
4 (Hardened)	450 minimum	3 minimum

The casting techniques and equipment used for low-gold alloys are similar to those used for conventional gold alloys. This, coupled with their acceptable properties, good clinical performance and lower cost compared to conventional gold alloys, has led to their widespread use.

7.7 Silver–palladium alloys

The silver–palladium alloys contain little or no gold and as their name suggests contain primarily silver and palladium. There is generally a minimum of 25% palladium along with small quantities of copper, zinc and indium, in addition to gold which is sometimes present in small quantities.

The silver–palladium alloys have significantly lower density than gold alloys, a factor which may affect castability. For a given volume of casting, there is a lower force generated by the molten alloy during casting. In this regard, there appears to be a significant variation amongst brands, indicating that small variations in composition can affect castability. Some silver–palladium alloys have castability characteristics which compare favourably with gold alloys. Attention must be paid to details such as casting temperature and mould temperature if the mould is to be adequately filled by the alloy.

Alloys containing large quantities of palladium have a propensity for dissolving oxygen in the molten state which may lead to a porous casting. Care must be taken to avoid overheating or oxidation of the melt during casting.

The properties of silver–palladium alloys are similar to those of type 3 gold (Table 7.5). Materials claiming compliance with the ISO Standard for casting alloys having a noble metal content of greater than 25% must meet the specification limits set out in Table 7.4. There are significant variations in properties between individual brands within each of the two groups. Whereas most gold alloys have high ductility as demonstrated by an elongation value

Table 7.5 Properties of a typical Ag/Pd alloy compared with a type 3 gold alloy.

Property	Ag/Pd	Gold (type 3)
Hardness (VHN)	120–220	120–160
Modulus of elasticity (GPa)	80–95	85
Proportional limit (MPa)	250	290
Elongation at break (%)	3–25	15–25
Melting range (°C)	900–1100	900–1000
Density (g cm^{-3})	11–12	15–16

above 15%, some silver–palladium alloys have much lower ductility. The corrosion resistance is not as good as for gold alloys but, provided the palladium content is above 25%, the amount of corrosion expected during service is negligible.

These alloys offer a suitable alternative to gold alloys provided that care is taken during casting. They offer a considerable saving in cost when compared to gold alloys.

7.8 Soldering and brazing materials for noble metals

Some larger restorations/appliances produced from cast alloys are produced in two or more parts which are then joined together by soldering or brazing. This approach is used to overcome distortions that may occur during cooling for metal frameworks for long span bridge work, and also when joining metal components formed from different alloys, e.g. a type 4 gold veneer crown may be joined to a precious metal porcelain bonding alloy structure for bridgework. In dentistry the terms soldering and brazing are used interchangeably. However, in normal metallurgical terms the two processes, although trying to achieve the same goal, are carried out at different temperatures, brazing being a process carried out at higher temperatures.

The definition of a dental brazing material given in ISO Standards is 'an alloy suitable for use as a filler material in operations in which dental alloy(s) parts are joined to form a dental restoration'.

The requirement of a brazing material for noble alloys is that it be capable of forming a strong, corrosion resistant joint between the two components being joined without changing their structure or properties. Hence, the tensile strength of the brazed joint is required to exceed the 0.2% proof stress for the weakest of the two components. There should be no visible signs of corrosion when a brazed joint is soaked in a solution of lactic acid and sodium chloride for 7 days. In order that the components being joined do not suffer from recrystallization, grain growth or distortion during the brazing procedure it is important that the brazing material has a *flow temperature* which is well below the melting point of the alloys being joined. The flow temperature is defined as the lowest temperature at which the filler material is fluid enough to flow into the gap and to wet the surface of the metallic parts. Solders for joining noble metal components are formulated from mixtures of gold, silver and copper designed to have low fusion temperatures. This is achieved through the eutectic nature of certain silver/copper alloys and through the addition of tin and zinc such that the fusion temperature of the solder is generally 50–100°C below that of the casting gold alloys.

Solders are susceptible to oxidation during the melting/softening procedure and the resulting oxides can weaken the soldered joint. Furthermore, the metal components being joined are often coated with a thin oxide film which can limit the ability to achieve proper jointing. Fluxes are employed to break down the surface oxide layers on metals and to prevent oxidation of the solder. Fluxes commonly used are fluoride salts and borax. Fluoride salts are particularly useful in breaking down the tenacious oxide film which forms on the surface of chromium containing alloys.

7.9 Noble alloys for metal-bonded ceramic restorations

Alloys of precious metals are commonly used for the fabrication of metal-bonded ceramic restorations. Their requirements are similar to those described in this chapter but with additional requirements related to the following:

(1) thermal stability during firing of the ceramic;
(2) bonding to the ceramic;
(3) compatibility with the ceramic;
(4) support for the ceramic.

For further information see Chapter 11.

Chapter 8
Base Metal Casting Alloys

8.1 Introduction

Base metal alloys contain no gold, silver, platinum or palladium. The two most commonly used base metal alloys in dentistry are the nickel–chromium (Ni/Cr) alloys which are commonly used for crown and bridge casting, including porcelain fused to metal (PFM) restorations, and the cobalt–chromium (Co/Cr) alloys which are commonly used for partial denture framework castings.

8.2 Composition

Cobalt–chromium alloys

The chemical composition of these alloys specified in the ISO Standard for Dental Base Metal Casting Alloys (Part 1) is as follows:

Cobalt	main constituent
Chromium	no less than 25%
Molybdenum	no less than 4%
Cobalt + nickel + chromium	no less than 85%

A typical material would contain 35–65% cobalt, 25–35% chromium, 0–30% nickel, a little molybdenum and trace quantities of other elements such as beryllium, silicon and carbon. Cobalt and nickel are hard, strong metals. The main purpose of the chromium is to further harden the alloy by solution hardening and also to impart corrosion resistance by the *passivating effect*. Chromium exposed at the surface of the alloy rapidly becomes oxidized to form a thin, passive, surface layer of chromic oxide which prevents further attack on the bulk of the alloy. The concentrations of the minor constituents have a greater effect on the physical properties of the alloys than do the relative cobalt–chromium–nickel concentrations. The minor elements are generally added to improve casting and handling characteristics and modify mechanical properties. For example, silicon imparts good casting properties to a nickel-containing alloy and increases its ductility. Likewise, molybdenum and beryllium are added to refine the grain structure and improve the behaviour of base metal alloys during casting. Carbon affects the hardness, strength and ductility of the alloys and the exact concentration of carbon is one of the major factors controlling alloy properties. The carbon forms carbides with any of the components and its concentration depends on both the amount added by the manufacturer and that which may be inadvertently introduced during casting if the alloy is melted with an oxyacetylene torch. The presence of too much carbon results in a brittle alloy with very low ductility and an increased danger of fracture. During crystallization the carbides become precipitated in the interdendritic regions which form the grain boundaries. The grains are generally much larger than those produced on casting gold alloys and it is possible for the precipitated carbides to form a continuous phase throughout the alloy. If this occurs the alloy becomes extremely hard and brittle as the carbide phase acts as a barrier to slip. A discontinuous carbide phase is preferable since it allows some slip and reduces brittleness. Whether a continuous or discontinuous carbide phase is formed depends on the amount of carbon present and on the casting technique. High melting temperature during casting favour discontinuous carbide phases but there is a limit to which this can be used to any advantage since the use of very high casting temperatures can cause interactions between the alloy and the mould.

Nickel–chromium alloys

The chemical composition of these alloys specified in the ISO Standard for Dental Base Metal Casting Alloys (Part 2) is as follows:

Nickel	main constituent
Chromium	no less than 20%

Molybdenum	no less than 4%
Beryllium	no more than 2%
Nickel + cobalt + chromium	no less than 85%

As for the Co/Cr alloys the concentrations of minor ingredients can have a profound effect on properties. The concentration of carbon and the nature of the grain boundaries are major factors in controlling the properties of these alloys.

8.3 Manipulation of base metal casting alloys

The fusion temperatures of the Ni/Cr and Co/Cr alloys vary with composition but are generally in the range 1200–1500°C. This is considerably higher than for the casting gold alloys which rarely have fusion temperatures above 950°C. Melting of gold alloys can readily be achieved using a gas–air mixture. For base metal alloys, however, either an acetylene–oxygen flame or an electrical induction furnace is required. The latter method is to be favoured since it is carried out under more controlled conditions. When using oxyacetylene flames the ratio of oxygen to acetylene must be carefully controlled. Too much oxygen may cause oxidation of the alloy whilst an excess of acetylene produces an increase in the metal carbide content leading to embrittlement.

Investment moulds for base metal alloys must be capable of maintaining their integrity at the high casting temperatures used. Silica-bonded and phosphate-bonded materials are favoured with the latter product being most widely used. Gypsum-bonded investments decompose above 1200°C to form sulphur dioxide which may be absorbed by the casting, causing embrittlement. This effect can be reduced by the incorporation of oxalate in the investment, however the problem is generally avoided by choosing an investment which is more stable at elevated temperatures.

The density values of base metal alloys are approximately half those of the casting gold alloys. For this reason the thrust developed during casting may be somewhat lower, with the possibility that the casting may not adequately fill the mould. Casting machines used for base metal alloys must therefore be capable of producing extra thrust which overcomes this deficiency. The problem may be aggravated if the investment is not sufficiently porous to allow escape of trapped air and other gases. Careful use of vents and sprues of adequate size is normally sufficient to overcome such problems.

The greatest expense involved in producing a Co/Cr dental casting is in the time required for trimming

and polishing. In the 'as cast' state, the alloy surface is normally quite rough, partially due to the coarse nature of some investment powders. Finer investments can be used to give a smoother surface requiring less finishing. One common technique involves painting the wax pattern with fine investment – this then forms the inner surface of the investment mould. The bulk of the mould is then formed from the coarser grade material.

Base metal alloys, and particularly the Co/Cr type, are very hard and consequently difficult to polish. After casting, it is usual to sandblast the metal to remove any surface roughness or adherent investment material as well as the green layer of oxide which coats the surface after casting. *Electrolytic polishing* may then be carried out. This procedure is essentially the opposite to electroplating. If a rough metal surface is connected as the anode in a bath of strongly acidic electrolyte, a current passing between it and the cathode will cause the anode to ionize and lose a surface film of metal. With a suitable electrolyte and the correct current density, the first products of electrolysis will collect in the hollows of the rough metal surface and so prevent further attack in these areas. The prominences of the metal surface will continue to be dissolved and in this way the contours of the surface are smoothed. Final polishing can be carried out using a high-speed polishing buff.

The process of electropolishing is not generally used for Ni/Cr alloy castings. These products are normally used for crown and bridge work and it is essential to maintain the accuracy of fit, particularly at the margins of crowns. This accuracy may be lost during polishing procedures and care is required to avoid such problems.

8.4 Properties

The properties of these alloys very from one brand to another but typical values are listed in Tables 8.1 and 8.2. The ISO standards for both materials require a minimum of 0.2% proof stress of 500 MPa and a minimum elongation after fracture of 3%. Hence an ability to withstand permanent deformation under stress and a reasonable ductility are deemed to be important characteristics of these alloys.

The Co/Cr and Ni/Cr alloys are very hard materials and although this makes the polishing of castings a difficult process the final polished surface is very durable and resistant to scratching. In addition, fine margins seem less likely to be lost during finishing of a base metal alloy.

Co/Cr and Ni/Cr alloys have very good corrosion resistance by virtue of the *passivating effect* (see

Section 2.7). The alloys are covered with a tenacious thin layer of chromic oxide which protects the bulk of the alloy from attack. Unlike chromium-plated metals, which lose their corrosion resistance if the surface layer becomes scratched, these alloys are permanently resistant to corrosion since the oxide layer immediately becomes replenished if the surface is damaged.

Co/Cr alloys have relatively low ductility, a fact which should be remembered when carrying out alterations to partial denture clasps. The ductility may be further reduced if the concentration of carbides becomes increased during melting with an oxyacetylene torch.

Although the ISO specification limits for Ni/Cr alloys are the same as those for Co/Cr alloys for both proof stress and elongation, some NiCr alloys are relatively ductile. This would suggest that restorations produced from some alloys can be burnished. However, their relatively high proportional limit values indicate that high stresses would be required for effective burnishing.

The proportional limit values of the Co/Cr alloys are somewhat higher than even the Ni/Cr alloys. They are able to withstand high stresses without undergoing permanent deformation.

The Ni/Cr alloys and Co/Cr alloys are both very rigid materials with high modulus of elasticity values.

8.5 Comparison with casting gold alloys

The properties of the two main groups of base metal casting alloys dictate that the Co/Cr alloys are primarily used for partial denture castings, where the high values of modulus of elasticity and proportional limit are of major importance whilst the Ni/Cr alloys are primarily used for small castings such as crowns and bridges. These two groups of base metal alloys offer alternatives to the casting gold alloys at potentially considerable savings in cost. Table 8.1 gives comparative properties of the Co/Cr alloys and the type 4 casting gold alloys. Table 8.2 gives comparative properties of the Ni/Cr alloys and type 4 casting gold alloys.

Cast partial denture alloys

The two major components of cast partial denture frameworks are the connectors and clasps. The connectors should be rigid (high value of modulus of elasticity required) and should not be permanently deformed by the action of mechanical stresses (high value of proportional limit required). It can be seen from Table 8.1 that the Co/Cr alloys most closely meet these two requirements. In addition, the lower density of the base metal alloys means that dentures constructed from this material

Table 8.1 Comparative properties of Co/Cr alloys and type 4 casting gold alloys for partial dentures.

Property (units)	Co/Cr	Type 4 gold alloy	Comments
Density (g cm^{-3})	8	15	More difficult to produce defect-free castings for Co/Cr alloys but denture frameworks are lighter
Fusion temperature	As high as 1500°C	Normally lower than 1000°C	Co/Cr alloys require electrical induction furnace or oxyacetylene equipment. Cannot use gypsum-bonded investments for Co/Cr alloys
Casting shrinkage (%)	2.3	1.4	Mostly compensated for by correct choice of investment
Tensile strength (MPa)	850	750	Both acceptable
Proportional limit (MPa)	700	500	Both acceptable; can resist stresses without deformation
Modulus of elasticity (GPa)	220	100	Co/Cr more rigid for equivalent thickness; advantage for connectors; disadvantage for clasps
Hardness (Vickers)	420	250	Co/Cr more difficult to polish but retains polish during service
Ductility (% elongation)	3	15 (as cast) 8 (hardened)	Co/Cr clasps may fracture if adjustments are attempted

Note: Values for gold alloy are for heat-hardened material except where indicated.

Table 8.2 Comparative properties of Ni/Cr alloys and type 3 casting gold alloys for small cast restorations.

Property (units)	Ni/Cr	Type 3 gold alloy	Comments
Density (g cm^{-3})	8	15	More difficult to produce defect-free castings for Ni/Cr alloys
Fusion temperature	As high as 1350°C	Normally lower than 1000°C	Ni/Cr alloys require electrical induction furnace or oxyacetylene equipment
Casting shrinkage (%)	2.0	1.4	Mostly compensated for by correct choice of investment
Tensile strength (MPa)	600	540	Both adequate for the applications being considered
Proportional limit (MPa)	500	290	Both high enough to prevent distortions for applications being considered; note that values are lower than for partial denture alloys (Table 8.1)
Modulus of elasticity (GPa)	220	85	Higher modulus of Ni/Cr is an advantage for larger restorations, e.g. bridges and for porcelain-bonded restorations
Hardness (Vickers)	300	150	Ni/Cr more difficult to polish but retains polish during service
Ductility (% elongation)	3–30	20	Relatively large values suggest that burnishing is possible; however, large proportional limit values suggest high forces would be required

are lighter, the more so if the connectors are of thinner section.

For clasps, a high value of proportional limit is required in order to prevent deformation. A lower value of modulus of elasticity would enable the clasp to engage relatively deep undercuts due to its increased flexibility. In addition, the alloy used to construct clasps should ideally be ductile so that adjustments can be made to clasps without fracturing. The gold alloys most closely match the requirements for clasps since they have adequately high proportional limits, lower values of modulus of elasticity than Co/Cr alloys and greater ductility. A clasp of the same cross-sectional area would be much stiffer in Co/Cr than in gold alloy. A greater force would therefore be required to flex it outwards past the most bulbous part of the tooth for a given undercut. The stress developed in the Co/Cr clasp would be more than double that in an equivalent gold alloy clasp. There is a greater chance of reaching the stress which is equivalent to the proportional limit in the Co/Cr clasp and therefore a greater risk of permanent deformation.

In practice, connectors and clasps are generally cast together from the same alloy. For reasons of cost, Co/Cr alloys are almost universally used despite their limitations. When designing partial denture frameworks due regard must be paid to the high modulus

values and low ductility of the Co/Cr alloys. Clasps should not be designed to engage deep undercuts and alterations by bending may result in fractures. A reduction in thickness of the Co/Cr alloy decreases the force necessary to push the clasp over the bulge of the tooth but leaves the clasp arm exposed to the dangers of deformation during cleaning and handling of the denture. By a reduction of the undercut to approximately half that engaged by a gold clasp, coupled with the use of a slightly thinner cross-section, a clasp of moderate retention and adequate functional life can be designed. The use of very small undercuts, however, requires precise positioning of the clasp arm and this is not always easy to achieve. Consequently, it is often found that Co/Cr clasps are either too retentive initially and slowly lose this retention due to permanent deformation or, alternatively, clasps may engage undercuts which are too small and give barely adequate retention.

The best of both worlds is to use Co/Cr alloy for the connectors and type 4 gold alloy for clasps. Whilst it is possible to solder these structures together, corrosion at the joint is not uncommon and, where possible, the gold clasp should be attached to the denture via the polymeric denture base material.

There has been an increased use of Ni/Cr alloys for partial denture framework castings. This is due to the relative ease of finishing and polishing compared with Co/Cr as a consequence of the lower hardness value (Tables 8.1 and 8.2).

Crown and bridge alloys

Alloys used for crown and bridge work should be hard, rigid and durable. Both Ni/Cr and gold alloys have adequate mechanical properties with the greater rigidity of the Ni/Cr alloys being an advantage for bridges, particularly those with large spans.

The success of crown and bridge alloys depends to a great extent on the accuracy with which the restorations can be cast. The gold alloys have a significant advantage from this point of view. They have greater density which results in better castability due to the high thrust which is generated by the alloy as it enters the mould. The gold alloys undergo less casting shrinkage (approximately 1.4%) when compared with the Ni/Cr alloys (2.0%). In the case of gold alloys, the shrinkage is well compensated for by dimensional changes in the investment mould. For Ni/Cr alloys the contraction is probably not as well compensated. This, occasionally, results in ill-fitting castings. One advantage of the Ni/Cr alloys, which results from their great hardness, is that the margins of the cast restoration are unlikely to be destroyed during polishing.

Clinically one difficulty with Ni/Cr alloys for crown and bridgework also relates to their hardness. It is common practice to make the occlusal (biting) surface of a porcelain fused to metal (PFM) crown from the cast metal. This helps to reduce tooth wear which may occur between tooth tissue and porcelain. Unfortunately the very hard surface of a cast Ni/Cr alloy makes it more difficult to perform occlusal adjustments than is the case with precious metal alloys, and they are themselves more likely to cause wear of the opposing dentition.

Base metal alloys for porcelain bonding

Ni/Cr alloys are rarely used for all-metal cast restorations but are widely used in bonded porcelain restorations. There are also some Co/Cr formulations which have been developed for porcelain bonding techniques. In all these cases compatibility of the alloy and porcelain is critical. These issues are addressed in Section 11.9.

8.6 Biocompatibility

Base metal casting alloys contain some components which should be regarded as either toxic or known to cause allergic reactions in some people.

Beryllium is a known animal carcinogen and poses a potential threat to dental personnel who inhale metal dust during polishing or grinding procedures. It is essential that areas in which such operations are carried out are kept well ventilated. Some base metal alloys do not contain beryllium – a trend which is likely to increase as the toxic effects of this metal are subjected to greater scrutiny.

For the patient, the most immediate biocompatibility risk concerns nickel and the risk of allergic contact dermatitis. It is known that nickel causes more contact dermatitis than all other metals combined and that relatively small nickel concentrations can be problematical. Nickel-free base metal alloys are available and are likely to gain fairly wide use as alternatives for those patients with known or suspected nickel allergy.

Titanium metal and alloys of titanium with other metals, for example vanadium, have excellent biocompatibility for dental applications in the future.

8.7 Metals and alloys for implants

Implants offer an alternative method of treatment for the replacement of missing teeth which can be used instead of dentures or fixed bridges. They generally have a structure which enables one part of the implant to be located beneath the oral soft tissues (mucosa) such that it can be stabilized by resting on the bone or by being embedded in the bone. The other part of the implant structure protrudes through the mucosa to provide a structure suitable for supporting a denture, crown or bridge. The requirements of implant materials encompass biocompatibility, acceptable stability in the medium-long term, acceptable function and ease of manufacture. Biocompatibility and stability are often seen as closely related in that some materials are known to encourage bone growth which produces a very intimate interface between bone and implant which helps to stabilize the latter. Function primarily depends upon the rigidity of the implant structure. This in turn is related to the dimensions and the modulus of elasticity of the material from which the implant is manufactured. The use of high modulus materials enables implants of smaller cross-sectional bulk to be used.

Dental implants are normally classified according to the way in which they are stabilized. The three most common types are: subperiosteal, blade-vent endosseous and osseointegrated. Subperiosteal implants consist of an open framework of cast alloy which rests on top of the bony ridge but beneath the mucosa. The variable geometry of the bony surface means that each implant must be fabricated individually. Cast cobalt–chromium alloys are most commonly used for these applications. The very high modulus of elasticity of these materials (Table 8.1) combined with reasonable castability are the main factors affecting this choice. Attempts have been made to improve the biocompatibility of the alloys by using hydroxyapatite coatings. Subperiosteal implants have now been superseded largely by osseointegrated implants embedded in bone. Their major cause of failure was that the oral mucosa grew to cover the whole of the surface of the implant, 'externalizing' it. Obviously the risks of infection in such a situation are high.

Blade-vent endosseous implants involve the use of a design in which one end of the implant (the blade) is embedded into the bone whilst the other end protrudes through the mucosa into the oral cavity. These implants are normally constructed from titanium which has excellent biocompatibility, although this characteristic cannot be used to the greatest effect in blade-vent implants because the implant has insufficient time to stabilize within the bone before it is placed under load. Also the techniques for preparation of the bony socket tend to be less well controlled. A critical factor for success in osseo-integration is careful bone surgery to minimize bone damage associated with heating. This necessitates the use of very low cutting speeds and copious cooling of the cutting instruments. Unlike the sub-periosteal implants, the blade-vent variety are commercially available in standardized shapes and sizes and casting is not required. The clinical success or failure of the blade-vent implants is a controversial issue. The most common cause of failure is due to the implant becoming loose.

Tooth-root implants constructed from titanium have been used with a considerable measure of success since 1965. The advantage of these implants over the blade-vent type is that for some systems their design enables a period of stabilization of the implant before it is subjected to load. The implants are supplied as a kit which contains various components. The initial stage of treatment involves implantation of a cylinder of titanium into the bone. These implants are available in a variety of forms from perforated threaded structures that are screwed into a prepared hole in the bone to smooth sided cylinders coated with hydroxyapatite which are a friction fit within the prepared socket. Clinical evidence would suggest that the coated implants are less successful than their pure titanium counterparts. The upper level of the cylinder is sealed at this stage with a cover screw and the whole implant is covered with the mucosa to allow post-operative healing and *osseointegration* to occur. The excellent biocompatibility of titanium combined with the unstressed state of the implant allows bone growth to occur which stabilizes the implant. After stabilization has been achieved the cover screw is removed during a second surgical stage from the upper end of the implant and replaced by a transmucosal element and ultimately a fixture which retains the crown, bridge or denture.

8.8 Suggested further reading

Albrektson, T., Jansoon, T. & Lekholm, U. (1986) Osseointegrated dental implants, *Dent. Clin. North Am.* **30**, 151.

Carter, T.J. & Kidd, J.N. (1965) The precision casting of cobalt–chromium alloy, parts I and II. *Br. Dent. J.* **118**, 383 and 431.

Kelly, J.R. & Rose, T.C. (1983) Nonprecious alloys for use in fixed prosthodontics: A literature review. *J. Prosthet. Dent.* **49**, 363.

Newman, S.M. (1986) The relationship of metals to the general health of the patient, the dentist and office staff. *Int. Dent. J.* **36**, 35.

Chapter 9
Casting

9.1 Introduction

Previous chapters have dealt with wax-pattern materials, investment materials and casting alloys. This chapter describes how the investment mould is formed and how the wax pattern is replaced by the alloy using a casting process. One of several methods can be used for casting depending upon the alloy which is to be used.

There are several faults which can occur in alloy castings, most of which can be traced to incorrect selection of materials or faulty technique.

9.2 Investment mould

The various components of a typical investment mould are illustrated in Fig. 9.1.

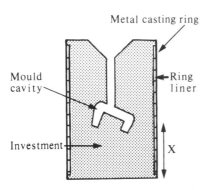

Fig. 9.1 Diagram illustrating components of an investment mould.

The mould cavity is formed by allowing the investment to set around the wax pattern and associated sprue former and sprue base (crucible). After allowing the investment material to set, the sprue base and former are removed and the wax pattern 'burnt out' to leave the completed mould cavity. The choice of investment material depends on the type of alloy which is to be cast. The casting ring liner serves a dual purpose. It forms a relatively pliable lining to the inner surface of the rigid metal casting ring. This allows almost unrestricted setting expansion and thermal expansion of the investment. In addition, its thermal insulating properties ensure that the investment mould does not cool rapidly and contract after removal from the 'burn out' oven.

The temperature to which the investment mould is heated during burn out deserves special mention since this controls the thermal expansion of the investment. For gold alloys, either a slow burn out at 450°C or a more rapid burn out at 700°C is commonly used with gypsum-bonded investments. For Ni/Cr alloys a temperature in the range 700–900°C is normal, whilst for Co/Cr alloys a burn out temperature of 1000°C is typical.

Heating of the investment mould should be carried out at a rate which enables steam and other gases to be liberated without cracking the mould. Also it is important that the temperature to which the mould is heated is adequate to enable thermal expansion and inversion to occur and that this temperature is not allowed to fall significantly before casting begins. Casting into a quartz-containing investment mould should be carried out with a mould temperature above 650°C if adequate expansion due to thermal expansion and inversion is to be achieved. This requires that the mould be heated to about 750°C to allow for cooling which may occur before casting commences. For cristobalite-containing investment moulds the mould temperature should be above 350°C at the time of casting and this requires heating to about 450°C to allow for cooling effects.

The balance between the molten alloy temperature and mould temperature is important in terms of producing a complete and accurate casting with a fine grain structure. The alloy should be hot enough to ensure that it is fully molten and remains so during casting into the mould, but should not be so hot that it begins to oxidize or that crystallization is delayed when it reaches the extremities of the mould cavity or causes damaging interactions with the mould walls. The mould temperature should be great enough to ensure complete expansion of the mould and to prevent premature crystallization leading to incomplete filling of the mould by alloy, but not great enough for crystallization to be delayed for so long that a coarse grain structure forms.

Factors such as length and diameter of the sprue and the distance of the mould cavity from the base of the mould all have an effect on the quality of the casting. For large castings, two or more sprues may be necessary in order to ensure that molten alloy is able to reach all parts of the mould cavity before solidifying.

9.3 Casting machines

Numerous types of casting machines are available, the aim of each being to cause molten alloy to completely fill the investment mould cavity. The three main variables which characterize the machines are as follows:

(1) The alloy may be melted in the mould sprue base (mould crucible) or in a separate crucible located in the casting machine.
(2) The alloy may be melted by one of several methods including gas–air torch, oxyacetylene torch, electrical induction heating or electrical resistance melting.
(3) The molten alloy may be driven into the mould by gravity, air pressure, steam pressure or by centrifugal force. The arm of the centrifugal casting machine is rotated either by a spring or by means of an electric motor.

Possibly the most popular system in current use is that in which the alloy is melted in a separate crucible using electrical induction heating and forced into the mould using centrifugal force.

The classical approach to centrifugal casting was to have the casting ring attached to a chain. The alloy was melted in the mould sprue base and forced into the mould cavity by swinging the casting ring around at the end of the chain.

9.4 Faults in castings

The faults which can occur in casting may be of four types.

(1) Finning and bubbling.
(2) Incomplete casting.
(3) Porosity in casting.
(4) Oversized or undersized casting.

Finning and bubbling: Finning occurs when the investment is heated up too rapidly in the furnace. This causes the investment to crack. Molten alloy flows into the cracks forming thin 'fins' on the casting in regions where the cracks have been located.

Bubbling effects on casting appear as spheres of excess material attached to the surface of the casting. These reflect the presence of surface porosities in the investment, a problem which can be overcome by vacuum investing.

Finning and bubbling increase the time required to finish a casting and if the defects occur in critical areas (e.g. near a crown shoulder) can result in a need to re-cast.

Incomplete castings: There are many possible causes of incomplete castings. In any casting the greater the number and thickness of the sprues, the more readily the metal will fill the mould. Against this, the sprues must be severed from the completed casting and an excessive number of sprues creates more work in finishing. Also, a larger weight of alloy is required for the casting and this presents difficulties in melting. It will be seen that the point of attachment of the sprues is a common site for defects and therefore an excessive number should be avoided.

The sprues should be attached at points of greatest bulk within the casting. This helps create a larger heat sink in these areas and prevents premature solidification which would cause incomplete filling of the mould. Placing sprues near to the bulky areas of the casting also aids the process of sprue removal and finishing without damaging the casting.

If the alloy is not properly melted, or if the mould temperature is too low, solidification occurs before the mould can be properly filled. The balance between molten alloy temperature and mould temperature plays an important part in ensuring complete filling of the mould as discussed in the previous section.

If there is insufficient thrust created during casting the alloy may not flow to all parts of the mould cavity. For centrifugal casting machines the thrust depends on the rotational speed of the casting arm, the length of the arm and the density of the alloy. The problem is therefore more significant for base metal alloys which have lower density and create less thrust.

Back pressure effects are caused by an inability of air or other gases within the mould to escape, making way for the alloy. To assist the escape of gases, the investment material between the casting and the end of the ring should be as thin as is consistent with strength, (distance X in Fig. 9.1). Also, the end of the ring should not be completely covered by any part of the casting apparatus. In all cases the plate of metal which supports the end of the ring must be perforated.

Permeability of investments varies with particle size distribution, but generally it decreases in the order of gypsum-, phosphate- and silica-bonded. A rather dense layer of investment material is often created at the base of the ring, particularly when the base of the ring has been closed temporarily by a sheet of metal or glass. This dense layer should be scraped away to facilitate the escape of gases. When using silica-bonded or fine-grained, phosphate-bonded investments a vent, 0.5 mm in diameter, should be provided to allow escape of gases towards the crucible end of the mould. A casting which has been subjected to back pressure is rounded at the edges and lacking in detail.

Defects may also be caused by cooling shrinkage. On solidification, the alloy contracts but the outer portions of the casting remain in contact with the internal walls of the mould.

The thinner sections, or those portions which are less effectively insulated against heat loss by the investment material, freeze first. As they solidify they contract and draw molten metal from the remaining portions. Voids or secondary pipe will be formed unless more metal can enter the mould. Local shrinkage defects are commonly seen in the casting at the base of the sprue (Fig. 9.2). It is preferable, therefore, that the casting should freeze by a wave of solidification traversing its mass, moving towards the sprue. A reservoir of metal is then present within the sprues if these are of sufficient thickness. One method is to thicken up a section of each sprue as near to the casting as possible. These round *sprue reservoirs* should freeze last of all and

any shrinkage porosity will be found in them, in the casting.

Porosity: Porosity may be seen as surface pitting on the casting or may be revealed within the cast metal on filing and polishing. Broken pieces of investment, or particles of dirt which have fallen down the sprue, may become embedded in the casting and produce pitting of the surface. For this reason all casting moulds should be handled with the sprue downwards.

Gaseous porosity in castings is produced by gases which become dissolved in the molten alloy. Copper, gold, silver, platinum, and particularly palladium, all dissolve oxygen in the molten state. On cooling, the alloys liberate the absorbed gases but some remain trapped when the alloy becomes rigid. This type of porosity may affect all parts of the casting. Its effects can be reduced by avoiding overheating of the alloy or casting in the atmosphere of an inert gas or vacuum.

Undersized or oversized castings: The final *fit* of a casting depends on a *balancing out* of expansions and contractions which occur during its construction. The major dimensional changes involved are the casting shrinkage of the alloy which should be compensated for by the setting expansion, thermal expansion and inversion of the investment. Faults in technique, for example not heating the investment mould to a high enough temperature, may produce insufficient compensation for casting shrinkage.

It should be remembered, however, that other factors such as the choice of impression material and impression technique may also influence the final result.

9.5 Suggested further reading

Hollenback, G.M. (1964) *Science and Technic of the Cast Restoration.* C.V. Mosby Co., Saint Louis.
Skinner, E.W. (1965) Casting techniques for small castings. *Dental Clin. North Am.* **March**, 225.

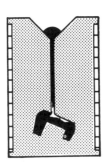

Fig. 9.2 Diagram illustrating a casting fault occurring at the base of the sprue.

Chapter 10
Steel and Wrought Alloys

10.1 Introduction

The previous chapters have dealt with casting alloys and casting techniques. Casting, however, is not the only way in which metals can be shaped. An alternative approach is to use *cold working*, in which the metal is hammered, drawn or bent into shape at temperatures well below the recrystallization temperature of the metal, often at room temperature. Metal or alloy structures produced in this way are said to have a wrought structure and often rely for their special properties on the work hardening which takes place during shaping.

Examples of the use of wrought alloys in dentistry include materials for making instruments and burs, wires, and occasionally, denture bases. Steel and stainless steel are the most widely used wrought alloys and are therefore worthy of some detailed discussion.

10.2 Steel

Steel is an alloy of iron and carbon in which the carbon content is less than 2%. Greater quantities of carbon produce a very brittle alloy which is unsuitable for cold working. In the solid state, steel is able to adopt a variety of structures depending on the carbon content and temperature. Above 723°C an interstitial solid solution of carbon in a face-centred cubic iron matrix is formed. This solid solution, termed *austenite*, is unstable below 723°C (the *critical temperature*) and the face-centred cubic iron matrix breaks down to form two phases. One phase consists of a very dilute solid solution of carbon in iron (up to 0.02% C), called *ferrite*. The other phase is a specific compound of iron and carbon with formula Fe_3C, called *cementite*. The mixture of ferrite and cementite is termed *pearlite*. These transitions are illustrated in the iron–carbon phase diagram given in Fig. 10.1.

It can be seen that certain aspects of the iron–

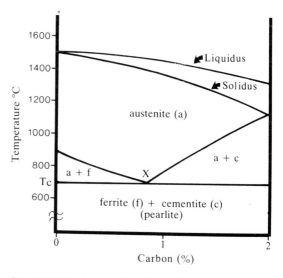

Fig. 10.1 The iron–carbon phase diagram (up to 2% carbon), slightly simplified for clarity.

carbon phase diagram resemble that for a eutectic alloy shown in Fig. 6.10. The critical temperature (Tc) for the iron–carbon system is equivalent to the eutectic temperature which characterized the eutectic alloys. In both cases, the temperature in question indicates the point at which the alloys undergo phase separation. Eutectic refers to the behaviour of an alloy of two mutually insoluble metals during crystallization. In the case of the iron–carbon system the transitions occur within the solid state. An alloy containing 0.8% carbon (corresponding to point X in Fig. 10.1) is known as the eutectoid alloy. Alloys with greater concentrations of carbon are called *hypereutectoid* alloys and those with smaller carbon contents, *hypoeutectoid* alloys. Both hypereutectoid and hypoeutectoid alloys consist of a mixture of ferrite and cementite at room temperature. The hypereutectoid alloys contain relatively greater amounts of cementite whilst the hypoeutectoid alloys contain greater amounts of ferrite.

Cementite is a very hard, brittle material whilst ferrite is softer and more ductile. Hence the hypereutectoid steels which contain greater quantities of cementite are commonly used to produce cutting instruments such as burs. The hypoeutectoids are used for the construction of non-cutting instruments such as forceps.

Steel can be further hardened by heat treatment. If an alloy is heated to a temperature above the critical temperature but below the solidus temperature it forms an austenitic solid solution as shown in Fig. 10.1. If the alloy is then quenched there is insufficient time for the alloy to undergo the transition from the austenitic structure to the pearlite structure. Instead, a very hard and brittle steel, called *martensite*, which has a distorted body-centered cubic lattice, is formed. Martensite is too brittle for most applications but its brittleness can be reduced by using a low temperature heat treatment, called *tempering*. The alloy is heated to a temperature in the range 200–400°C, at which martensite partially converts to ferrite and cementite. The degree of conversion depends on the tempering temperature and the tempering time. Thus, the hardness and brittleness can be controlled quite accurately by choosing suitable heat treatment conditions. The process of heat treatment hardening and tempering is illustrated in Fig. 10.2.

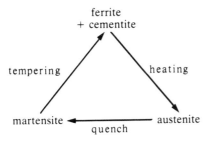

Fig. 10.2 Diagram illustrating the hardening and tempering cycle of heat treatments which can be used on steel.

The ability to be hardened by heat treatments is one of the major advantages of steel. Probably its main disadvantage is its susceptibility to corrosion.

10.3 Stainless steel

In addition to iron and carbon the stainless steels contain chromium which improves corrosion resistance. This is achieved by the *passivating effect* in which the chromium exposed at the surface of the alloy is readily oxidized to form a tenacious surface film of chromic oxide. This film resists further attack from aqueous media thus preventing corrosion. Nickel is also present in many stainless steels. It contributes towards corrosion resistance and helps to strengthen the alloy.

The addition of chromium and nickel to steel causes the critical temperature (Tc) (see Fig. 10.1) to be lowered. If sufficient quantities of these two metals are incorporated, the austenitic structure remains even at room temperature. One of the most commonly used stainless steels contains 18% chromium and 8% nickel (termed *18/8 stainless steel*). This alloy has a critical temperature below the point at which atomic movements are possible and is therefore sometimes referred to as *austenitic stainless steel*. It is not possible to harden these stainless steels by heat treatment because the solid–solid transitions occur below the temperature at which atomic diffusions are possible. Hence, 18/8 stainless steels are used in applications where heat hardening is not necessary, for example, for non-cutting instruments, wires and occasionally as denture bases. These applications involve a degree of *cold working* since the alloy is shaped by either bending, drawing or swaging, all of which result in the formation of a wrought structure. Alloys having wrought structures tend to have much higher values of proportional limit than equivalent alloys which have not been cold worked. It is this property coupled with a relatively high modulus of elasticity which makes wrought stainless steel wires suitable for orthodontics and wrought stainless steel sheets suitable for denture bases. Whilst these alloys cannot be hardened by heat treatments they can be softened if inadvertently overheated and recrystallized. This destroys the fibrous grain structure which results in a marked reduction in yield stress and proportional limit.

When smaller quantities of chromium and nickel are incorporated into steel it is possible to produce an alloy which has adequate corrosion resistance but which can be hardened by heat treatment. An alloy with these characteristics may, typically, contain about 12% chromium and little or no nickel. This alloy is capable of forming a martensitic structure and is therefore sometimes referred to as *martensitic stainless steel*. This type of alloy is commonly used to construct cutting instruments and probes which can be hardened by heat treatment, using a technique similar to that previously described for steel.

10.4 Stainless steel denture bases

Stainless steel denture bases are formed from very thin pressed/rolled sheets of wrought stainless steel. The method used for forming a stainless steel denture base deserves special mention. A thin sheet of 18/8 stainless steel (approximately 0.2 mm thick) is pressed between an alloy or epoxy resin die and counter die. The method of applying the pressure required for *swaging* may vary. Traditionally, a hydraulic press was used but modern techniques involve the use of a sudden pressure wave which adapts the sheet of alloy to the die very quickly. The pressure wave may be generated by using a controlled explosion or a sudden, controlled release of hydraulic pressure. These techniques are known as explosion forming and hydraulic forming respectively.

The wrought stainless steel sheets have high values of modulus of elasticity and proportional limit. This enables sufficient rigidity to be achieved with a very thin sheet of material. The weight of the denture can thus be kept to a minimum. Care must be taken not to overheat the wrought appliance since this may cause re-crystallization and a marked reduction in proportional limit.

A further advantage of stainless steel denture bases is that they conduct heat rapidly through the thin metallic sheet, thus ensuring that the patient retains a normal reflex reaction to hot and cold stimuli. The main disadvantages are the lack of surface detail on the swaged plate and, perhaps more significantly, the involved technique required for swaging, attaching retention tags by welding and processing of the acrylic parts of the denture.

10.5 Wires

Wires are commonly used for the construction of orthodontic appliances and occasionally as wrought clasps and rests on partial dentures. Orthodontic wires are designed to function such that they apply forces to malaligned teeth in order to change their positions/arrangements and to approximate more closely an ideal dental arch. The main variables involved in wire selection are related to the extent of movement required and the speed at which movement should occur. The aim of the orthodontist is to maximize the rate of tooth movement whilst minimizing the potential for pathological change. Wires are normally produced by drawing an ingot of alloy through dies of gradually decreasing cross-section to produce a circular, ovoid or square section wire in which the grain structure is highly fibrous in nature (see p. 49).

Requirements

The requirements of wires relate to their springiness, stiffness, ability to be bent without fracturing, corrosion resistance and an ability to be simply joined by soldering or welding. The springiness of a wire is a function of its fibrous grain structure which is incorporated during drawing of the wire. The 'springback' ability of a wire is a measure of its ability to undergo large deflections without permanent deformation. In terms of mechanical properties this is given by the ratio of yield stress to modulus of elasticity as follows:

$$\text{Springback potential} = \frac{\text{Yield stress}}{\text{Modulus of elasticity}}$$

A more approximate form of this equation uses proportional limit in place of yield stress.

A wire should have a value of stiffness, as indicated by its modulus of elasticity, which enables it to apply a suitable force for tooth movement during orthodontic treatment. This requirement varies considerably, since it is sometimes necessary to carry out rapid movements using stiff wires, whilst on other occasions it is necessary to apply small forces with flexible wires in order to bring about slow movements. Most wires are produced in circular cross-section and the stiffness of such wires is markedly dependent on thickness, being a function of the fourth power of the radius. Thus increasing the thickness of a wire from 0.6 mm to 0.7 mm increases stiffness by a factor of 1.86. Treatment strategy may involve the initial use of a relatively stiff wire capable of applying a large force in order to move teeth rapidly. Such wires may need to be replaced regularly if they have limited springback ability. A different strategy may be required if the teeth are very badly aligned. In this case it may be difficult to adapt a stiff wire to the teeth so a more flexible wire is used and the resulting tooth movement will be slower. When flexibility is required one approach is to use wires of smaller radius, although these can cause problems relating to tilting in the bracket slots so a better approach may be to choose a wire which is inherently more flexible.

Orthodontic wires are generally shaped by bending and the wire should possess sufficient ductility to resist fracture during this bending procedure. The amount of residual ductility remaining in a wire depends in part on the ductility used up in its manufacture. Hence, manufacturers can supply wires with varying ductility depending upon the extent to which they have been work hardened and/or recrystallized during production.

Wires often remain in the oral cavity for several months, whether they be part of a fixed or a removable orthodontic appliance. The wire should therefore have good corrosion resistance in order that it can withstand attack from oral fluids.

Finally, it is sometimes necessary to join two parts of an appliance together and, ideally, wires should be capable of being easily joined either by soldering or by welding, without impairing the mechanical properties of the wire or reducing the corrosion resistance. The importance of this property is reduced in alloys which can be easily bent into loops as a means of joining.

Available materials

Table 10.1 lists the commonly used wires and summarizes their main properties.

Stainless steel: Stainless steel wires are constructed from the 18/8 austenitic type of stainless steel – containing less than 0.15% carbon. The wires most commonly used are designated as types 302 and 304 by the American Iron and Steel Institute. They have a high value of modulus compared with some other alloys used to construct wires and are therefore used to apply relatively high forces. Lower forces can be achieved by using a wire of smaller diameter. 18/8 stainless steel has a relatively high value of yield stress and the springback properties are thus adequate for most applications.

Stainless steel wires have sufficient ductility to allow bending without fracture. They can be obtained in three grades, often referred to as soft, half-hard and hard, ranging from very ductile (soft) to less ductile (hard). The type of wire is chosen according to the amount of bending which must be carried out. Following bending, a stress relief anneal can be carried out in order to relieve internal stresses. This involves heating the wire to 450°C for about 10 minutes. The annealing procedure should be carried out only with 'stabilized' stainless steel wires which contain small quantities of titanium. Unstabilized wires become brittle during annealing due to reaction between chromium and carbon.

Joining of stainless steel wires can be accomplished either by soldering or by welding. Silver solders are normally used for soldering. They contain silver and copper with small quantities of other elements to lower the fusion temperature. Care must be taken during soldering not to overheat the wires since this may cause recrystallization of the grain structure with a subsequent lack of springiness. In addition, overheating may cause the chromium to react with carbon, forming carbides, a phenomenon referred to as *weld decay*. This results in a loss of corrosion resistance around the soldered joint and the introduction of a degree of brittleness. The solder itself, of course, is a source of potential corrosion being of a eutectic-type composition.

Welding is accomplished by pressing two pieces of wire together between two electrodes then passing an electric current, sufficient to melt the wires at the point of contact joining them together. The temperature rise ($\triangle T$) at the joint when a current passes is given by the function

$$\triangle T \alpha I^2 R t$$

where I is the current passing, R is the electrical resistance at the junction of the two wires and t is the time for which the current passes.

High temperatures, sufficient for welding, can only be achieved with alloys giving relatively high values of electrical resistance at the junction. Thus, welding is not a suitable technique for joining gold wires. The electrical current and the time for which the current flows must be controlled such that adequate welding is achieved without overheating the rest of the wire. This would lead to weld decay and a degree of recrystallization, causing loss of the fibrous grain structure.

Table 10.1 Summary of properties of commonly used wires.

Material	Stiffness	Springback ability	Ductility	Ease of soldering or welding
Stainless steel	High	Good	Adequate	Reasonable
Gold alloy	Medium	Adequate	Adequate	Easy to solder
Co/Cr alloy	High	Adequate following heat treatment	Good in soft state	Difficult
Ni/Ti alloy	Low	Excellent	Poor	Difficult
β-Ti	Medium	Good	Adequate	Joined by welding

Gold alloys: Traditionally, two types of wrought gold alloy wires have been used in the past – classified as high gold and low gold. High gold materials contain greater than 75% gold and platinum group metals. Low gold alloys contain smaller quantities of noble metals. A typical material contains 60% gold, 15% silver, 15% copper and about 10% platinum or palladium. The high platinum or palladium content raises the melting point and recrystallization temperature of the wires making them more amenable to soldering operations. Gold alloy wires have a lower value of modulus of elasticity than the stainless steel variety and therefore apply lower forces. An advantage of the gold alloy wires is that they are easily soldered using normal gold solders. Gold alloy wires are rarely used nowadays due to their cost.

Cobalt–chromium alloys (elgiloy): These alloys contain cobalt, chromium, nickel, iron and molybdenum in approximate proportions 40:20:15:16:7. They have the unique characteristic of being supplied in a softened state which has excellent ductility. Following bending, the wires can be hardened by heat treating at 480°C. The precipitation hardening that occurs introduces the required springback properties into the wire.

The modulus of elasticity of the wire is similar to that for stainless steel, indicating a similar performance in terms of tooth movement. These wires are difficult to join by soldering.

Nickel–titanium alloys (nitinol): These alloys contain almost equal amounts of nickel and titanium with small quantities of other metals. They are flexible wires with low modulus values and are used to apply relatively low forces. The low modulus coupled with high yield stress indicates excellent springback properties and they are particularly useful for carrying out large tooth movements using low forces over along period of time. Nitinol wires have limited ductility and are not easy to bend without fracturing. They are not amenable to joining operations such as soldering or welding.

Nitinol wires possess a rather unique shape-memory property which enables a plastically deformed wire to return to its original shape following an appropriate heat treatment. This behaviour has not yet been used to good effect in any dental applications of the wires.

β-Titanium: These alloys consist mainly of titanium with some molybdenum. They are ductile, allowing good formability, and have springback characteristics similar to those of stainless steel. They have a lower modulus value than stainless steel and therefore apply lower forces, and they can be joined by welding.

10.6 Suggested further reading

Reisbick, M.H. (1978) Orthodontic wires. In *An Outline of Dental Materials and Their Selection* (W.J. O'Brien & G. Ryge, eds), pp. 307–319. W.B. Saunders Co., Philadelphia.

Waters, N.E. (1975) Properties of wires. In *Scientific Aspects of Dental Materials* (J.A. von Fraunhofer, ed.), pp. 2–15. Butterworths, Sevenoaks.

Chapter 11
Ceramics and Porcelain Fused to Metal (PFM)

11.1 Introduction

The word ceramic is derived from the Greek word *keramos* which literally means 'burnt stuff' but which has come to mean more specifically a material produced by burning or firing. The first ceramics fabricated by man were earthenware pots used for domestic purposes. This material is opaque, relatively weak and porous and would be unsuitable for dental applications. It consisted mainly of kaolin. The blending of this with other minerals such as silica and feldspar produced the translucency and extra strength required for dental restorations. Material containing these additional important ingredients was given the name porcelain.

Fused porcelain has long been used in the construction of works of art. It can be produced in almost every shade or tint and its translucency imparts a depth of colour unobtainable by other materials. Although the technique or porcelain fusing is exacting it can be initially moulded by hand as a paste and alterations can be made at various stages of the work. It is not surprising, therefore, that dentistry has turned to porcelain for the production of artificial teeth, crowns, bridges and veneers.

Although the favourable aesthetic properties and excellent biocompatibility of porcelain has never been in doubt, its use is somewhat restricted by the relatively brittle nature of the material and the large shrinkage which occurs during processing. Some recent developments offer a potential for overcoming these problems.

11.2 Composition of traditional dental porcelain

The compositions of the various types of porcelain are summarized in Table 11.1. It can be seen that there are considerable differences in composition

Table 11.1 Composition of porcelains.

Material	Components (%)			
	Clay (kaolin)	Silica	Binder (feldspar)	Glasses
Decorative porcelain	50	25	25	0
High-fusing dental	4	15	80	0
Low-fusing dental	0	25	60	15

between the dental porcelains and decorative porcelain. Indeed, the dental porcelains contain little or no clay and, possibly, would be more aptly described as dental glasses.

Kaolin is a hydrated aluminosilicate, $Al_2O_3 \cdot 2SiO_2 \cdot 2H_2O$. The set decorative porcelain is essentially a mixture of this with silica, bound together by a flux or binder such as feldspar which is a mixture of potassium and sodium aluminosilicates, $K_2O \cdot Al_2O_3 \cdot 6SiO_2$ and $Na_2O \cdot Al_2O_3 \cdot 6SiO_2$. Feldspar is the lowest fusing component and it is this which melts and flows during firing, uniting the other components in a solid mass. The fusion temperature of feldspar may be further reduced by adding to it other low-fusing fluxes such as borax.

Of the two types of dental porcelain, the high-fusing materials fuse in the range 1300–1400°C whilst the low-fusing materials fuse in the range 850–1100°C. The latter materials are by far the more commonly used products.

The precise formulations of dental porcelains vary among the variable products from the proportions given in Table 11.1; however the general trend towards the use of less kaolin (clay) with an increase in the feldspar content in order to improve translucency suggests that dental porcelains should be more correctly described as glasses. The large glassy phases developed by compositions of low kaolin content require closely controlled firing times and temperatures in order to produce an acceptable result.

The powders supplied to the dentist or technician are not just mixtures of the various ingredients. During manufacture the constituents are mixed together and then fused to form a *frit*. This is broken up, often by dropping the hot material into cold water. It is then ground into a fine powder ready for use.

In the fusion process which takes place during manufacture the flux reacts with the outer layers of the grains of silica, kaolin or glass and partly combines them together. When the technician fuses the porcelain powder, during the production of a crown for example, he simply remelts the fluxes without causing any significant increase in reaction between the flux and the other components.

Porcelain powders are sometimes pigmented in order that natural tooth shades can be matched. The *pigments* used are normally metal oxides which are stable at the fusion temperature.

Some feldspathic porcelains are supplied as *opalescent porcelains*. Opalescence is a light scattering effect achieved by the addition of very small amounts of metallic oxides having a higher refractive index and a particle size near to that of the wavelength of light. Since natural teeth can display some opalescence the availability of opalescent porcelains adds further to the ability to match natural tooth appearance in every way.

The use of uranium compounds in dental porcelains to simulate tooth fluorescence is now considered inadvisable. It is not only unnecessary but can give an unnatural appearance under ultraviolet light and, in addition, may create a potential health hazard.

A low-fusing, transparent glass may be used as a *glaze* over the completed body of the porcelain restoration. The glaze gives the crown an impervious, smooth surface and imparts greater translucency.

A smooth surface can be obtained without using a glaze. By careful control of the furnace temperature, the surface of the normal porcelain will flow and glaze with only a slight rounding of the contours of the restoration. Unfortunately, any overheating will cause gross distortions of the shape.

The porcelain powders are mixed with water to produce a plastic mass of material which can be moulded and carved before firing. To improve the working properties a *binder* such as sugar or starch is added to some powders.

11.3 Compaction and firing

The aqueous plastic mass of porcelain particles is compacted as much as possible onto a platinum foil matrix. This reduces the size of the spaces between the particles and thus reduces firing shrinkage. Powders consisting of a mixture of particle sizes compact more easily than those with particles of one size only.

The moulded crown may be lightly vibrated, thus helping to settle the powder particles and bring excess water to the surface, where it is blotted by an absorbent cloth. Alternatively, the powder may be 'patted' with a spatula to achieve the same effect.

A well-compacted crown not only reduces firing shrinkage but also shows a regular contraction over its entire surface, thus maintaining the original form on a slightly reduced scale.

Following compaction, the next stage involves porcelain 'firing'. A porcelain furnace consists, essentially, of an electrically heated muffle with a pyrometer which indicates the temperature in that part of the muffle where the porcelain is placed. Most modern porcelain furnaces allow firing under vacuum. This has the effect of reducing the porosity within the finished material from around 4.6% to about 0.5%.

If the freshly compacted, wet structure is placed directly into a hot furnace it will evolve steam rapidly and crumble or even explode. The normal procedure, therefore, is to dry the wet structure in a warm atmosphere before placing into the hot furnace.

At the elevated temperatures of the furnace, the starch or sugar binder ignites and the surface of the structure blackens. The door of the furnace is left slightly ajar during this stage to allow the products of combustion to escape. The furnace door is then closed and firing is completed. Shrinkage takes place as the fluxes bind the particles together causing a uniform inward contraction of the whole mass. Further additions of fresh material may be made at this stage before glazing. Whenever porcelain work is heated or cooled the process must be carried out slowly. Porcelain is a poor conductor of heat and is brittle. Rapid cooling would result in cracking and loss of strength.

The accuracy of fit is maintained by building up the porcelain on a platinum foil which has been closely adapted to the die. The firing shrinkage which occurs does not therefore cause a great discrepancy in the accuracy of fit, since the shrinkage occurs inwards towards the platinum foil and the foil itself is not affected by firing. Before cementation, the platinum foil is removed from the inner surface of a crown to create about 25 μm of space for cementation.

The porcelain surface is generally glazed as mentioned in Section 11.2. This has the dual effect of improving appearance and removing surface imperfections, particularly porosities, which may adversely affect mechanical properties. The use of porcelain for constructing inlays is a most exacting technique because, in this case, firing shrinkage has a direct effect on the fit of the inlay. For this reason the porcelain inlay was a very rare restoration. This situation has changed with the development of castable ceramics, shrink-free materials, the more widespread availability of refractory materials on which porcelain restorations can be manufactured, and CAD–CAM systems.

11.4 Properties of porcelain

Aesthetically, porcelain is an almost perfect material for the replacement of missing tooth substance. It is available in a range of shades and at various levels of translucency such that a most life-like appearance can be achieved. The inner layer of the porcelain crown, for example, is normally constructed from a fairly opaque 'core' material. This is overlaid with a more translucent 'dentine' material with a final coating of translucent 'enamel' porcelain forming the outermost layer.

Porcelain is a very rigid, hard and brittle material whose strength is reduced by the presence of surface irregularities or internal voids and porosities. Fine-grained powders give more uniform surfaces than coarser grains, and firing at reduced pressures can reduce porosity. The formation of superficial cracks due to thermal stresses are best avoided by slow cooling from the firing temperature. Fracture can be initiated from small surface scratches caused by grinding and these should be eliminated by smoothing or by further fusing. Cracks in porcelain crowns invariably emanate from the inner, unglazed fitting surface and propagate outwards towards the exposed surface material as illustrated in Fig. 11.1. The brittleness of dental ceramics is compounded by their tendency to undergo *static fatigue*. This is a time-dependent decrease in strength, even in the absence of any applied load. The process is thought to occur through alkaline hydrolysis of Si–O groups within the porcelain structure. Alkalinity within the

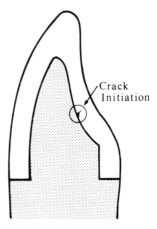

Fig. 11.1 Diagram illustrating the initiation and propagation of a crack from the inner surface of a porcelain crown.

material results from a solubilization of Na_2O and K_1O which forms part of the feldspathic component of porcelain. The weakening is further accelerated by dynamic mechanical loading and the whole process has been likened to stress corrosion cracking which can occur with metals and alloys. Attempts to overcome some of these problems involved reducing the proportions of Na_2O and $K_2)O$ within the materials.

Tooth preparation for all porcelain crowns needs to be designed to reduce the possibility of producing areas of high stress within the finished restoration. All internal line angles should be rounded and care is required to ensure that there are no areas of sudden change in thickness of porcelain. The gingival finishing margin should be a smooth shoulder (i.e. without steps) and the finishing angle should be 90° to the root surface.

As we have said earlier, fracture in ceramic materials occurs through crack initiation and propagation from surface flaws. In order for cracks to grow the material in the region of the crack tip must be placed under tension. Hence, one method of strengthening ceramics is to generate compressive stresses in these regions. This can be achieved by one of two mechanisms. First, ion strengthening can be used. This involves soaking the fired material in a molten salt in order to allow ion exchange at the surface. If sodium ions are partially replaced by potassium ions, the latter occupy a greater volume and effectively create compressive stresses in the surface layer of the material. Such procedures can be carried out in a dental laboratory using an ion-exchange paste which is painted onto the surface.

The ion-exchange procedure is achieved by placing the treated ceramic material in a dental laboratory oven in order to create the conditions under which diffusion can occur.

A second method for strengthening involves putting the outer layer into compression through thermal strengthening. During firing the outer layer solidifies first as it cools more rapidly. The poor thermal conductivity of the material dictates that the inner part of the material remains liquid for longer. When the inner material finally solidifies it shrinks and sets up a compressive stress in the outer layer. This method of strengthening can occur during the initial firing of the ceramic or during subsequent heat tempering.

The relatively poor mechanical properties of porcelain can be improved using alumina, or metal supporting structures. These are discussed in the next sections.

The hardness of porcelain (Table 2.1) contributes to its ability to resist forces of abrasion but may give rise to some concern over the potential for porcelain restorations to abrade the opposing teeth. It has been shown, however, that the wear of enamel by ceramic restorations cannot easily be predicted by the hardness of the ceramic. Some extremely hard ceramics seem to produce lower enamel wear compared with softer materials. The shape of crystalline inclusions within the ceramic appears to be an important factor in determining the abrasive potential of a ceramic material. The appearance of ceramic restorations depends in part on the surface gloss which can be produced using a glaze or by polishing. The hardness of porcelain dictates that polishing using abrasives should be difficult. However, different porcelains respond differently to abrasive polishing. Carefully controlled polishing with a fine abrasive such as pumice can give a satisfactory surface with some materials. From a clinical standpoint a polished porcelain surface will accumulate more plaque than a glazed surface. Hence porcelain at crown margins should be glazed whenever possible.

Porcelain has excellent thermal properties and is a particularly good thermal insulator. This fact is of importance when gross amounts of enamel and dentine are to be replaced and the residual layer of dentine may be of minimal thickness.

Correctly formulated porcelain is very resistant to chemical attack, being unaffected by the wide variations of pH which may be encountered in the mouth.

11.5 Alumina inserts and aluminous porcelain

The major disadvantage of porcelain is brittleness and this is the factor which most limits its use. Several methods are available which are aimed at preventing the formation or propagation of cracks on the inner surface of porcelain restorations.

One approach is to use a core of pure alumina on which the porcelain crown is constructed. Alumina is a very hard, opaque material which is less susceptible to crack propagation than porcelain. Another approach to strengthening involves the use of pure alumina inserts. These may be in the form of small sheets of alumina which are generally placed palatally in a crown in order to strengthen without impairing the appearance.

Powdered alumina may be added to porcelain in order to achieve a significant strengthening. The mechanism of strengthening is that the alumina particles act as 'crack stoppers' preventing the propagation of a crack throughout the body of the porcelain (Fig. 11.2a). This improvement of properties is achieved not only as a result of the good mechanical properties of alumina but also due to the compatibility of alumina with porcelain. The two materials have closely matching values of coefficient

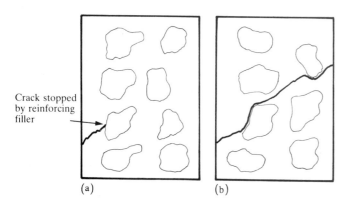

Crack stopped by reinforcing filler

(a)   (b)

Fig. 11.2 Diagram illustrating how the propagation of a crack can be halted by a reinforcing particle. (a) Alumina particle acting as a crack stopper. (b) A crack propagating around a filler particle.

of thermal expansion and modulus of elasticity. This ensures that the interface region between the alumina particles and the porcelain is virtually stress-free and not likely to encourage crack propagation around the alumina particles. Attempts to improve the properties of porcelain with materials which are not compatible have been unsuccessful since the cracks propagate around the 'reinforcing' material as illustrated in Fig. 11.2b.

Porcelain which contains alumina is referred to as aluminous porcelain and the alumina content is normally around 40%. Although aluminous porcelain has definite advantages in terms of mechanical properties, it is opaque and therefore can only be used to construct the inner core region of a porcelain crown. This is generally acceptable, since it is the inner region from which cracks propagate and which is therefore the area in need of reinforcement. A matched expansion veneering porcelain is baked onto the surface of the high alumina material to give the finished restoration. Flexural strength values of aluminous porcelains are typically in excess of 110 MPa compared to only about 80 MPa for unreinforced materials (Table 11.2).

Table 11.2 Flexural strength values (MPa) of some dental ceramics.

Unreinforced porcelain	70–120
Aluminous porcelain	120–180
Cast glass ceramic	100–150
Sintered alumina core ceramic	400–600
Pressed glass with leucite	120–180
Minimum for core ceramic (ISO Standard)	100
Minimum for dentine/enamel ceramic (ISO Standard)	50

11.6 Sintered alumina core ceramics

The use of alumina additions to strengthen porcelain has been taken a stage further with the introduction of sintered alumina cores. For one such system (Inceram) the first stage in producing the restoration involves the formation of a duplicate die using a 'special' plaster. An alumina slip prepared from alumina powder and water is then painted on to the die. The moisture from the slip is absorbed by the plaster leaving a layer of alumina powder which should ideally be at least 0.5 mm thick. This is then sintered by firing at 1120°C for 2 hours. The firing causes the die material to shrink, making the removal of the sintered alumina core quite easy. The outer surface of the core is painted with a slurry of a

glass powder and firing at 1100°C is carried out to liquefy the glass which flows to fill all the spaces between the sintered alumina particles. The glass used is a lanthanum aluminosilicate glass. The lanthanum reduces viscosity and assists infiltration. It also increases the refractive index of the glass and improves the translucency of the ceramic. After microblasting to remove gross excesses of glass a re-firing at 960° is performed to ensure proper infiltration of the alumina with glass.

On completion of the core firing procedures, the dentine and enamel layers are built up in the traditional manner. The extremely high flexural strength of the sintered alumina system (Table 11.2) gives rise to some optimism that these materials may be suitable for the production of multi-unit restorations which have previously required the use of cast-metal substructures. *Spinel*-based cores of magnesium aluminate have been used instead of alumina. These produce improved translucency but are not as strong as sintered alumina cores.

11.7 Injection moulded and pressed ceramics

These materials were first reported in 1983 for the production of all-ceramic, single, anterior or posterior crowns. The first commonly used commercial system based on this principle (Cerestore) involved the production of crown cores by injection moulding, potentially eliminating the need for the use of a platinum foil and improving marginal adaptation of the crown. The non-shrink properties are achieved by incorporating significant quantities of magnesium oxide into the ceramic frit. This reacts with the alumina during firing to form a mixed metal oxide, called a spinel. The spinel is less dense than the original mixture of oxides and its formation results in an expansion which compensates for firing shrinkage.

The technique for fabricating ceramic copings from this type of material involves the formation of a wax pattern on an epoxy resin die. A variation of the lost wax technique is used to maintain the correct shape and size in the ceramic material. The mixed material, containing magnesium and aluminium oxides, glass, kaolin, calcium stearate and wax is injected under pressure at 180°C into the prepared mould. Firing is then carried out in a special furnace using controlled temperatures up to 1300°C during which formation of the spinel occurs. Veneer porcelains are baked onto the surface of the coping to produce the finished crown.

It was hoped that these ceramic copings would

offer the possibility of constructing all-ceramic crowns for molars with the attendant improvement in aesthetics which this would bring. The strength of the material is however, not much different from that of ordinary aluminous porcelain and the complexity of the process involving the need for special equipment has limited its use.

A further development of this idea of injection moulding involved the introduction of a material (IPS Empress) in which a molten feldspathic type glass is pressed into a pre-formed mould formed using a high temperature investment material and a wax pattern (see Section 9.2). After the molten glass has been forced into the mould under pressure, it is allowed to cool under controlled conditions which allows reinforcing leucite crystals to form. The properties of the material are similar to those of the cast glass ceramics.

One of two methods can be used for characterization. For anterior crowns a layering technique is normally used to achieve the best possible appearance. A fully sized crown is first produced from a wax pattern. This structure is then 'cut back' in those areas where conventional layered porcelains are used to give optimal aesthetics to give adequate space for the veneering material. During the firing of the outer veneer layer of porcelain further strengthening of the pressed ceramic core may occur as the concentration of leucite crystallites increases.

For posterior crowns, inlays or labial veneers where either aesthetics are not considered so important or where layering would be impossible due to insufficient thickness, characterization is achieved by the application of surface stains.

11.8 Cast glass ceramics

Techniques now exist for producing cast ceramic restorations by the lost wax technique in much the same way that alloy castings are produced. At present the use of the material is limited to single anterior or posterior crowns.

Crowns are formed from wax patterns which are invested in a phosphate-bonded investment. The wax burn-out and heat soak of the investment is carried out at about 950°C. The molten ceramic is cast centrifugally into the mould at around 1350°C. This results in a transparent glass crown which is then heat treated in an oven at 1075°C for 10 hours. This heat treatment or *ceramming* causes partial crystallization to form mica-like crystals (containing K, Mg and Si oxides along with significant quantities of fluoride) which have a dual effect. They slightly reduce the translucency of the previously clear

material and significantly increase the strength. Table 11.2 shows that the strength of these cast ceramics can match that of aluminous porcelain.

Colour matching is achieved by applying a series of the appropriate tinted porcelains to the surface and re-firing. This procedure may be circumvented with the development of new candidate materials in which the shading can be incorporated within the body of the crown. Further improvements in appearance are achieved by selecting the correct shade of luting cement. The surface glazes used to provide colour to cast glasses can produce a very realistic result. Unfortunately, if there is a need to undertake any adjustment of the shape of the crown they are rapidly removed, resulting in poor aesthetics unless the crown is re-glazed.

The technique of casting offers the ability to produce accurately fitting, all-ceramic crowns which may be strong enough for use in the posterior region without the need of an alloy substructure. The need for some specialist equipment may be considered a disadvantage.

11.9 CAD–CAM restorations

CAD–CAM stands for computer aided design–computer aided manufacture. This is a hi-tech approach to providing patients with durable tooth-coloured restorations. It involves recording an optical impression from which a restoration can be designed using a computer. The design details are then used to construct the restoration using a milling machine which cuts the desired shape from a monolithic block of ceramic under the control of the computer. Great care must be taken during tooth preparation to take due account of the limitations of the type of shape which can be cut by the milling machine. The optical impression is recorded using a miniature video camera which scans the prepared tooth for about 5 minutes. The recording of a suitable image can be assisted by applying an opaque white powder over the area to be scanned. For the sake of accuracy it is important that this layer is uniform and kept as thin as possible.

The design of the restoration on the computer screen takes about 5 to 15 minutes. At this stage it is again important that the limitations of the milling machine are considered. Milling of the restoration takes about 5 minutes. Until recently only the fitting surface could be milled, but improvements in software and milling equipment now allow the whole restoration to be milled. The restoration is tried in and adjusted if necessary. It is then normal to silane treat the fitting surface to aid retention before final cementation using a dual cured resin cement. A final polishing can be performed in situ.

An alternative to the chairside CAD–CAM approach is the use of a mechanical copy milling technique in the laboratory. The clinical stages are identical to those for a conventional inlay. A pattern is produced in the laboratory and then a replica of that pattern produced in a ceramic using a copy-milling device. The commercially available systems are capable of reproducing both relatively intricate fitting surfaces and the occlusal surface of the inlay.

Materials used to form the ceramic block from which the restoration is cut include conventional feldspathic porcelains and glass ceramics. It has recently been shown that restorations can be cut from sintered alumina blocks which can be infiltrated with glass to form In-ceram like CAD–CAM restorations.

One advantage of CAD–CAM systems is that the ceramic manufacturing processes including forming and heat treating are under the control of the manufacturer and are taken away from the dental laboratory, maximizing the physical properties of the ceramic itself. Cementation of CAD–CAM restorations normally involves the use of dual cured composite cements. The cement is potentially the weak link in the restoration as it is much softer than either the ceramic restoration or the tooth enamel (i.e. 20 VHN compared with >300 VHN). Cement margins surrounding CAD–CAM restorations are typically 60–150 µm wide, but are sometimes reported to be even wider. The cement can undergo rapid wear to a depth of about half the value of the width. It is therefore not unusual to find a 50 µm deep defect surrounding the restoration. Improvements in marginal fit which will come as impression and milling techniques develop will help to overcome this problem.

11.10 Porcelain veneers

Porcelain veneers offer a means of improving the appearance of stained or discoloured teeth. The veneer consists of a thin shell-like structure which is ideally fabricated in such a way that it can be closely adapted to the prepared tooth. There is some controversy as to whether the veneers can be attached to unprepared teeth – a technique which would obviously conserve sound tooth substance, or whether some reduction in the tooth contour is necessary. Most authorities do advise the removal of about 0.5 mm of labial enamel.

The veneers which are normally 0.5–0.8 mm thick, may be constructed from feldspathic porcelain, glass ceramic, pressed ceramic or CAD–CAM techniques and are bonded to the tooth enamel using a composite resin luting agents. The bonding is achieved by etching the enamel with a phosphoric acid solution or gel. The fitting surface of the veneer is etched with a solution of hydrofluoric acid, then dried and treated with a silane coupling agent to aid bonding to the composite resin.

The appearance of the veneered tooth depends on the colour of the underlying tooth structure, the aesthetic qualities of the ceramic and the use of the correct shade of luting composite which may be required to mask any discoloration in the underlying tooth and give a natural appearance. The use of a light activated luting composite is normal. These materials offer the advantage of an extended working time during which the veneer can be placed accurately.

An accurate assessment of the shade of a porcelain veneer cannot be made at trial without 'coupling' the veneer to the underlying tooth. This process involves optically linking the veneer to the underlying tooth to see what effect the colour of the tooth has on the finished restoration. In its simplest form this can be achieved using water, but a better alternative is a water-soluble trial paste. This commercial product has similar colour characteristics to the luting resin but can be washed off the veneer surface with water prior to luting the veneer in place.

In some respects the apparent clinical success which has been achieved with porcelain veneers is surprising. The technique involves the support of a very thin, rigid and brittle material, the veneer, by a more flexible material, the luting composite. It would be expected that cracking of the ceramic would be a frequent occurrence under such circumstances. The fact that this does not appear to be a major problem suggests that stresses generated are not great enough to cause a strain of 0.1%, the critical strain above which most ceramic materials will fracture.

Alternatives to the use of porcelain veneers involve the use of pre-formed acrylic veneers or polishable composite resin veneers. The ceramic materials have the advantage of being more durable, probably related to their greater hardness (see Table 2.1). The technique of fabrication is however more time consuming than the direct method of using a veneering composite. The preformed acrylic veneers seem to offer few advantages. They combine an involved clinical and laboratory technique with poor durability.

11.11 Porcelain fused to metal (PFM)

Porcelain fused to metal restorations involve a marrying of the good mechanical properties of cast dental alloys with the excellent aesthetic properties of porcelain. Generally, the restorations consist of an alloy substructure with bonded porcelain veneers as shown in Fig. 11.3.

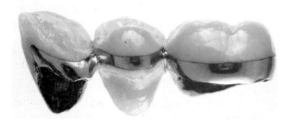

Fig. 11.3   Photograph showing a metal-bonded porcelain restoration. Porcelain is built up on an alloy substructure.

A major requirement of the materials used in PFM restorations is compatibility of the metal and ceramic used. Feldspathic porcelains used for PFM work normally contain significant amounts of leucite. This increases the coefficient of thermal expansion of the porcelain to a value which is closer to that for the metal. This helps to prevent the development of thermal stresses during cooling from the firing temperature. The presence of leucite also helps to strengthen the ceramic. The minimum flexural strength requirement for PFM ceramics as specified in ISO Standards is 50 MPa, which is equivalent to the requirement for dentine/enamel porcelains used in all-ceramic restorations.

The requirements of the alloy used to form the substructure are similar to those for non-porcelain bonding work with additional requirements as follows

(1)   The alloy, having been previously cast into the desired shape, should be capable of withstanding porcelain firing without melting or suffering creep. Hence the alloy must have a high fusion temperature.

(2)   The alloy should be sufficiently rigid to support a very brittle porcelain veneer otherwise fracture of the veneer is inevitable.

(3)   The alloy should be capable of forming a bond with the porcelain veneer in order that the latter does not become detached.

(4)   The alloy should have a value of coefficient of thermal expansion similar to that for the porcelain to which it is bonded.

There are four types of alloy currently available for porcelain bonding. These are (a) high-gold alloys, (b) low-gold-content alloys, (c) silver–palladium alloys and (d) nickel–chromium alloys. Table 11.3 gives a summary of the comparative properties of the four alloys.

High-gold alloys

The composition of a typical high-gold-content porcelain-bonding alloy is shown in Table 11.4. The major differences between these alloys and the non porcelain-bonding alloys are the high platinum/palladium content, the absence of copper and the presence of small amounts of base metals such as tin and indium.

The high platinum/palladium content raises the melting temperature of the alloy, reducing the risk of softening and creep during porcelain firing. In addition, these two metals decrease the coefficient of thermal expansion of the gold alloy to a value closer to that for porcelain. Copper is absent from porcelain-bonding gold alloys since, when present, it imparts a green hue to the porcelain veneer. The minor quantities of base metals such as tin and indium are essential in promoting bonding between the alloy and the overlying veneer. The base metals become oxidized at the surface and the oxide layer forms a chemical bond with porcelain during firing.

The high-gold alloys have two disadvantages when used for porcelain bonding. Despite the high

Table 11.3   Properties of alloys used for porcelain bonding.

Alloy	Castability	Creep resistance during firing	Modulus	Bond strength	Biocompatibility
High-gold	+++	−	+	+	++
Low-gold	++	+	++	+	+
Silver–palladium	−	+	++	+	+
Nickel–chromium	− −	++	+++	−	− − −

Table 11.4 Composition of a typical high-gold-content porcelain-bonding alloy.

Metal	Percentage
Gold	85
Platinum	10
Palladium	3
Silver	1
Tin	0.5
Indium	0.5

platinum/palladium content, the melting range is still sufficiently low that there is a risk of alloy 'sag' during porcelain firing. Secondly, the modulus of elasticity of the high-gold alloys is less than ideal. Subsequently, *copings* must be produced in fairly thick section in order to prevent flexing which would result in porcelain fracture. The requirement of a minimum copying thickness of around 0.5 mm results in the risk of an over-contoured restoration and gingival irritation.

Low-gold alloys

Low-gold porcelain-bonding alloys contain approximately 50% gold, 30% palladium to raise the melting temperature and lower the coefficient of thermal expansion, 10% silver and 10% indium and tin for porcelain bonding.

The mechanical properties of the low-gold alloys are similar to those for the high-gold materials. They have a slightly greater modulus of elasticity which is an advantage for porcelain bonding. The higher melting range produces better creep resistance for these materials during porcelain firing.

Good properties and a significant cost saving compared with high-gold alloys account for the widespread use of these materials for bonded porcelain work.

Silver–palladium alloys

These alloys contain about 60% palladium, 30% silver and 10% indium and/or tin to aid porcelain bonding. They have the advantages of a higher modulus value and a higher melting range than the high-gold alloys. They offer a suitable alternative to the high-gold materials for bonded porcelain work at a considerable saving in cost, providing care is taken during casting to avoid defects and gas inclusions.

The taking up of a green hue in some ceramics in contact with high silver content alloys (silver green-

ing) has been reported, although this appears to be as much a feature of the composition of the ceramic as the composition of the alloy.

Nickel–chromium alloys

Nickel–chromium casting alloys typically contain 70–80% nickel and 10–25% chromium with small quantities of other metals such as molybdenum, tungsten and beryllium. Porcelain bonding is to the layer of ceramic oxide which forms on the surface of the alloy.

These alloys have the advantages of a very high modulus and high melting temperature. Their disadvantages are as follows.

(1) A high casting shrinkage which may affect accuracy of fit if not fully compensated by the investment.
(2) A tendency for poor castability, with voids in the castings.
(3) A bond strength with porcelain which does not compare with that achieved with the other alloys.

Indeed, fractures in Ni/Cr–porcelain systems invariably occur through the oxide layer whereas fractures in the other systems generally occur cohesively in the porcelain. In addition, these alloys are suspect from the biocompatibility point of view, as discussed on p. 67.

Tooth preparation for PFM restorations

During tooth preparation it is necessary to allow about 1.5 mm in thickness for a metal coping (0.3–0.5 mm) and the porcelain veneer (1.0 mm) to achieve optimal aesthetics. If this space is not available then the technician will either produce an overly bulky restoration with reasonable appearance or the opaque layer of porcelain used to mask the metal coping will 'shine through' the surface layers of porcelain producing an opaque white or cream spot. For this reason preparations for PFM crowns need to be designed to give adequate space for the technician to produce an appropriate restoration. The margin configuration for a PFM crown is a flat shoulder where there is porcelain and a chamfer or bevel where this is a metal finishing line. The appearance of the margins of PFM crowns has been revolutionized by the development of *shoulder porcelains*. These porcelains have adequate *substantivity* so that they do not flow significantly during firing. This allows the technician to cut the metal coping back from the edge of the tooth, leaving an adequate bulk of porcelain to give a reasonable marginal fit with much improved aesthetics.

11.12 Capillary technology

The capillary technology (or Captek™) system is an alternative means of producing porcelain–metal restorations. The metal substructure is produced in two stages. Firstly, a wax strip loaded with powdered, high palladium content metal is adapted to the cast. This is fired in order to burn off the wax and sinter the metal, forming a three-dimensional capillary network. A second wax strip, heavily loaded with almost pure gold (97% pure), is applied to the surface of the sintered layer and, during a second firing, the wax is again burnt off and the molten gold infiltrates the capillary network to form a metal substructure with a composite structure. A thin layer of veneer porcelain is finally baked onto the surface. It is claimed that this layer need only be about 35μm thick as there is no dark oxide layer of material to cover. The bonding between the metal and porcelain is achieved through mechanical attachment.

11.13 Bonded platinum foil

A problem with the metal-bonded porcelain restoration is that a considerable thickness of tooth substance must be removed to allow space for the metal coping and the porcelain veneer. An alternative approach, which does not produce such a robust result but which may be adequate in some circumstances, is to make a porcelain crown which is bonded to a platinum foil.

The technique involves laying down two platinum foils on the working die as opposed to the normal single foil (Fig. 11.4). The surface of the outer foil is then tin plated and the porcelain crown constructed and fired on top of the tin-plated surface. Porcelain bonds to the layer of tin oxide on the tin-plated

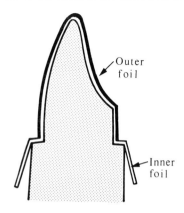

Fig. 11.4 Diagram illustrating two layers of closely adapted platinum foil on a die prior to tin plating and porcelain build-up.

surface. The inner platinum foil is removed prior to cementation of the crown whilst one platinum foil remains bonded to the inner surface of the crown. This foil helps to prevent crack formation on the inner surface.

11.14 Suggested further reading

Fan, P.L. & Stanford, J.W. (1987) Ceramics: their place in dentistry. *Int. Dent. J.* **37**, 197.

Kelly, J.R., Nishimura, I. & Campbell, S.D. (1996) Ceramics in dentistry: Historical roots and current perspectives. *J. Pros. Dent.* **75**, 18–32.

McLean, J.W. (1979/1980). *The Science and Art of Dental Ceramics*, vols. I and II. Quintessence Publishing Co., New Malden.

McLean, J.W. (1988) Ceramics in clinical dentistry. *Br. Dent. J.* **164**, 187.

O'Brien, W.J. (ed.) (1985) Ceramics. *Dent. Clin. North Am.* **29**(4).

Preston, J.D. (ed.) (1988) *Perspectives in Dental Ceramics.* Quintessence Publishing Co., New Malden.

Chapter 12
Synthetic Polymers

12.1 Introduction

Synthetic polymers have been of importance for 60 years or more and find use in almost every sphere of modern life. Prior to the realization of the importance of such products they were often discarded as unwanted byproducts of other chemical processes.

Polymers are high molecular weight, chain-like molecules. A polymer chain does not consist of a random arrangement of atoms, but of distinct repeating groups of atoms, derived from the small molecules or *monomers* from which the chain is built up. The process by which monomers are converted into polymers is called polymerization.

Monomers are generally liquids or gases and during the process of polymerization they become converted to crystalline or amorphous solids. These may vary from being very rigid at one extreme to being soft and rubbery at the other.

12.2 Polymerization

The conversion of monomer molecules into polymers may proceed by either an *addition* reaction or a *condensation* reaction.

Addition polymerization

An addition reaction simply involves the joining together of two molecules to form a third, larger molecule. For example, ethylene reacts with bromine under the correct conditions to form dibromoethane, as follows.

$$CH_2 = CH_2 + Br_2 \rightarrow CH_2Br - CH_2Br$$

Addition polymerizations involve the addition of a reactive species with a monomer to form a larger reactive species which is capable of further addition with monomer. In simplified terms the reaction may be visualized as follows:

$$R* + M \rightarrow R - M*$$
$$R - M* + M \rightarrow R - M - M*$$
$$R - M - M* + M \rightarrow R - M - M - M* \text{ etc.}$$

The initial reactive species is represented by R* and the monomer molecules by M. It can be seen how monomer molecules are added during each stage of the polymerization reaction and eventually a long-chain molecule is produced.

The reactive species which is involved in the addition reaction may be ionic in nature or it may be a free radical. *Free radical addition polymerization* is very commonly used for the synthesis of polymers and is the method used in many dental polymers. The free radicals are produced by reactive agents called *initiators*. These are, generally, molecules which contain one relatively weak bond which is able to undergo decomposition to form two reactive species each carrying an unpaired electron. One very popular initiator, which is used extensively in dental polymers, is benzoyl peroxide. Under certain conditions the peroxide linkage is able to split to form two identical radicals as shown in Fig. 12.1. The decomposition of benzoyl peroxide may be accomplished either by heating or by reaction with a chemical *activator*. The use of a chemical activator allows polymerization to occur at low temperatures. Activators commonly used with peroxide initiators are aromatic tertiary amines such as N, N' dimethyl-p-toluidine (Fig. 12.2).

An alternative activation system involves the use

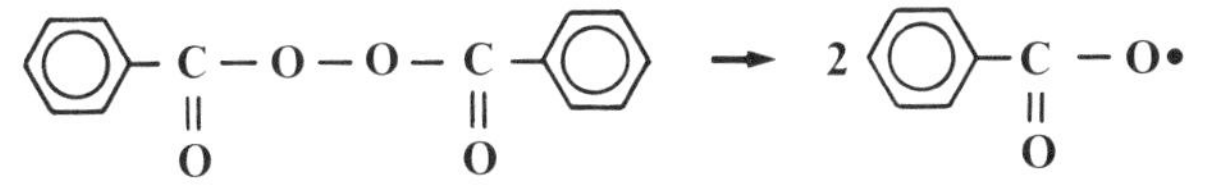

Fig. 12.1 Benzoyl peroxide readily splits to form two identical free radicals which can initiate polymerization.

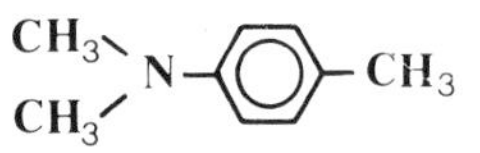

$$\begin{array}{c} CH_3 \\ \diagdown \\ CH_3 \diagup \end{array} N - \bigcirc - CH_3$$

Fig. 12.2 *N, N'* dimethyl-*p*-toluidine – a tertiary amine which is capable of activating peroxide initiators.

of radiation to cause decomposition of a suitable radiation-sensitive initiator. For example, benzoin methyl ether decomposes to form free radicals when exposed to ultraviolet radiation. Certain ketones, when exposed to radiation in the visible spectrum range and in the presence of a tertiary amine, are capable of forming active radicals which can initiate polymerization.

The majority of monomers which can be polymerized by a free radical addition mechanism are of the alkene type. That is, they contain a carbon–carbon double bond. These monomers can be represented by the general formula given in Fig. 12.3. Some of the familiar monomers which can be obtained by substituting for X and Y in the figure are also given. Methylmethacrylate and other closely related monomers are of particular importance in dentistry.

The polymerization processes follow a well-documented pattern which consists of four main stages – *activation, initiation, propagation* and *termination.*

Activation: This involves decomposition of the peroxide initiator using either thermal activation (heat), chemical activators or radiation of a suitable wavelength if a radiation-activated initiator is present. For

benzoyl peroxide the activation reaction is represented by the equation given in Fig. 12.1. In simplified, general germs it may be expressed as follows:

$$R - O - O - R \rightarrow 2RO \cdot$$

where R represents any organic molecular grouping.

Initiation: The polymerization reaction is initiated when the radical, formed on activation, reacts with a monomer molecule. This is illustrated for the specific case of the benzoyl peroxide radical and the methacrylate monomer in Fig. 12.4. The reaction may be given in simplified general terms as follows:

$$RO \cdot + M \rightarrow RO - M \cdot$$

where the symbol M represents one molecule of monomer. It can be seen from the above equation and from Fig. 12.4 that the initiation reaction is an addition reaction producing another active free radical species which is capable of further reaction.

Propagation: Following initiation, the new free radical is capable of reacting with further monomer molecules. Each stage of the reaction produces a new reactive species capable of further reaction, as illustrated in the following equations:

$$RO - M \cdot + M \rightarrow RO - M - M \cdot$$
$$RO - M - M \cdot + M \rightarrow RO - M - M - M \cdot$$
$$RO - M - M - M \cdot + M \rightarrow RO - M - M - M - M \cdot$$

A general equation for the propagation reaction may be written as follows:

$$RO - M \cdot + nM \rightarrow RO - (M)_n - M \cdot$$

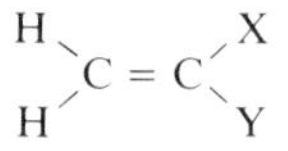

$$\begin{array}{c} H \\ \diagdown \\ H \diagup \end{array} C = C \begin{array}{c} \diagup X \\ \diagdown Y \end{array}$$

X	Y	Monomer	Polymer
H	H	Ethylene	Polyethylene
H	Cl	Vinyl chloride	Polyvinylchloride (PVC)
H	Phenyl	Styrene	Polystyrene
H	$-CH=CH_2$	Butadiene	Polybutadiene
H	$-CO_2CH_3$	Methylacrylate	Polymethylacrylate
CH_3	$-CO_2CH_3$	Methylmethacrylate	Polymethylmethacrylate

Fig. 12.3 General formula for alkene molecules which are capable of polymerizing to form polymers. Examples of some specific monomers are given.

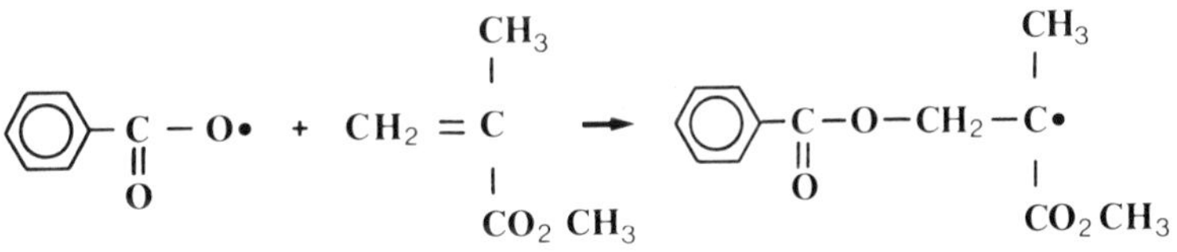

$$\text{\}$$

Fig. 12.4 The reaction of a benzoyl peroxide radical with methylmethacrylate to form a new radical species. This is the initiation reaction in free radical polymerization of methylmethacrylate.

where the value of n defines the number of monomer molecules added and hence the length of the chain and the molecular weight.

Termination: It is possible for the propagation reaction to continue until the supply of monomer molecules is exhausted. In practice however, other reactions, which may result in the termination of a polymer chain, compete with the propagation reaction. These reactions produce *dead* polymer chains which are not capable of further additions.

One example of termination is the combination of two growing chains to form one dead chain as follows:

$$RO - (M)_n - M \cdot + RO\ (M)_x - M \cdot \rightarrow$$
$$RO - (M)_n - M - M - (M)_x - OR$$

Other examples of termination involve the reactions of growing chains with molecules of initiator, dead polymer, impurity or solvent, if present.

Factors which have an important influence on the properties of the resulting polymer are *molecular weight* and the degree of *chain branching* or *cross-linking*.

Molecular weight: Within any addition polymerization system, activation, initiation, propagation and termination reactions occur simultaneously and the resulting polymer is therefore composed of chains of varying lengths. Thus, it is not possible to define a precise molecular weight for polymers and they are normally characterized in terms of an average molecular weight.

Chain branching and cross-linking: Addition polymerization reactions generally lead to the production of *linear polymers*. This does not imply that the chains form straight lines but simply that there are no branches off the main polymer chain and that the chains are not linked together.

Chain branching may result if a growing chain undergoes *chain transfer* with a polymer molecule. This involves termination of the growing chain, but a new reactive radical is formed along the side of a polymer molecule. Growth of a fresh chain from this site produces a branched polymer. This is illustrated in Fig. 12.5.

Cross-linking is accomplished by adding *cross-linking agents* to the polymerizing monomer. In the case of free radical addition polymerizations these agents are invariably difunctional alkenes in which each of the two double bonds present is able to become polymerized into a separate chain, thus effectively linking two chains together. Figure 12.6 shows the general formula for a typical cross-linking agent and the way in which this gives a cross-linked polymer when it becomes involved in a polymerization reaction. Figure 12.7 gives the structural formula of ethylene glycol dimethacrylate, a cross-linking agent which is commonly used for methacrylate polymers.

Chain branching and cross-linking can have important effects on the properties of polymers.

Condensation polymerization

A condensation reaction involves two molecules reacting together to form a third, larger molecule

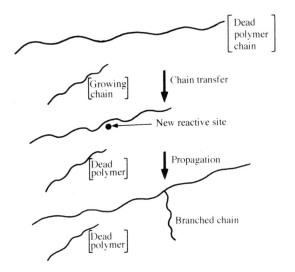

Fig. 12.5 Diagram showing the production of branched polymer chains by chain transfer.

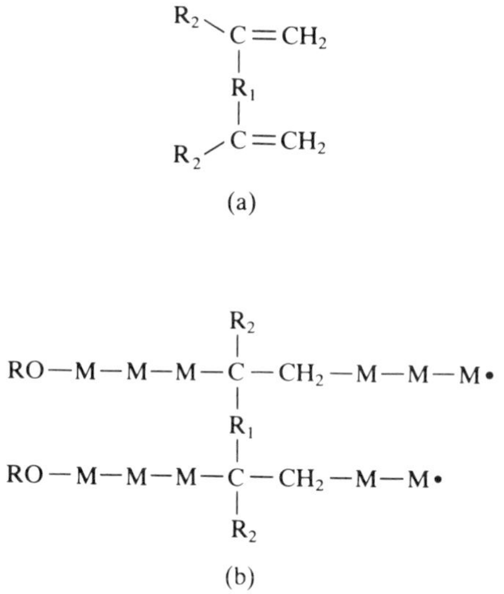

$$R_2 \diagdown C = CH_2$$
$$|$$
$$R_1$$
$$|$$
$$R_2 \diagup C = CH_2$$

(a)

$$\begin{array}{c} R_2 \\ | \\ RO-M-M-M-C-CH_2-M-M-M \cdot \\ | \\ R_1 \end{array}$$

$$\begin{array}{c} R_1 \\ | \\ RO-M-M-M-C-CH_2-M-M \cdot \\ | \\ R_2 \end{array}$$

(b)

Fig. 12.6 (a) General formula of a difunctional molecule which is capable of acting as a cross-linking agent. (b) The incorporation of the cross-linking agent into two polymer chains causes linking.

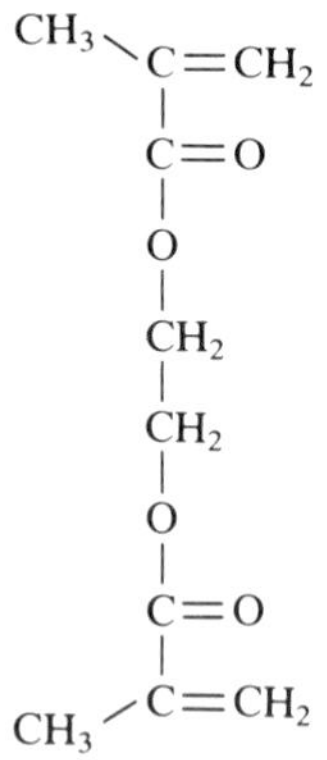

$$CH_3 \diagdown C=CH_2$$
$$|$$
$$C=O$$
$$|$$
$$O$$
$$|$$
$$CH_2$$
$$|$$
$$CH_2$$
$$|$$
$$O$$
$$|$$
$$C=O$$
$$|$$
$$CH_3 \diagup C=CH_2$$

Fig. 12.7 The structural formula of ethylene glycol dimethacrylate, a commonly used cross-linking agent.

with the production of a byproduct which is normally a small molecule such as water. A simple example of a condensation reaction is an esterification reaction in which an organic acid and an alcohol react together to form an ester with the evolution of water. This reaction may be illustrated by the reaction between acetic acid and ethyl alcohol to form ethyl acetate:

$$CH_3CO_2H + C_2H_5OH \rightarrow CH_3CO_2C_2H_5 + H_2O$$

In order for such a reaction to result in the formation of a polymer, each reacting molecule should have at least two reactive groups so that the reaction product is capable of undergoing further condensation reactions.

A simple generalized reaction sequence for condensation polymerization for two monomers, $X–M_1–X$ and $Y–M_2–Y$, with reactive groups X and Y can be written as follows:

$$X - M_1 - X + Y - M_2 - Y \rightarrow$$
$$X - M_1 - M_2 - Y + XY$$
$$X - M_1 - M_2 - Y + X - M_1 - X \rightarrow$$
$$X - M_1 - M_2 - M_1 - X + XY$$
$$X - M_1 - M_2 - M_1 - X + Y - M_2 - Y \rightarrow$$
$$X - M_1 - M_2 - M_1 - M_2 - Y + XY \text{ etc.}$$

This series of condensation reactions can be related to the simple esterification reaction shown above if X is a carboxylic acid group and Y is an alcohol group. The reaction product, XY, produced as a result of every condensation reaction then becomes water for that specific example.

It can be seen that at each stage of the reaction the chain grows by one monomer unit and there is one molecule of byproduct XY evolved. In addition, the growing polymer chain retains two reactive groups at each stage. The resulting polymer is a *regular copolymer* of the monomers M_1 and M_2 which are arranged in sequence along the chain. Chain branching and cross-linking can be produced by introducing some trifunctional monomer, e.g.

$$\begin{array}{c} X \\ | \\ X - M_1 - X \end{array}$$

into the reaction.

By using a monomer which carries two reactive groups it is possible to produce a homopolymer as follows:

$$X - M_1 - Y + X - M_1 - Y \rightarrow$$
$$X - M_1 - M_1 - Y + XY$$
$$X - M_1 - M_1 - Y + X - M_1 - Y \rightarrow$$
$$X - M_1 - M_1 - M_1 - Y + XY$$
$$X - M_1 - M_1 - M_1 - Y + X - M_1 - Y \rightarrow$$
$$X - M_1 - M_1 - M_1 - M_1 - Y + XY \text{ etc.}$$

Examples of the use of condensation polymerization include the production of nylon 6,6 as illustrated in Fig. 12.8, the production of nylon 6, as illustrated in Fig. 12.9, and the synthesis of polydimethysiloxane (silicone rubber) as illustrated in Fig. 12.10. The latter example illustrates the simplest type of condensation polymerization, in which each molecule contains two identical reactive groups (hydroxyl groups in this case) which are capable of reacting to eliminate water.

$$H_2N(CH_2)_6 \ NH_2 + \ HO_2C(CH_2)_4 \ CO_2H$$

$$\swarrow -H_2O$$

$$H_2N(CH_2)_6 \ NH \ CO(CH_2)_4 \ CO_2H + H_2N(CH_2)_6 \ NH_2$$

$$\swarrow -H_2O$$

$$H_2N(CH_2)_6 \ NH \ CO(CH_2)_4 \ CO \ NH(CH_2)_6 \ NH_2 + \ HO_2C(CH_2)_4 \ CO_2H$$

$$\swarrow -H_2O$$

$$H_2N(CH_2)_6 \ NH \ CO(CH_2)_4 \ CO \ NH(CH_2)_6 \ NH \ CO(CH_2)_4 \ CO_2H$$

$$\swarrow$$

etc.

Fig. 12.8 Schematic representation of the condensation reaction between hexamethylene diamine and adipic acid to produce nylon 6,6.

$$H_2N \ (CH_2)_5 \ CO_2H + \ H_2N \ (CH_2)_5CO_2H$$

$$\swarrow -H_2O$$

$$H_2N \ (CH_2)_5 \ CO \ NH \ (CH_2)_5 \ CO_2H + H_2N(CH_2)_5 \ CO_2H$$

$$\swarrow -H_2O$$

$$H_2N \ (CH_2)_5 \ CO \ NH \ (CH_2)_5 \ CO \ NH \ (CH_2)_5 \ CO_2 + \ H_2N \ (CH_2)_5 \ CO_2H$$

$$\swarrow -H_2O$$

$$H_2N(CH_2)_5 \ CO \ NH(CH_2)_5 \ CO \ NH(CH_2)_5 \ CO \ NH(CH_2)_5 \ CO_2H \ \ etc.$$

Fig. 12.9 Schematic representation of the formation of nylon 6 by the condensation of hydrolysed caprolactam.

12.3 Physical changes occurring during polymerization

Phase changes: Most monomers are gases or liquids at normal temperatures and pressures. Some liquid dental monomers are mixed with inert fillers, such as glass powders, to form pastes which can be easier to handle than the monomer alone. In addition, the filler often has a very beneficial effect on the properties of the set material. During polymerization, as the average molecule weight increases and chain entanglement occurs, the viscosity begins to increase.

This is most noticeable when polymerization is being carried out in the absence of solvents, which is the case for the vast majority of dental polymers. When the polymerization has reached an advanced stage the chain entanglements may become so great that the material develops a degree of rigidity and effectively behaves more like an amorphous solid than a liquid. At this stage the rate of conversion of monomer declines rapidly for two reasons. First, the quantity of unreacted monomer is now very small. Secondly, the rate of diffusion of the monomer through the highly viscous material to the reactive

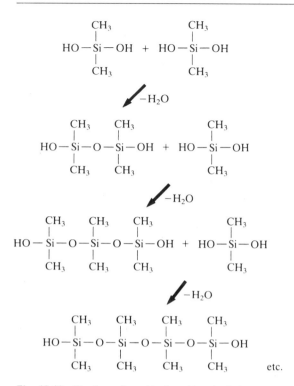

Fig. 12.10 The formation of hydroxyl-terminated polydimethylsiloxane by condensation of hydrolysed dimethylsiloxane.

polymerization sites becomes very slow. The result is that polymer produced as a result of the reaction inevitably contains a small concentration of unreacted or residual monomer. The majority of dental polymers have amorphous structures. Other polymers are capable of forming crystalline structures in which the chains are arranged in regular patterns.

Temperature changes: The majority of polymerization reactions are exothermic in nature and cause a marked increase in temperature of the polymerizing material. This temperature rise may have important consequences for both industrial polymers and dental polymers.

Industrial polymers are generally produced in large quantities using huge reaction vessels. An uncontrolled increase in temperature in such a vessel could be catastrophic. The heat liberated will cause an acceleration in the rate of polymerization which causes heat to be liberated more rapidly and so on. If such a process continues an explosion may result. At the very least, the polymer may solidify in the reaction vessel causing the requirement for a massive cleaning operation or the scrapping of the reaction

vessel. Naturally, attempts are made to avoid such events which may be both dangerous and expensive. One of the most effective ways of dissipating heat during polymerization is to either dissolve the monomer in a suitable solvent or to form a suspension of the monomer in water (suspension polymerization). The heat of polymerization is dissipated through the solvent or water. The resulting polymer, normally in the form of a powder, may be collected either by precipitation from the solvent or by sieving beads from the water. Suspension polymers formed in this way are normally moulded into the required shape by softening the polymeric moulding powder with heat and shaping under pressure (e.g. injection moulding). Condensation polymers are often cured in bulk in the absence of water or solvent. The reaction is allowed to proceed under controlled conditions and is halted (e.g. by cooling) when only a small proportion of the reactive groups of the monomer have been converted. At this stage the partially polymerized monomer is still relatively fluid and can be moulded. Polymerization is completed during the moulding stage.

Dental polymers are used in much smaller quantities than industrial polymers and temperature rises are therefore much smaller and less likely to cause the reaction to go out of control. Polymerization in bulk is therefore possible and this enables the conversion of monomer to polymer to be carried out *in situ* (e.g. in the mouth) in many cases. Due consideration must still be given to the temperature rise during polymerization however, as a relatively small increase in temperature within a filling material may damage the dental pulp. Another occurrence in some materials is that elevated temperatures during polymerization cause vaporization of some unconverted monomer producing spherical voids, known as gaseous porosity, in the set material.

Dimensional changes: Each addition or condensation reaction which takes place during polymerization results in a small contraction since the resulting species occupies less space than the two initial reacting species. Since many hundreds of reactions of this type take place during polymerization, the overall shrinkage which takes place can be very marked. For example, when methylmethacrylate is converted to polymethylmethacrylate a volumetric shrinkage of about 21% occurs. Dimensional changes of this magnitude are unacceptable for most dental applications and methods are normally sought to reduce the shrinkage.

Common methods involve blending the monomer with an inert material such as glass powder or polymer (e.g. polymethylmethacrylate beads in the case of methylmethacrylate), overfilling moulds to allow for some contraction, polymerizing under pressure and using monomers which undergo less polymerization contraction. The latter method is based on the principle that if larger monomer molecules are used the concentration of reactive groups within them is decreased and the subsequent contraction is less. Inspection of Fig. 22.4, for example, shows that the concentration of reacting carbon–carbon double bonds in Bis-GMA is much lower than in the equivalent amount of methylmethacrylate. The polymerization shrinkage for Bis-GMA is therefore considerably lower than that for methylmethacrylate. In some urethane acrylates and methacrylates the space between the two terminal reactive double bonds is greater still, effectively diluting them further and reducing the shrinkage to a greater extent.

12.4 Structure and properties

Factors which control the structure and therefore the properties of polymers include:

(1) The molecular structure of the repeating units including the use of copolymers.
(2) The molecular weight or chain length.
(3) The degree of chain branching.
(4) The presence of cross-linking and the *cross-link density*.
(5) The presence of *plasticizers* or *fillers*.

Two basic properties which characterize polymers are *glass transition temperature* (Tg) and *melting temperature* (Tm). Crystalline polymers exhibit both a glass transition temperature and a melting temperature. Amorphous polymers, on the other hand, exhibit only a glass transition temperature. The latter materials are more widely used in dentistry. The glass transition temperature is the temperature at which molecular motions become such that whole chains are able to move. This temperature is close to the *softening temperature*, which can be observed in practice for amorphous polymers. The glass transition temperature can be estimated mechanically by noting the temperature at which a sudden change in elastic modulus occurs.

Amorphous polymers below their glass transition temperature generally behave as rigid solids whilst above the glass transition temperature they may behave as viscous liquids, flexible solids or rubbers, depending on the molecular structure and the degree of branching or cross-linking.

From a practical point of view the value of Tg has great significance. For example, if a denture were constructed from a polymer which had a Tg value of 60°C, the denture would be rigid at normal mouth temperature but might soften and become flexible on taking a hot drink at 70°C.

Molecular structure is the factor which, naturally, has the greatest influence over polymer properties. For example, polymer backbones which contain phenyl groups are more rigid than those which contain only carbon–carbon bonds whilst backbones with silicon–oxygen bonds tend to be even more flexible. Hence the introduction of a phenyl group into a polymer backbone has the effect of increasing Tg whilst the introduction of carbon–oxygen links has the reverse effect. It is not only the atomic groups forming the backbone of the polymer chain which have an effect on Tg. Pendant groups may have an equally marked effect. This is illustrated by considering the Tg values of a series of poly N-alkyl methacrylates where the alkyl group can be methyl, ethyl, propyl or butyl (Table 12.1). It can be seen that altering the pendant group in this series of polymers has a significant effect. Polymethylmethacrylate is rigid at mouth temperature whereas polybutylmethacrylate is relatively soft and flexible.

Table 12.1 Glass transition temperatures of N-alkyl methacrylate polymers.

Polymer	Tg (°C)
Polymethylmethacrylate	105
Polyethylmethacrylate	65
Polypropylmethacrylate	35
Polybutylmethacrylate	20

Molecular weight is another factor which affects Tg. The two properties are related by an equation of the type

$$Tg = Tg_0 - \frac{K}{M}$$

where K is a constant, M is the average molecular weight and Tg_0 is the glass transition temperature for a polymer of infinite molecular weight. It can be seen that the value of Tg increases with increasing molecular weight. As M becomes large Tg approaches Tg_0. The reduction of the average molecular weight of a polymer by low molecular weight chains or residual, unreacted monomer may have a considerable effect on the Tg value and hence on material performance. In addition to influencing the glass transition temperature, molecular weight has an effect on other fundamental properties, such as modulus of elasticity. Many polymers exhibit a linear relationship between molecular weight and modulus up to fairly high values of molecular weight (10^5 or above) then reach a plateau region in which further increases in molecular weight have little or no effect.

Optimizing mechanical properties often involves producing polymers with a high value of average molecular weight and a low concentration of residual monomer. Chain branching may have an effect on polymer properties. Increasing the concentration of branches generally lowers the glass transition temperature. The mechanism of this lowering is probably related to the fact that chain branches prevent adjacent chains from drawing close enough together to undergo interchain attraction and the formation of interchain bonds. This can be viewed as an extension of the trend seen in Table 12.1, where the pendant alkyl groups can be viewed as small chain branches. Unsuccessful attempts to form cross-links can result in a branched structure if only one end of a difunctional monomer becomes polymerized into a chain. The other end of the monomer is left unreacted and may have the opposite effect to that which would be expected.

The effect of cross-linking is of considerable practical importance. Increasing the number of cross-links increases the glass transition temperature. In addition, alteration of the cross-link density can have a considerable effect on mechanical properties. A material with a low value of Tg and a small cross-link density may behave as a rubber at room temperature. On the other hand, a very high cross-link density normally produces a rigid, brittle polymer in which it is not possible to detect a glass transition since the material often decomposes thermally before softening. An example of this behaviour is the effect of cross-linking on the properties of natural rubber. When natural rubber (polyisoprene) is lightly cross-linked (vulcanized) it has rubbery, elastic properties. When the same material is highly cross-linked however, it becomes hard, rigid and brittle. This highly cross-linked material, vulcanite, has been used as a denture base material.

Certain additives such as plasticizers and fillers can have a profound effect on the properties of polymers. Plasticizers such as di-*n*-butylphthalate (Fig. 12.11) have an effect on both the glass transition temperature and the modulus of elasticity of some polymers. They are said to 'lubricate' the movements of polymer chains and are sometimes added to help moulding characteristics. They also lower the Tg and elastic modulus. For this reason the inclusion of plasticizers is a common method used by manufacturers to produce 'soft' polymers.

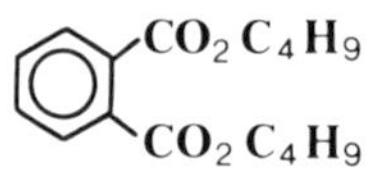

$$\underset{\text{CO}_2\text{C}_4\text{H}_9}{\overset{\text{CO}_2\text{C}_4\text{H}_9}{\bigcirc}}$$

Fig. 12.11   Structural formula of di-*n*-butylphthalate, a commonly used plasticizer.

The inclusion of particulate or fibrous inorganic fillers has an equally significant effect on polymer properties. The modulus of elasticity and strength are generally increased although, in the case of fibre-filled polymers, a degree of *anisotropy* may exist; that is, the strength depends on the orientation of the fibres in the polymer.

Particulate fillers are often used to increase the hardness of a resin and improve its resistance to abrasion. In addition, these fillers may have an important effect on thermal properties, since the added fillers are commonly glasses, ceramics or quartz which have lower values of coefficient of thermal expansion than organic polymers.

Crystalline polymers are normally formed when polymer chains are able to undergo orientation. Crystallites often take the form of polymer chains in rows, held together by Van der Waals forces or hydrogen bonds. The crystals may consist simply of straight chains or of folded chains as illustrated in Fig. 12.12. In order to form crystals of this type the chains must be able to come into close proximity with the neighbouring chain. Hence, the presence of bulky pendant groups and and regular chain branching are factors which decrease the possibility of crystallite formation.

In nylon, the chains take up a helical form in which hydrogen bonding is responsible for both intra-molecular and intermolecular links in the crystals.

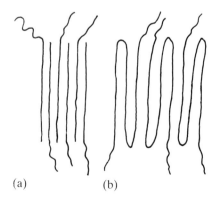

(a)   (b)

Fig. 12.12   Crystalline polymers may take one of several possible structural forms. Two examples are: (a) straight chains forming crystallites; (b) folded chains forming crystallites.

Crystalline polymers have limited use in dentistry because they tend to be opaque and are not amenable to polymerization under ambient conditions of temperature and pressure.

12.5 Methods of fabricating polymers

Some polymers are produced in powder form and fabricated at a later stage by softening and moulding. Techniques for moulding include *injection moulding*, *vacuum forming* and *blow mouldikng*. Polymers which can be fabricated in this way are described as *thermoplastic polymers*, that is, they can be softened on heating and re-hardened on cooling. Providing care is taken not to overheat the polymer, causing decomposition, the process can be repeated many times.

Other polymers are described as *thermosetting resins* – these are generally condensation polymers which are partly polymerized before moulding to produce a viscous liquid. During heating and moulding, generally into simple shapes such as flat sheets, the polymerization and cross-linking are completed. These resins are generally highly cross-linked polymers which cannot be softened without causing thermal degradation.

A method commonly used for dental polymers is to blend the monomer with an inert filler to form a paste. The paste is then split into two halves to which initiator and activator are added respectively. On mixing the two pastes the polymerization reaction begins and, for dental restorative materials, is completed *in situ*.

The technique of *dough moulding* is very important to dentistry, particularly for the fabrication of denture bases. Powdered polymer, normally as beads, containing some initiator is mixed with monomer to form a 'dough'. The dough is packed into a preformed mould and the monomer cured by applying heat. Alternatively, if the monomer contains a chemical activator the polymerization of monomer will occur at room temperature.

12.6 Suggested further reading

Billmeyer, F.W. (1984) *Textbook of Polymer Science*, 3rd edn. John Wiley Co, Chichester.

Chapter 13
Denture Base Polymers

13.1 Introduction

The denture base is that part of the denture which rests on the soft tissues and so does not include the artificial teeth. Prior to 1940 vulcanite was the most widely used denture base polymer. This a highly cross-linked natural rubber which was difficult to pigment and tended to become unhygienic due to the uptake of saliva. Nowadays acrylic resin is used almost universally for denture base construction.

The acrylic denture base is normally fabricated in a two-part gypsum mould. The mould is produced by investing wax trial dentures on which the artificial teeth have been mounted. After 'boiling out' of the wax the gypsum mould is treated with an alginate mould-sealing agent. This is a viscous solution of sodium alginate which is rapidly converted to calcium alginate on contact with the gypsum. It forms a thin 'skin' over the surface of the mould, preventing monomer in the acrylic 'dough' from entering the gypsum. The space remaining after removal of wax is filled with acrylic dough which may be heat cured or allowed to cure at room temperature depending on the material being used. During curing the acrylic resin denture base becomes attached to the artificial teeth. The formation of the denture base by this technique is known as the *dough moulding method*. Acrylic denture bases may also be produced by *injection moulding* or by using a *pourable resin technique*, although the latter methods are not commonly used.

13.2 Requirements of denture base polymers

The requirements of a denture base material can be conveniently listed under the headings of physical, mechanical, chemical, biological and miscellaneous properties.

Physical properties: An ideal denture base material should be capable of matching the *appearance* of the natural oral soft tissues. The importance of this requirement varies considerably, depending on whether the base will be visible when the patient opens his mouth.

A polymer which is used to construct a denture base should have a value of *glass transition temperature* (Tg) which is high enough to prevent softening and distortion during use. Although the normal temperature in the mouth varies only from $32°C$ to $37°C$, account must be taken of the fact that patients take hot drinks at temperatures up to $70°C$ and, despite advice, sometimes clean dentures in very hot or even boiling water.

The base should have good *dimensional stability* in order that the shape of the denture does not change over a period of time. In addition to distortions which may occur due to thermal softening, other mechanisms such as relief of internal stresses, continued polymerization and water absorption may contribute to dimensional instability.

The material should, ideally, have a low value of *specific gravity* in order that dentures should be as 'light' as possible. This reduces the gravitational displacing forces which may act on an upper denture.

A high value of *thermal conductivity* would enable the denture wearer to maintain a healthy oral mucosa and to retain a normal reaction to hot and cold stimuli. If the base is a thermal insulator it is possible that the patient may take a drink which he would normally detect as being 'too hot to bear', and undergo a painful experience as the drink reaches the throat and gut.

The denture base should, ideally, be *radiopaque*. It should be capable of detection using normal diagnostic radiographic techniques. Patients occasionally swallow dentures and may even inhale fragments of dentures if involved in a violent accident, such as a car crash. Early radiological detection of the denture or fragment of denture is of immense help in deciding the best course of treatment.

Mechanical properties: Although opinion varies slightly, most clinicians consider that the denture base should be rigid. A high value of *modulus of elasticity* is therefore advantageous. A high value of *elastic limit* is required to ensure that stresses encountered during biting and mastication do not cause permanent deformation. A combination of a high modulus and high value of elastic limit would have the added advantage that it would allow the base to be fabricated in relatively thin section.

Fractures of upper dentures invariably occur through the midline of the denture, due to flexing (Fig. 13.1). The denture base should have sufficient *flexural strength* to resist fracture. The method of measuring flexural strength or transverse strength is described in Section 2.2.

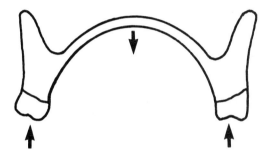

Fig. 13.1 Diagram illustrating how an upper denture may flex about the midpoint of the palate. This fatigue process may eventually cause fracture.

Fracture of the denture base *in situ* often occurs by a fatigue mechanism in which relatively small flexural stresses, over a period of time, eventually lead to the formation of a small crack which propagates through the denture, resulting in fracture. The base material should therefore have an adequate *fatigue life* and a high value of *fatigue limit*.

When patients remove dentures for cleaning or overnight soaking, there is a danger of fracture if the denture is accidentally dropped onto a hard surface. The ability of a denture base to resist such fracture is a function of the *impact strength* of the material. Impact fracture of the denture may occur *in situ* if the patient is involved in a violent accident involving the facial region, for example, of the head hits a windscreen during a motor accident. The fragments of denture may then become embedded into soft tissue or may be inhaled.

Denture base materials should have sufficient *abrasion resistance* to prevent excessive wear of material by abrasive denture cleansers or foodstuffs. Wear is a complex phenomenon which may depend

on many material properties. For abrasive wear it is thought that surface hardness of the substrate is of primary importance.

Chemical properties: A denture base material should be chemically inert. It should, naturally, be insoluble in oral fluids and should not absorb water or saliva since this may alter the mechanical properties of the material and cause the denture to become unhygienic.

Biological properties: In the unmixed or uncured states the denture base material should not be harmful to the technician involved in its handling. The 'set' denture base material should be non-toxic and non-irritant to the patient. In the previous section it was mentioned that the base should, ideally, be impermeable to oral fluids and this would certainly be an ideal property. If a degree of absorption occurs however, the base should not be able to sustain the growth of bacteria or fungi.

Miscellaneous properties: An ideal denture base material should be relatively inexpensive and have a long shelf life so that material can be purchased in bulk and stored without deteriorating. The material should be easy to manipulate and fabricate without having to resort to using expensive processing equipment. If fractures do occur they should be easy to repair.

13.3 Acrylic denture base materials

Acrylic resin is the most widely used material for construction of dentures. Polymeric denture base materials are classified into five groups (or types), as shown in Table 13.1. Types 1 and 2 are the most widely used products and are described in more detail below.

Table 13.1 Classification of denture base polymers according to ISO 1567.

Type	Class	Description
1	1	Heat-processing polymers, powder and liquid
1	2	Heat-processed (plastic cake)
2	1	Autopolymerized polymers, powder and liquid
2	1	Autopolymerized polymers (powder and liquid pour type resins)
3	—	Thermoplastic blank or powder
4	—	Light-activated materials
5	—	Microwave-cured material

Composition of type 1 and type 2 materials

Most materials are supplied as a powder and liquid, details of the composition of which are given in Table 13.2. The major component of the powder is beads of polymethylmethacrylate with diameters up to 100 μm. (Fig 13.2) These are produced by a process of *suspension polymerization* in which methylmethacrylate monomer, containing initiator, is suspended as droplets in water. Starch or carboxymethylcellulose can be used as thickeners and suspension stabilizers, but have the disadvantage of potentially contaminating the polymer beads. The temperature is raised in order to decompose the peroxide and bring about polymerization of themethylmethacrylate to form beads of polymethylmethacrylate which, after drying, form a free-flowing powder at room temperature.

Table 13.2 Composition of acrylic denture base materials.

Powder	Polymer	Polymethylmethacrylate beads
	Initiator	A peroxide such as benzoyl peroxide (approximately 0.5%)
	Pigments	Salts of cadmium or iron or organic dyes
Liquid	Monomer	Methylmethacrylate
	Cross-linking agent	Ethyleneglycoldimethacrylate (approximately 10%)
	Inhibitor	Hydroquinone (trace)
	Activator*	N N'-dimethyl-p-toluidine (approximately 1%)

* Only in self-curing materials.

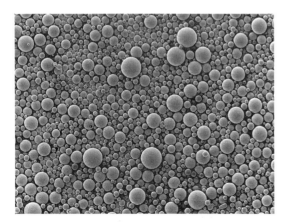

Fig. 13.2 Scanning electron microscope view of polymethylmethacrylate beads used in acrylic denture bases (× 60).

The initiator present in the powder may consist of peroxide remaining unreacted after the production of the beads, in addition to extra peroxide added to the beads after their manufacture.

Polymethylmethacrylate is a clear, glass-like polymer and is occasionally used in this form for denture base construction. It is more normal, however, for manufacturers to incorporate pigments and opacifiers in order to produce a more 'lifelike' denture base. Sometimes, small fibres coated with pigment are used to give a veined appearance. Pink pigments used in denture base resins are traditionally salts of cadmium. These pigment have good colour stability and have been shown to leach cadmium from the denture base in only minute amounts. Fears over the toxicity of cadmium compounds, however, have led to the gradual replacement of cadmium salts with other 'safer' substances.

The major component of the liquid is methylmethacrylate (MMA) monomer. This is a clear, colourless, low-viscosity liquid with a boiling point of 100.3°C and a distinct odour exaggerated by a relatively high vapour pressure at room temperature. MMA is one of a group of monomers which are very susceptible to free radical addition polymerization (see Fig. 12.3). Following mixing of the powder and liquid components and activation by either heat or chemical means, the *curing* of the denture base material is due to the polymerization of MMA monomer to form polymethylmethacrylate.

The liquid normally contains some cross-linking agent. The substance most widely used is ethyleneglycoldimethacrylate, the structural formula of which is given in Fig. 12.7. This compound is used to improve the physical properties of the set material.

The inhibitor is used to prolong the *shelf life* of the liquid component. In the absence of inhibitor, polymerization of monomer and cross-linking agent would occur slowly, even at room temperature and below, due to the random occurrence of free radicals within the liquid. The source of these free radicals is uncertain, but once formed they cause a slow increase in viscosity of the liquid and may eventually cause the liquid component to set solid.

The inhibitor, which is commonly a derivative of hydroquinone, works by reacting rapidly with radicals formed within the liquid to form stabilized radicals which are not capable of initiating polymerization. This is illustrated in Fig. 13.3 in which the product radical (z) is a relatively stable species which will not initiate polymerization of MMA at room temperature. The stability of the radical (z) is explained by the fact that the unpaired electron is

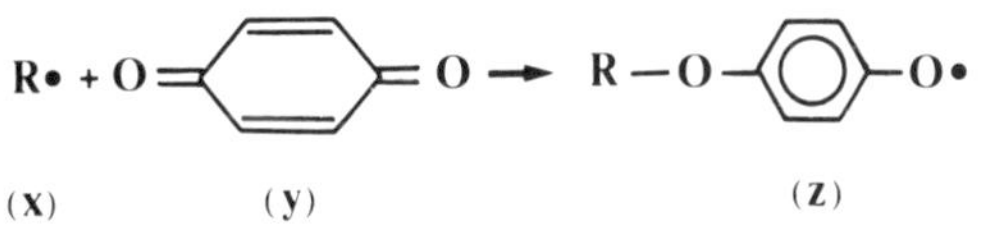

Fig. 13.3 The inhibitor (hydroquinone) (y), works by reacting with active radicals (x), to form stable radicals (z).

not isolated in the oxygen atom but may occupy several sites around the ring, as shown in Fig. 13.4.

One way of reducing the occurrence of unwanted radicals in the liquid is to store the material in a can or in a dark-brown bottle. Visible light or ultra-violet radiation may activate compounds which are potentially capable of forming radicals. Eliminating the source of radiation is therefore beneficial.

The activator is present only in those products which are described as *self-curing* or *autopolymerizing* materials and not in *heat curing* denture base materials. The function of the activator is to react with the peroxide in the powder to create free radicals which can initiate polymerization of the monomer.

Mixing and curing (heat curing materials)

Mixing: The manipulation of acrylic denture base materials involves the mixing of powder and liquid to form a 'dough' which is packed into a gypsum mould for curing. The ratio of powder to liquid is important since it controls the 'workability' of the mix as well as the dimensional change on setting. MMA monomer undergoes a volumetric polymerization shrinkage of 21% on conversion to polymer. This shrinkage is considerably reduced by using a mix with a high powder/liquid ratio. If the powder/liquid ratio is too high however, the mix becomes 'dry' and unmanageable and the mixture will not flow when placed under pressure in the gypsum mould. In addition, there is insufficient monomer in a dry mix to bind all the polymer beads together. This may produce a granular effect on the denture surface which is normally referred to as *granular porosity*.

In order to produce a workable mix, whilst maintaining shrinkage at a low level, a powder/liquid ratio of 2.5:1 by weight is normally used. This gives a

volumetric polymerization shrinkage of around 5–6%.

Proportioning is normally carried out by placing a suitable volume of liquid into a clean, dry mixing vessel followed by slow addition of powder, allowing each powder particle to become *wetted* by monomer. The mixture is then stirred and left to stand until it reaches a consistency suitable for packing into the gypsum mould. During this standing period a lid should be placed on the mixing vessel to prevent evaporation of monomer. Loss of monomer during this stage could produce *granular porosity* in the set material. This is characterized by a blotchy, opaque surface.

Immediately after mixing, a material of rather 'sandy' consistency is produced. After a short period of time this becomes a 'sticky' mass which forms 'strings' of material sticking to the spatula, if an attempt is made to carry out further mixing. The next stage is the 'dough' stage. Here, the material is more cohesive and has lost much of its 'tackiness'. It can be moulded like plasticine and does not adhere to the sides of the mixing vessel. The material should be packed into the mould at this stage. If packing is delayed the material may become quite tough and rubbery and eventually becomes quite hard.

The transitions from 'sandy' to 'stringy' to 'dough' and eventually rubbery and hard stages are due to physical changes occurring within the mix. Smaller polymer beads dissolve in monomer causing a gradual increase in viscosity of the liquid phase. Larger beads absorb monomer and swell, thus depriving the liquid phase of monomer and causing a further increase in viscosity. During this period the monomer remains unpolymerized.

The time taken to reach the dough stage is called the *doughing time* whilst the time for which the material remains at the dough stage and is mouldable is termed the *working time*. Manufacturers aim to combine a short doughing time with a long working time. They do this by controlling such factors as bead size and molecular weight of the powder. Smaller beads, with lower molecular weight, dissolve more rapidly in the polymer.

The dough is packed into a two-part gypsum mould, which has previously been treated with a

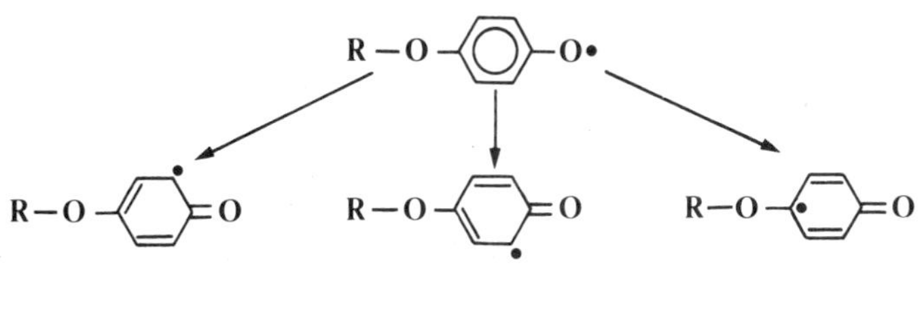

Fig. 13.4 The stability of the radical (z) formed in Fig. 13.3 is explained by the way in which the unpaired electron can occupy several sites in the molecule.

mould-sealing compound (Fig. 13.5). Excess dough is used and a *trial closure* is performed causing excess material to form a 'flash' at the point where the two halves of the flask meet. The flask is opened and the flash removed. The flask is then closed again under pressure using a threaded bench press and maintained under pressure during curing using a spring-loaded clamp. The applied pressure has three important functions. It ensures that dough flows into every part of the mould. It enables excess dough to be used, thus causing an effective reduction in the polymerization shrinkage and it prevents the formation of a 'raised bite' on the denture by giving a base which is too thick.

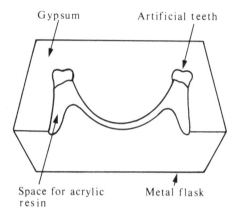

Fig. 13.5 Diagrammatic representation of two-part split mould used for acrylic denture construction.

The use of insufficient dough to create an excess in the mould or the application of insufficient pressure during curing can lead to porosity voids dispersed throughout the whole mass of the denture base. This is known as *contraction porosity*.

Occasionally, the dough is forced into the mould by *injection moulding*. A sprue hole and a vent hole are formed in the gypsum mould and the metal flask is constructed such that it will adapt to the injection moulding equipment. During processing, the equipment is normally arranged so that a 'wave' or curing propagates from the part of the flask which is furthest from the sprue and vents. This enables shrinkage during curing to be compensated by taking up extra material from the sprue reservoir. Materials processed in this way are sometimes provided in the form of a premixed dough or 'plastic cake', i.e., type 1 class 2.

Curing: Having filled the mould with dough, the next stage is to polymerize the monomer to produce the final 'processed' denture. Curing is normally carried out by placing the clamped flask in either a water bath or an air oven. Whichever type of system is used, many 'curing cycles' are available. When choosing which curing cycle to use, attention should be paid to certain facts.

(1) Benzoyl peroxide initiator begins to decompose rapidly to form free radicals above 65°C.

(2) The polymerization reaction is highly exothermic.

(3) The boiling point of the monomer is 100.3°C and if the temperature of the dough is raised significantly above this, the monomer will boil, producing spherical voids in the hottest part of the curing dough. These will be apparent as *gaseous porosity* in the cured denture base (Fig. 13.6).

(4) It is important to get a high degree of conversion from monomer to polymer and to produce a polymer with high molecular weight. Residual monomer and low molecular weight polymer result in poor mechanical properties as well as possible adverse tissue reactions.

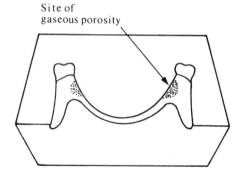

Fig. 13.6 Diagram illustrating the normal sites of gaseous porosity in an upper denture.

Taking the above points into account, manufacturers often recommend curing cycles which they feel are appropriate for their brand of denture base material.

One popular method is to heat the flask containing the dough for seven hours at 70°C followed by three hours at 100°C. Most of the conversion of monomer to polymer occurs during the seven hours at 70°C stage, during which time the temperature of the dough itself may approach 100°C due to the polymerization exotherm (Fig. 13.7a). The final three hours at 100°C ensure almost complete conversion of monomer in those thinner areas of the denture base

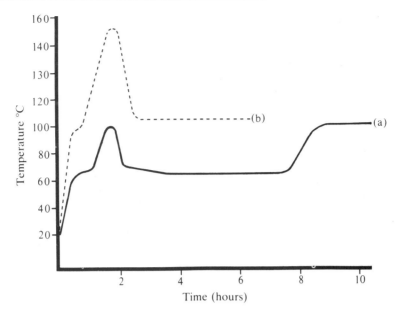

Fig. 13.7 Curing cycles (temperature versus time) for heat curing acrylic denture resins. (a) The curing flask is placed in an oven or water bath at 70°C for 7 hours. The temperature is raised to 100°C for 1 hour. (b) The curing flask is placed directly into an oven or water bath at 100°C. Temperature of the acrylic dough is indicated.

where the effect of the exothermic heat of reaction is less pronounced. There are many other curing cycles which manufacturers recommend and it is not possible to list all of them. One other example is to place the flask in a bath of cold water. The water is gradually brought to the boil over a period of one hour, allowed to boil for one hour and then allowed to cool slowly. Very few manufacturers recommend that the flask, containing dough, is placed directly into boiling water since this, couple with the exothermic heat of reaction, can cause the dough to reach temperatures in excess of 150°C as shown in Fig. 13.7b. This would, undoubtedly, result in gaseous porosity being produced in the thicker parts of the denture.

Before deflasking the processed denture the flask is cooled to room temperature. This may lead to the setting up of internal stresses within the denture base since the coefficient of thermal expansion of acrylic resin is about ten times greater than that of the gypsum mould material. These internal stresses may be compounded with those caused by polymerization shrinkage, although the latter are normally eliminated by plastic flow when the polymerization takes place at elevated temperatures. Internal stresses may lead to warpage of the denture base at a later stage if the denture is placed in warm water for cleaning. The magnitude of the stresses can be reduced by allowing the flask to cool slowly from the curing temperature.

Mixing and curing (autopolymerizing materials)

When constructing a denture base from an autopolymerizing material, powder and liquid components are mixed together just as for the heat curing products. Mixing is followed by a gradual increase in viscosity until the dough stage is reached. This increase in viscosity is due to a combination of physical and chemical changes occurring in the mix. Smaller acrylic beads are dissolved in the monomer, whilst the larger beads absorb monomer and become 'swollen'. In addition, when peroxide from the powder and chemical activator from the liquid meeting during mixing the polymerization of monomer is initiated. Thus, conversion of monomer to polymer contributes to the increase in viscosity. Generally, these materials reach the 'dough' stage quite quickly and remain workable for only a short period of time. Within a few minutes of attaining a dough consistency, the rate of polymerization increases rapidly causing a large temperature rise and the material becomes hard and unmanageable. The time available for carrying out a trial closure of the processing flask is minimal and, if the viscosity has increased beyond a certain point at the time of final closure, there is a danger of increased vertical height in the denture. These problems, coupled with the inferior mechanical properties and higher residual monomer content of the cold curing resins, generally restrict their use to *repairing and relining* of dentures. For repairing, a very fluid mix of cold cure resin is used. The large excess of monomer ensures adequate 'wetting' of the fragments being repaired.

Some cold cure resins, known as *pourable resins*, are occasionally used for denture base construction. These materials are mixed to a very fluid consistency using a low powder/liquid ratio. The mixed material is poured into a hydrocolloid mould and allowed to cure at or just above room temperature. The advantage of this technique is that the cured denture can be removed from the flexible hydrocolloid mould with a minimum of time and effort and the denture base needs little further finishing. The disadvantages are high residual monomer levels coupled with inferior mechanical properties of the base and the possibility of distortions arising from the use of a flexible mould. One development of this technique is to use a pour-type resin which is heat cured in a hydrocolloid mould under the dual influence of vacuum (to help adaptation of the denture base to the flask) and pressure (to increase the degree of conversion and reduce the effects of shrinkage).

Other new developments take advantage of the use of high-intensity visible radiation to activate polymerization in much the same way that composite resins are activated (but using a light box instead of a fibre-optic) and also microwave ovens which can concentrate heat within the confines of the curing denture and may therefore be more efficient than conventional ovens.

The light activated materials typically contain a blend of urethane dimethyacrylate monomer (similar to that used in resin matrix composites), sub-micron particles of silica and some polymethylmethacrylate beads as an organic filler. Small quantities of light sensitive initiators (e.g. camphoroquinone) and activators (amines) are present in order to provide a source of free radicals after light activation. The material is normally supplied premixed in the form of a flexible sheet packaged in a light-proof sachet. These materials obviously cannot be cured under pressure in a mould – they are exposed to activating radiation in a specialist oven at normal atmospheric pressure. The surface of the material is coated with a non-reactive barrier compound (e.g. carboxymethyl cellulose) to prevent inhibition of polymerization by oxygen. These light-activated products are very useful when trying to produce hollow denture bases (commonly used for large obturators after ablative surgery for cancer). The box can be relatively easily made from sheet base material and the end product is both durable and light.

Structure of the set material

The structure of the material is quite complex. It can be considered as a type of composite system in which residual polymethylmethacrylate beads, which initially formed part of the powder, are bound in a matrix of freshly polymerized material (Fig 13.8). The extent to which the two parts of the composite structure are bound together affects the mechanical properties of the materials. During mixing and the 'dough' stage, monomer from the liquid is able to penetrate the outer layers of the beads. The latter are susceptible to this since they are generally produced in uncross-linked or only lightly cross-linked form and are thus soluble in, or readily softened by, the monomer. On polymerization of the monomer the bead and matrix phases become inextricably bound together by inter-penetrating networks of polymers. The extent to which interpenetrating networks are formed depends on factors such as molecular weight of bead polymer, polymer/monomer ratio and the time for which polymer and monomer are in contact before polymerization causes a depletion of the amount of monomer. The type 1 class 2, 'plastic cake' materials may have little or no residual bead structure and the mixed monomer and polymer may be in contact for months before processing. The molecular weight of the bead polymer is normally quite high (5 $\times$ 10^5) and only the surface layers of the larger beads become impregnated with monomer. Some of the smaller beads can, however, become totally dissolved in monomer. The use of beads containing highly cross-linked polymer would greatly reduce the extent to which they become penetrated by monomer. Increasing the monomer content of the polymer/monomer mixture would be one way of increasing the extent of penetration of beads by

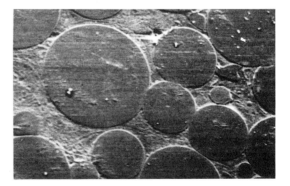

Fig. 13.8 Microstructure of set acrylic material showing the residual bead structure bound together in a matrix consisting of a mixture of freshly polymerized monomer and dissolved bead polymer ($\times$ 220).

matrix material; however any advantage gained from this would be more than off-set by the increase in setting contraction which would result. It should be remembered however that a dry mix, with insufficient monomer, will result in a structure having only weak links between bead and matrix areas. The time, during and after mixing, that the beads and monomer remain in contact before the monomer becomes consumed by polymerization is important. For heat curing materials the material often remains in the dough state for many minutes before being packed into the mould ready for curing. This gives adequate time for penetration of beads by monomer. For cold curing materials however the monomer begins to polymerize immediately after mixing the powder and liquid. A rapid rate of polymerization may leave insufficient monomer to cause penetration of polymer beads. Cold curing materials having a slower rate of polymerization allow more time for interpenetration before the monomer becomes consumed.

Curiously, the matrix phase of the set material is often reported to be weaker than the bead phase, having a lower average molecular weight. This is not strictly true since the matrix phase is normally cross-linked and this makes measurement of molecular weight difficult. In one sense it is reasonable to state that the cross-linked material has a greater effective molecular weight than the uncross-linked material. One way in which this is readily demonstrated is that beads of polymethylmethacrylate denture material are readily soluble in a solvent such as chloroform, whereas the cross-linked matrix material is not soluble and will only swell when exposed to the same solvent. It is known, on the other hand, that the matrix phase contains more low molecular weight material and residual monomer and this must have a marked effect on the properties of the materials.

Properties

Some of the minimum requirements for denture base polymers are set out in ISO specification 1567 and are reproduced in Table 13.3. It is clear that the autopolymerizing materials (type 2) are expected to have inferior properties when compared to the other products. As with all standards the values set out in Table 13.3 indicate minimum levels of acceptability. The quality of a cured denture base can be improved markedly by careful processing.

Physical properties: From the point of view of appearance the acrylic denture base materials are adequate. The materials are available in a variety of shades and opacities and can be veined or unveined. Characterization 'kits' containing various pigments allow tissue colour matching for patients of various races.

The value of Tg may vary from one product to another depending on the average molecular weight and the level of residual monomer. A typical value of Tg for a heat curing material is 105°C. This is somewhat higher than any temperature which the base should reach during 'normal' service. The value of modulus of elasticity decreases and the potential for creep increases considerably at temperatures approaching Tg however, and patients may cause distortions by soaking dentures in boiling water. Tg values for cold curing resins are generally lower than those for heat curing products. A value of about 90°C would be typical. Thus, there is a greater chance of these products suffering distortions in hot water. The use of water at temperatures above approximately 65°C should be avoided for soaking dentures. This not only ensures that the Tg of the resin is not approached but also that the relief of internal stresses, accompanied by distortions, is minimized. The Tg value may be reduced to 60°C or lower if large quantities of low molecular weight material or residual monomer are present. This may occur if the material is not properly cured and is most commonly observed in cold curing materials. The light-activated materials tend to have higher values of Tg than conventional acrylic products.

Acrylic resins have relatively low values of specific gravity (approximately 1.2 g cm^{-3}) because they are composed of groups of 'light' atoms, for example, carbon, oxygen and hydrogen. The 'lightness' of the resulting denture is beneficial, since the gravitational forces causing displacement of an upper denture are

Table 13.3 Requirements of denture base polymers as given in ISO 1567.

Type	Flexural strength (MPa)	Flexural modulus (GPa)	Residual monomer (% wt)	Water sorption (µg/mm^3)	Solubility (µg/mm^3)
1, 3, 4, 5	65 min	2.0 min	2.2 max	32 max	1.6 max
2	60 min	1.5 min	4.5 max	32 max	8.0 max

minimized. Dentures constructed from acrylic resin are radiolucent because C, O and H atoms are poor X-ray absorbers. This is a serious disadvantage of these materials. If a patient swallows or inhales a denture or fragment of a denture it is difficult to detect using simple radiological techniques.

Acrylic resin may be considered a good thermal insulator. Its thermal conductivity is some 100–1000 times less than the values for metals and alloys. This is a disadvantage for a denture base because the oral soft tissues are denied normal thermal stimuli which help to maintain the mucosa in a healthy condition. In addition, the patient may partially lose the protective reflex responses to hot and cold stimuli. This may result in some painful experiences, for example, when taking hot drinks.

Mechanical properties: Compared with alloys such as Co/Cr and stainless steel, acrylic resins would be classified as soft, weak and flexible materials (Table 13.4). Providing the denture base is constructed in sufficient thickness however, rigidity and strength are adequate. Dentures are subjected to bending forces and the flexural stress required to cause fracture depends on the square of the thickness of the denture (p. 6). Thus, if the thickness of the base is doubled, the stress required to fracture is increased fourfold. Although this factor is important it can be applied to only a limited extent when designing an acrylic denture base since a thick base may be more difficult for the patient to tolerate and will further increase the degree of thermal insulation. The transverse strength of acrylic is generally sufficient to resist fracture caused by the application of a high masticatory load. Fractures of dentures, *in situ*, do occur however, as a result of fatigue. This is often the result of a patient wearing an ill-fitting or badly designed denture which flexes considerably with each masticatory load. Acrylic resin has a relatively poor resistance to fatigue fracture, a fact which is mainly responsible for the large number of denture repairs which are carried out annually.

Acrylic resin also has a relatively poor impact strength and if a denture is dropped onto a hard surface there is a high probability of fracture occurring. Impact strength is essentially a measure of the toughness of the material as it measures the energy required to initiate and propagate a crack through a specimen of known dimensions. For a sample of acrylic denture base material both the crack initiation and propagation components of energy make a significant contribution to the total energy and the impact strength of the material can be reduced markedly if a specimen is pre-notched (Section 2.2). Materials of this type are referred to as *notch sensitive*. Avoiding the presence of notches can reduce the risk of fracture by impact and fatigue. Unfortunately, the design of denture bases often requires the presence of notch-like anatomical structures (e.g. to accommodate the labial frenum and muscle insertions). If these notches cannot be avoided they should be produced in rounded as opposed to sharp form in order to reduce the likelihood of crack propagation.

Crazing may sometimes appear on the surface of an acrylic denture. This is a series of surface cracks which may have a weakening effect on the base. The cracks may arise by one of three mechanisms. If the patient develops the habit of frequently removing his denture and allowing it to dry out, the constant cycle of water absorption followed by drying may develop sufficient tensile stresses at the surface to cause crazing. Thus, patients are instructed to keep their dentures moist at all times. The use of porcelain teeth may cause crazing of the base in the region around the tooth neck due to differences in the coefficient of thermal expansion between porcelain and acrylic resin (ratio about 1:10). Thirdly, crazing may arise during denture repair when MMA monomer contacts the cured acrylic resin of the fragments being repaired. One function of the cross-linking agent is to reduce the degree of crazing by binding polymer chains together.

A process of denture whitening, occasionally described as bleaching, is occasionally reported by patients. This has traditionally been blamed on certain types of denture cleansers such as alkaline peroxides and hypochlorites (household bleach). It is now known that the cleanser plays no direct role in the process and that whitening is probably caused by a combination of circumstances, such as the use of water at too great a temperature for soaking dentures, exposure of the dentures to solvents such as acetone which can sometimes occur naturally in

Table 13.4 Mechanical properties of acrylic resin (a comparison with certain alloys).

	Modulus of elasticity* (GPa)	Tensile strength* (MPa)	Hardness* (VHN)
Acrylic resin	2.5	85	20
Co/Cr	220	850	420
Stainless steel	220	1000	400

* Values given are typical values. There may be significant variations between products.

saliva and the use of acrylic materials in which interpenetrating networks between beads and matrix phase is not properly developed. The process is not strictly a bleaching process and occurs just as readily in clear unpigmented bases as in pink ones. Microscopy shows that the whitening is almost certainly due to a structural change in the matrix phase resulting in a mismatch in refractive index between the bead polymer and the matrix polymer (Fig 13.9).

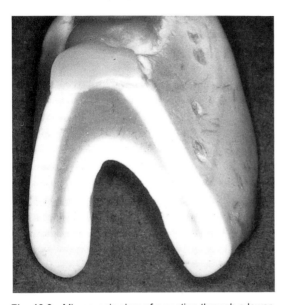

Fig. 13.9 Microscopic view of a section through a lower denture which has been whitened by cleaning in very hot water.

Vickers hardness numbers (Table 13.4) indicate that acrylic polymers are relatively soft, especially when compared with alloys. This predisposes the acrylic denture base to wear, caused by abrasive foodstuffs and particularly abrasive dentifrice cleansers. Wear of the denture base arises as a serious problem on very few occasions however and cannot be considered as a major disadvantage of acrylic resin denture materials. Dentifrices can be graded in terms of abrasivity depending on the type and particle size of the abrasive used. Whilst it would seem prudent to select a dentrifice of low abrasivity for cleaning dentures, it should be realised that some abrasive power is required in order to achieve adequate cleaning.

Chemical and biological properties: Acrylic resin slowly absorbs water and an equilibrium value of about 2% absorption is reached after a period of several days or weeks depending on the thickness of the denture. Loss or gain of water in the surface layers may occur quite rapidly however – a fact which contributes towards surface crazing.

Absorption of water causes a dimensional change, although this may be considered insignificant. This has never been demonstrated as a major cause of ill-fitting dentures in the presently available materials.

Associated with water absorption is the ability of certain organisms to colonize the fitting surface of an acrylic denture. It is not clear whether organisms, such as *Candida albicans*, exist entirely *on* the surface of the denture or whether they penetrate the outer layers of resin. Frequent cleansing, coupled with the practice of soaking dentures overnight, is normally sufficient to prevent the growth of these unwanted organisms and their associated clinical problems, such as *denture stomatitis*.

A very small minority of patients are reported to be *allergic* to acrylic resin and in particular to the residual MMA monomer which may exist within the base. When such cases can be proved genuine, it is necessary to use an alternative material. Patients who are not allergic may, nevertheless, suffer *irritation* if very high levels of monomer exist in, say, an undercured denture base. The ISO Standard for denture bases contains a requirement for the upper limit of the residual monomer concentration (Table 13.2). The limits of 2.2% for types 1, 3, 4 and 5 materials and 4.5% for type 2 materials are quite generous and it is accepted that residual monomer levels of this magnitude could be problematical for some denture wearers. Another requirement of the standard therefore is to request manufacturers to recommend a curing cycle that can achieve a monomer content of less than 1%. Reduced monomer content very much depends upon the type of curing regime used. Short cures involving minimal or no terminal boil generally produce higher monomer concentrations (and inferior properties). Longer cures involving a terminal boil of 2–3 hours can reduce the residual monomer concentration to well below 1%. High residual monomer concentrations can be associated with a relatively high solubility. Type 2 materials with higher residual monomer levels tend to have greatest solubility (Table 13.3).

Acrylic resin should be treated with respect and handled with care by technicians involved in its manipulation. Levels of acrylic powder dust and MMA monomer in the atmosphere should both be kept to a minimum since both may be potentially harmful.

13.4 Modified acrylic materials

The majority of acrylic resin is used in the unmodified form as discussed in Section 13.3. Some products have been developed, however, in which attempts have been made to improve impact strength, fatigue resistance or radiopacity.

The impact strength of acrylic polymers can be improved significantly by the incorporation of elastomers. The elastomer is able to absorb energy on impact and thus protect the acrylic resin from fracture. An alternative of the direct addition of elastomers is the use of acrylic–elastomer copolymers. These are, typically, methylmethacrylate–butadiene or methylmethacrylate–butadiene-styrene copolymers which are now available in certain commercial products. Despite the fact that impact strength can be increased almost tenfold in this way, these polymers are not widely used, mainly because of their greater cost.

One attempt to improve the fatigue resistance of acrylic denture polymers has involved the use of carbon fibre inserts. If the fibres are correctly positioned they may have a beneficial effect. They stiffen the denture, reducing the degree of flexing and the possibility of fatigue fracture. They also considerably increase the flexural strength. The technique is not in widespread use however, for several reasons. In order to gain benefit from the fibres, the positioning is critical. They must be placed in that part of the denture which is under a tensile stress. Bonding between the fibres and the acrylic resin may be difficult to achieve and if bonding is not achieved the fibres may 'weaken' the denture. The technique adds a complicating factor to the denture construction process and, finally, the appearance of the denture is adversely affected because the carbon fibres are black. Other reinforcing fibres, including Kevlar and ultra high modulus polyethylene are currently under investigation.

There have been many attempts to incorporate a degree of radiopacity into acrylic denture base materials. Table 13.5 summarizes the methods which have been suggested. Each method involves the incorporation of atoms of higher atomic number than the C, H and O atoms of which acrylic resin is comprised. One commercially available product contained 8% barium sulphate. This did not produce sufficient levels of radiopacity. Increasing the barium sulphate content to a level of 20% gives sufficient radiopacity but unfortunately has a deleterious effect on the mechanical properties of the resin. The most promising materials under development appear to be those in which

Table 13.5 Radiopaque denture base materials.

Radiopaque additive	Comments
Metal inserts or powdered metals	May weaken base and appearance is poor
Inorganic salts such as barium sulphate	Insufficient radiopacity at low concentrations Weaken base at high concentrations
Co-monomers containing heavy metals, e.g. barium acrylate	Polymer has poor mechanical properties
Halogen-containing co-monomers or additives, e.g. tribromophenylmethacrylate	Additives may act as plasticizers Co-monomers are expensive

bromine-containing additives or comonomers are used to give radiopacity. Figure 13.10 shows chest radiographs in which a segment of a denture has been placed over the lower right chest area. In the case of a conventional denture base material the denture segment is not visible on the radiograph. A material with a bromine-containing additive is clearly visible.

13.5 Alternative polymers

The major alternatives to acrylic polymers or modified acrylics are the polycarbonates and certain vinyl polymers. These may be considered when the patient has a proven allergy to acrylic resin or when greater impact strength is required. The polycarbonates and some of the vinyl polymers are processed by injection moulding and so can only be used when the specialist equipment is available.

Polycarbonates have T_g values around 150°C and are generally moulded at temperatures well in excess of this. Consequently, the moulded bases may have internal stresses after moulding and is likely to distort if placed in hot water. Some of the vinyl resins, on the other hand, have very low softening temperatures, as low as 60°C in some cases. These must obviously be handled with care if distortions are to be avoided.

The other alternative to acrylic resin is vulcanite. The equipment required for processing a vulcanite denture is now a rarity, however, and the material can no longer be considered as a serious alternative.

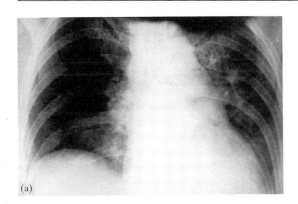

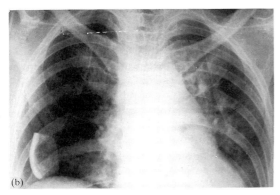

Fig. 13.10 Chest radiographs in which a segment of denture base has been placed over the lower right half of the chest: (a) for a radiolucent denture base material; (b) for a radiopaque denture base material. (From *Journal of Dentistry* (1976) vol. **4**, p. 214, with permission.)

13.6 Suggested further reading

McCabe, J.F. (1982) Characteristics of denture base polymers. In *Biocompatibility of Dental Materials* (D.C. Smith & D.F. Williams, eds), p. 123. CRC Press, Florida.

Robinson, J.G., McCabe J.F. & Storer, R. (1987) Denture bases: the effects of various treatments on clarity strength and structure. *J. Dent*, **15**, 159.

Stafford, G.D., Bates, J.F., Huggett, R. & Handley, R.W. (1980) A review of the properties of some denture base polymers. *J. Dent*, **8**, 292.

Chapter 14
Denture Lining Materials

14.1 Introduction

Denture lining materials are of several types and are used for a variety of reasons. Occasionally, the fitting surface of an acrylic denture needs replacement in order to improve the fit of the denture. In this case, there are two options. Either the whole of the denture base can be replaced with fresh heat curing acrylic resin, or a lining of a self-curing resin may be applied to the fitting surface of the existing base.

Sometimes it is necessary to apply a very soft material to the fitting surface of a denture in order to act as a 'cushion' which will enable traumatized soft tissues to recover before recording an impression for a new denture.

Some patients are unable to tolerate a 'hard' denture base and must be provided with a 'permanent' soft cushion on the fitting surface of the denture.

The materials which satisfy the various requirements listed above can be classified into three groups:

(1)   Hard reline materials;
(2)   Tissue conditioners;
(3)   Soft lining materials.

14.2 Hard reline materials

The materials discussed in this section are those products which are used to provide a chairside reline to the denture. The method should be distinguished from laboratory relining and *rebasing* techniques which involve replacing most of the denture base resin with fresh, heat cured polymer.

Composition: The materials are generally supplied as a powder and liquid which are mixed together. Table 14.1 gives the composition of the two types of material in common use. The major difference between the two types is that the liquid in the type 1 material contains methylmethacrylate monomer,

Table 14.1   Composition of typical hard reline materials.

Type 1	*Powder*	
	Polymer beads	Polymethylmethacrylate
	Initiator	Benzoyl peroxide
	Pigments	Probably inorganic salt
	Liquid	
	Monomer	Methylmethacrylate
	Plasticizer	Di-*n*-butylphthalate
	Chemical activator	Tertiary amine
Type 2	*Powder*	
	Polymer beads	Polyethylmethacrylate
	Initiator	Benzoyl peroxide
	Pigments	Probably inorganic salt
	Liquid	
	Monomer	Butylmethacrylate
	Chemical activator	Tertiary amine

whilst the liquid of the type 2 material contains butylmethacrylate monomer. Both type 1 and type 2 materials may be classified as autopolymerizing resins and will readily polymerize at room temperature or mouth temperature.

Manipulation: The normal procedure is to 'relieve' the fitting surface of the denture by grinding away some of the hard acrylic denture base. The powder and liquid of the hard reline material are then mixed in the recommended proportions to give a fluid mix of material. This is applied to the fitting surface of the denture which is seated in the patient's mouth whilst still fluid. The reline procedure must be undertaken using a 'closed mouth' technique in which the patient's denture or dentures are inserted into the mouth and the patient is then asked to close into gentle contact. Care needs to be taken to ensure that the dentures maintain an appropriate relationship to the underlying alveolar ridge. Both of these steps are designed to prevent major positional or occlusal errors being produced in the relined dentures. The reline material soon becomes rubbery and the impression of the patient's soft tissues is recorded. The denture is then removed from the patient's mouth and allowed to bench cure. Setting may be accelerated by placing the denture in warm water or using a combination of warm water and pressure in an appropriately designed pressure vessel. The materials are not allowed to remain in the patient's mouth throughout setting since the exothermic heat of reaction may cause an unbearably high temperature rise. The relined denture is normally ready for trimming and polishing within 30 minutes.

Properties: The major disadvantage of the type 1 materials is that they involve direct contact between the oral soft tissues and a fluid mixture of reline material containing methylmethacrylate monomer. The latter material is known to be irritant and may also sensitize patients who may then suffer allergic responses in the future. The advice offered by some manufacturers, to smear the soft tissues with petroleum jelly prior to recording the impression, is probably inadequate.

The type 2 materials contain butylmethacrylate monomer in the liquid component. This is known to be a far less irritant substance than methylmethacrylate.

Both type 1 and type 2 materials have low values of glass transition temperature (Tg). The reasons for this are the presence of plasticizer in type 1 materials and the use of higher methacrylates (ethyl and butyl) in the type 2 materials. This may lead to increased dimensional instability in the relined denture, particularly if the existing hard base has been significantly relieved in order to accommodate the lining.

The reline materials are often porous due to air inclusions during mixing of the powder and liquid. The initial fluidity of the mix, coupled with a relatively rapid increase in viscosity during setting at atmospheric pressure, ensure that it is difficult to eliminate voids. This is often considered unsightly and may affect patient acceptance. In addition such a porous surface will be more likely to become contaminated with oral debris and be colonized by micro-organisms including *Candida albicans*, and will be more difficult to clean.

One criticism of the direct reline materials is that the dentist has little control over the thickness of the lining achieved and therefore over the 'height' of the denture. A reline to the fitting surface is usually undertaken to improve denture stability/retention, not to correct an occlusal error nor to modify the vertical relationship between the dentures. The

'cushion' of relining material can result in a marked increase in thickness of the denture base and infringement of the freeway space that is normally present between the dentures with the jaws at rest. Furthermore, there is no guarantee, even when using a closed mouth technique, that an antero-posterior positional error or lateral cant is not produced during this procedure, either as a result of poor operator technique or a greater bulk of lining material on one side of the mouth compared with the other. Such errors are highly undesirable.

A final problem is an increase in thickness of the 'palate' of an upper denture using this technique which patients often find unacceptable.

It follows that the direct reline materials should be considered as only a temporary or at best semipermanent solution to the problem of an ill-fitting denture.

14.3 Tissue conditioners

Tissue conditioners are soft denture liners which may be applied to the fitting surface of a denture. They are used to provide a temporary cushion which prevents masticatory loads from being transferred to the underlying hard and soft tissues. These materials should undergo a degree of plastic flow for 24–36 hours after mixing to allow for soft tissue changes once 'trauma' has been removed and to capture the shape of the supporting tissues in function as opposed to a static or unloaded relationship.

Tissue conditioners have several applications. For example, when the soft tissues have become traumatized due to wearing an ill-fitting denture the dentist would like the tissue to recover before recording impressions for new dentures. Ideally, the patient would refrain from wearing his denture for a period, but this is not popular. In these circumstances, a layer of a cushioning tissue conditioner on the fitting surface of the denture will enable the soft tissue to recover without depriving the patient of their dignity.

Tissue conditioners are often applied to the dentures of patients who have undergone surgery. This reduces pain and helps prevent traumatization of the wound. They are also useful when a tooth or teeth are being added to a denture as an immediate procedure (very shortly after the extraction). The dental technician modifies the cast of the patient's mouth by removing the teeth that will be extracted and by estimating the amount of change in soft tissue contour. If this estimate is wrong there can be a large gap between the denture base and the socket. A tissue conditioner can be used to fill this gap to assist with stabilization of the prosthesis at the time of insertion of the immediate denture.

Another application of tissue conditioners is as *functional impression materials*. A layer of tissue conditioner in the fitting surface of the denture enables a functional impression to be obtained over a period of a few days.

Requirements: Tissue conditioners should remain *soft* during use in order to maintain an adequate cushioning effect on the underlying soft tissues. The material should be *resilient* in order that masticatory loads are absorbed without causing permanent deformation of the lining. Paradoxically, when the materials are being used to obtain a functional impression a degree *permanent deformation* under load is required. This enables the impression of the soft tissues to be altered during normal function.

Composition: The materials are normally supplied as powder and liquid components which are mixed together. Table 14.2 gives the composition of a typical product. The relative amounts of solvent and plasticizer as well as the type of plasticizer used vary significantly from one product to another. These variations control the softness and elasticity of the set material. Commercial products contain from 7.5% to 40% alcohol in the liquid component, whilst the plasticizer is normally a phthalate or benzoate ester. The powder may be pigmented to give a pink coloured lining similar to that of a pink denture base. It is more common, however, for the powder to be unpigmented, giving a white lining which is easily distinguished from the pink denture base.

Table 14.2 Composition of a tissue conditioner.

Powder	
Polymer beads	Polyethylmethacrylate
Liquid	
Solvent	Ethyl alcohol
Plasticizer	Butylphthalyl butylglycolate

It is important to note that the liquid component contains no monomer and the powder no initiator. When the powder and liquid are mixed together, a purely physical process occurs. The solvent dissolves the smaller polymer beads and the larger beads become swollen with solvent which acts as a carrier for the plasticizer. The final 'set' material is gel-like, with swollen, platicized spheres being cemented together with a matrix which is a saturated solution of polymer in a solvent/plasticizer mixture. The 'softness' of the set material is a function of the use of a higher methacrylate, ethyl methacrylate, coupled with considerable quantities of plasticizer and solvent.

Manipulation: Tissue conditions are used in chairside techniques in which the freshly mixed material is applied to the fitting surface of the denture. The denture is then seated in the patient's mouth, whilst the conditioner is still in a fluid state, in order to obtain an impression of the soft tissues. This stage of the procedure is important, since the aim is to form a cushion of reasonable thickness so that it will be effective, but not to increase the 'height' of the denture unduly compared to the unlined denture. On completion of setting ideally the tissue conditioner should form a regular layer over the whole of the fitting surface of the denture. It is normal practice to inspect the denture and the patient's soft tissues after 2–3 days to ascertain whether the tissue conditioning has been successful or, alternatively, whether an adequate functional impression has been obtained.

Properties: Tissue conditioners are initially very soft and viscoelastic. When loaded slowly they undergo permanent deformation even under moderate to low loads. A cylindrical sample of a tissue conditioner can be observed to slump under its own weight if allowed to stand unsupported on a bench top. The lack of a well defined elastic behaviour makes the measurement of rigidity difficult. Under rapid loading a modulus of elasticity value of 0.05 MPa has been estimated. This compares with a value of 2000 MPa for a typical hard acrylic denture base material. The property of *compliance* is often used to define the deformation-load characteristics of these materials. When this term is used the difference between elastic and viscoelastic strains is often ignored so its scientific value is questionable, although it can give some 'feel' for the perceived softness of a material.

The materials do not remain permanently soft since the alcohol and plasticizer are leached rapidly into saliva. The time taken for the materials to become so hard that they no longer give adequate cushioning varies from a few days to a week or two, depending upon the product used. Those materials which are softer initially, harden more rapidly and vice versa. For adequate conditioning, with a very soft material, the conditioner should be replaced with fresh material every 2–3 days until the tissues have recovered.

The materials are able to perform the functions of both a tissue conditioner and functional impression material due to their *viscoelastic* properties. The apparent paradox of requiring an elastic material for one purpose and a plastic one for the other is overcome in this way. The viscoelastic properties of the materials may be described by the Maxwell and Voigt models in series as discussed on p. 13 and illustrated in Fig. 2.15. The elastic nature of the products is extremely time-dependent. Under the influence of dynamic forces which are applied for a second or less during mastication, the materials are essentially elastic and provide a cushioning effect. Each application of force does, however, cause a small permanent deformation which helps to record the functional impression. Under the influence of smaller, resting loads, further permanent deformation occurs.

One of the most important properties of these materials is that they are non-irritant due to the absence of acrylic monomers from the liquid component.

14.4 Temporary soft lining materials

These materials are very similar to the tissue conditioners. They are supplied as a powder and liquid, the composition of which is equivalent to that given in Table 14.2. The materials are not as soft as the tissue conditioners immediately after setting but they retain their softness for longer, taking up to a month or two to harden. Like the tissue conditioners, they are viscoelastic in nature and give a cushioning effect under dynamic conditions of loading.

The method of manipulation of these products is similar to that discussed for tissue conditioners, but because they take longer to harden they do not require replacing as frequently.

Care should be exercised when selecting a denture cleanser to use with a denture carrying a temporary soft lining or tissue conditioner. The oxygenating-type cleansers, in particular, cause surface degradation and pitting of the materials.

Temporary soft liners are often used in place of tissue conditioners in cases where it is not practicable to replace the conditioner every 2–3 days. In addition, they may be used as a means of temporarily improving the fit of an ill-fitting denture until such a time as a new denture can be constructed. Another use of the products is as a diagnostic aid to ascertain whether the patient would benefit from a permanent soft lining.

Both tissue conditioners and temporary soft lining materials will go hard. When this occurs the surface is both rough and irregular, increasing the risk of trauma. In addition these materials can be relatively easily colonized by *Candida* in this hardened state, increasing the risk of a denture-induced stomatitis. Care must be taken by a patient when cleaning a denture with a temporary soft lining or tissue conditioner. Simple rinsing with water does least damage, whilst the use of a proprietary peroxide-based denture cleanser is highly damaging. It is possible to soak such dentures overnight in dilute sodium hypochlorite to help to mitigate infection risk.

14.5 Permanent soft lining materials

Permanent soft lining materials are most commonly used for patients who cannot tolerate a hard base. This problem generally arises if the patient has an irregular mandibular alveolar ridge covered by a thin and relatively non-resilient mucosa. Not surprisingly it may be very painful when a masticatory load is applied through a hard base on to this type of supporting tissue. In such cases, a soft lining on the denture will help to relieve the pain and increase patient acceptance of the denture.

Requirements: The requirements of a permanent soft lining are more critical than those of the tissue conditioner and temporary lining materials since they are expected to function over a much longer period of time.

The materials used should be permanently soft, ideally for the lifetime of the denture. They should be elastic in order to give a cushioning effect and prevent unacceptable distortions during service. The lining should adhere to the denture base. The materials should be non-toxic, non-irritant and incapable of sustaining the growth of harmful bacteria or fungi.

Available materials: Figure 14.1 indicates the types of materials which are available for use as permanent soft linings. Those products described as cold curing acrylic materials are in fact temporary soft lining materials. These materials harden within a period of a few weeks or at best a few months and cannot therefore be seriously considered as permanent soft linings since they would require regular replacement. One advantage of these materials is that they can be readily applied to an existing denture, by the dentist, in a chairside technique.

The heat curing acrylic materials are processed in the laboratory and are normally applied to a new denture at the time of production. They are supplied as a powder and liquid, the composition of which vary from one product to another. They rely, for

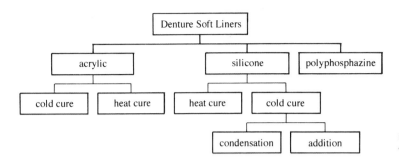

Fig. 14.1 Soft lining materials. An indication of the type of materials which are available.

softness, on the combined use of a higher methacrylate and a plasticizer. A typical powder consists of beads of polyethyl- or polybutylmethacrylate along with some peroxide initiator and pigment. The liquid is likely to be a mixture of butylmethacrylate and plasticizer. Powder and liquid are mixed to form a type of 'dough' which is heat processed simultaneously with the hard acrylic base.

A similar technique is used when applying a heat curing silicone soft lining. These products are supplied as a single paste which consists of a polydimethylsiloxane polymer with pendant or terminal vinyl groups through which cross-linking takes place. The liquid polymer is formulated into a paste by adding inert fillers such as silica. The paste also contains a free radical initiator such as a peroxide which breaks down on heating to initiate the cross-linking reaction.

The structure of the vinyl terminated liquid silicone polymer can be viewed as being similar to that for the hydroxyl terminated material (Fig. 19.4), except that the terminal hydroxyl groups in Fig. 19.4a are replaced by vinyl groups. These vinyl groups undergo chain extension and cross-linking by the mechanism described in Section 12.2. The chain extension reactions cause an increase in viscosity of the liquid polymer, whilst cross-linking causes the material to develop elasticity.

Two types of cold curing silicone elastomers are used as soft lining materials. They are analogous to the two types of silicone elastomers used as impression materials (Sections 19.3 and 19.4), i.e. condensation curing silicones and addition curing silicones. The condensation curing types are generally supplied as a paste and liquid.

The paste contains a hydroxyl-terminated polydimethylsiloxane liquid polymer (Fig. 19.4a) and inert filler. The liquid contains a mixture of a cross-linking agent, such as tetraethyl silicate (Fig. 19.4b) and a catalyst which is normally an organo-tin compound such as dibutyl tin dilaurate. On mixing the paste and liquid a condensation cross-linking reaction takes place. Alcohol is produced as a byproduct of this reaction (Fig. 19.4c). Cross-linking causes the paste to be converted to a rubber. The addition curing silicones have only recently become available as denture soft lining materials. They are very similar to the equivalent products used for recording impressions (Section 19.4). They are supplied as two pastes which are proportioned and mixed using a cartridge/gun system (Fig. 19.6). The setting reaction for these products is described in Section 19.4.

Although the cold curing silicones are cured at room temperature, they are generally processed in the laboratory. The method normally used is to pour casts into the dentures. The casts with dentures are then mounted on an articulator and the fitting surface of the dentures is relieved to make space for the lining. The paste and liquid are mixed together and the fluid mix applied to the fitting surface of the dentures. The dentures are then repositioned on the casts, the articulator closed into occlusion and the material allowed to set. An alternative method is to use an overcast instead of an articulator.

Polyphosphazine fluoroelastomers have recently become available for use as denture soft lining materials. They are supplied in sheet form and are manipulated in a similar manner to the heat cured silicone products. Recommended curing is either at 74°C for 8 hours or 74°C for $2\frac{1}{2}$ hours, followed by 100°C for 30 minutes. There is very little detailed information available on the composition of these products.

Properties: The ISO Standard for 'long-term' resilient lining materials (ISO 10139-2) utilizes a penetration test to evaluate the softness and elastic properties of the materials. A 4 mm thick specimen of material is indented with a 2 mm diameter probe under a load of 100 g for 30 seconds. Depth of penetration is monitored as a function of time to produce a result of the type shown in Fig. 14.2. The depth of penetration after 5 seconds loading is used to characterize softness. Materials are described as stiff, medium or soft depending on the extent of penetration. The elastic or viscoelastic properties of the materials are defined by the time dependence of the penetration. For elastic materials (Fig. 14.2a) penetration is essentially independent of time – it increases immediately on application of load and recovery is instantaneous after removal of the load. The penetration ratio, which is the ratio of the penetration after 30 seconds of loading to that at 5 seconds of loading, is close to one for these materials. For viscoelastic materials (Fig. 14.2b) penetration under load is time dependent and the ratio of the penetration at 30 seconds to that at 5 seconds is greater than unity. The limits set out in the ISO Standard are shown in Table 14.3.

The acrylic products tend to have behaviour which can be described by Fig. 14.2b, i.e. they tend to be materials which exhibit a low resistance to flow, whilst the silicone and polyphosphazine materials behave in a manner depicted in Fig. 14.2a, i.e. they have a high resistance to flow and are more elastic.

Table 14.3   Limits of penetration and penetration ratio (30 s : 5 s, Fig. 14.2b) set out in ISO 10139-2: Resilient Lining Materials for Removable Dentures – Long-term materials.

Description	Penetration (P) (mm)	Penetration (R) ratio
Type A stiff	$0.2 \leqslant P < 0.4$	—
Type B medium	$0.4 \leqslant P < 0.8$	—
Type C soft	$0.8 \leqslant P < 2.5$	—
Class I high resistance to flow	—	$R \leqslant 1.1$
Class II low resistance to flow	—	$1.1 < R < 1.75$

All types of soft lining material are sufficiently soft on insertion to give an adequate cushioning effect. The softest of the four materials initially are the cold curing acrylic materials. These products harden, however, through rapid loss of alcohol and slow leaching of plasticizer. These materials should not be considered suitable for anything other than short term use. Softness of the other products varies from brand to brand even within specific classes of materials. Some acrylic products are classified as stiff and others as soft, depending on the type and amount of plasticizer used. The heat curing acrylic products, though not as soft as the cold curing products initially, retain their softness for longer. They too eventually become hard due to gradual leaching of plasticizer into the oral fluids. The silicone materials remain permanently soft and the modulus of elasticity value may, in fact, decrease due to water absorption. This may cause problems with some silicones since water absorption may be followed by bacterial or fungal growth in the soft lining. The silicones have good elastic properties and retain their shape after setting despite being subjected to masticatory loading. The acrylic materials, on the other hand, are viscoelastic and gradually become distorted. There is a tendency for the materials to 'flow away' from areas of greatest stress causing the cushioning effect to be lost.

The durability of the bond between the denture base and the soft lining is adequate for the acrylic materials and the heat cured silicone products. In the case of the cold curing silicone material, however, there is a tendency for the lining to peel away from the base. This occurs despite the use of an adhesion primer supplied by the manufacturers. The problem is often reduced by 'boxing in' the soft lining. Clini-

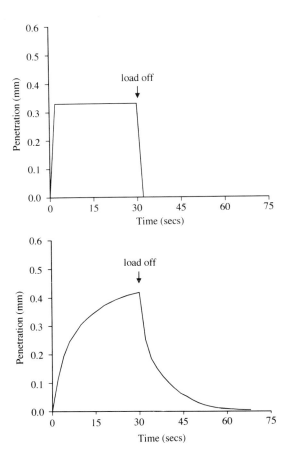

Fig. 14.2   Penetration under load for (a) an elastic material and (b) a viscoelastic material.

cally the techniques used to add a soft lining vary according to the material chosen. The acrylic based materials can either be added to an existing denture, using a technique analogous to that used when relining the denture with hard acrylic, or they can be incorporated into the denture base when making a new prosthesis. The results in terms of both resilience and durability are similar. Conversely, whilst the silicone rubber materials can be processed onto an existing denture, the quality of the attachment between the acrylic and the rubber is much better if it is processed against 'fresh' acrylic.

The cushioning effect of a soft lining depends on the thickness of the soft material. The greater the thickness of the soft material the greater the cushioning effect perceived by the patient. There are limits to the total thickness of the combined denture base and soft lining and this means that the use of a soft lining inevitably involves the use of a thinner residual acrylic denture base. Since a thickness of soft lining of 2–3 mm is required for adequate cushioning the residual hard acrylic base may become more flexible and weakened such that the occurrence of fracture is increased compared to dentures constructed solely from hard acrylic material.

Some soft linings are adversely affected by denture cleansers. Oxygenating cleansers may cause surface pitting in acrylic linings whilst brushing accelerates the rate at which silicone soft linings become detached. Soaking in a very *dilute* solution of hypochlorite is an acceptable way of achieving denture hygiene without damaging the soft lining.

None of the soft lining materials can be considered truly permanent in nature since none could be expected to last the full lifetime of a denture. Therefore, regular reviews of patients with soft linings are essential.

14.6 Self-administered relining materials

Several types of lining materials are available which enable the patient to attempt to improve the fit of ill-fitting dentures or to provide a soft cushioning effect to the fitting surface. Such products are generally available for purchase at many retail outlets such as supermarkets or chemists shops. The products normally contain methacrylate or vinyl polymers such as polymethyl-, polyethyl-, or polybutylmethacrylate or vinyl acetate along with a plasticizer such as butyl phthalate and a solvent such as acetone, ethanol or toluene. The claim for such products is that they improve the fit or comfort of a denture without having to visit the dentist. Most authorities agree however that the use of these products should be firmly discouraged, for all but short term emergency use. Long term use of these products can lead to harmful effects on the hard and soft oral tissues. Cases of irritation, severe bone loss and tumors, related to the use of self-administered denture lining materials, have been documented.

14.7 Suggested further reading

Brown, D. (1988) Resilient soft liners and tissue conditioners. *Br. Dent. J.* **164**, 357.

Dootz, E.R., Koran, A. & Craig R.G. (1993) Physical property comparison of 11 soft denture lining materials as a function of accelerated ageing. *J. Prosthet. Dent* **69**, 114.

Kalachandra, S., Minton, R.J., Taylor, D.F. & Takamata, T. (1995) Characterisation of some proprietary soft lining materials. *J. Mat. Sci.* **6**, 647.

Wright, P.S. (1976) Soft lining materials: their status and prospects. *J. Dent* **4**, 247.

Chapter 15
Artificial Teeth

15.1 Introduction

Chapters 13 and 14 have dealt with materials which are used to form the denture base and to line the fitting surface of the denture base. The other main components of a denture are the artificial teeth themselves. The materials most widely used for manufacturing artificial teeth are acrylic resin and porcelain.

15.2 Requirements

The most important requirement of artificial teeth is good appearance. They should, ideally, be indistinguishable from natural teeth in shape, colour and translucency. Good matching often requires that the shade and translucency of the artificial tooth should vary from the tip of the crown to the gingival area.

There should be good attachment between the artificial teeth and the denture base. The introduction of artificial teeth into the base should not adversely affect the base material. That is, the artificial tooth and base materials should be compatible.

It is an advantage for the artificial teeth to be of low density in order that they do not increase the weight of the denture unduly. The artificial teeth should be strong and tough in order to resist fracture. They should be hard enough to resist abrasive forces in the mouth and during cleaning, but should allow grinding with a dental bur so that adjustments to the occlusion can be made by the dentist at the chairside.

15.3 Available materials

The two materials which are commonly used for the production of artificial teeth are acrylic resins and porcelain.

Acrylic resins

Acrylic resin artificial teeth are produced in reusable metal moulds using either the *dough moulding* technique, described for denture base construction (Chapter 13), or by *injection moulding* in which the acrylic powder is softened by heating and forced into the mould under pressure.

The resins used are highly cross-linked in order to produce artificial teeth which are resistant to crazing. The main difference between the materials and those used for denture base construction is the incorporation of tooth-coloured pigments rather than pink ones.

Porcelain

The composition and manipulation of porcelain are dealt with in Chapter 11. Artificial porcelain teeth are produced to standard shapes and sizes by using moulds which are approximately 30% larger than required, in order to allow for shrinkage during firing. Small holes or metal pins are incorporated in the base of the porcelain teeth during their production. These are used to give mechanical attachment to the denture base.

15.4 Properties

Both acrylic and porcelain teeth can be made to give a realistic appearance. The slightly greater translucency and depth of colour achieved with porcelain possibly gives this material a slight advantage in terms of aesthetics. Both materials are produced to a variety of shapes, sizes, colours and shades which enable selection of teeth to suit most individuals.

One aspect of porcelain teeth which is sometimes unpopular with patients is the 'clicking' sound which is made when two porcelain teeth come into contact.

Attachment of the teeth to the base is through a chemical union in the case of acrylic teeth and by mechanical retention for porcelain teeth. For both materials, adequate bonding is achieved only if all traces of wax from the trial denture are removed from the teeth during the 'boiling out' stage.

Chemical bonding of the acrylic teeth depends on the softening of the resin at the base of the teeth with monomer from the 'dough' of denture base material. Some manufacturers encourage this process by constructing the base and core of the artificial teeth from uncross-linked or only lightly cross-linked resin which is more readily softened. The outer 'enamel' layers of the tooth are constructed from highly cross-linked resin to prevent crazing. Unfortunately it may be necessary to remove these lightly cross-linked areas when trimming denture teeth to fit into the space available within the dentures. It can then be very difficult to achieve an adequate attachment to the remaining highly cross-linked material.

Despite efforts to ensure bonding between the artificial teeth and the denture base, it has been reported that 33% of all denture repairs are required due to debonding of teeth. For acrylic teeth, bonding to heat-cured resins is more effective than bonding to autopolymerizing resins. The bond to autopolymerizing resin can be improved by grinding grooves into the teeth or through grinding followed by the use of a solvent/monomer mixture to soften the tooth base and impregnate it with methylmethacrylate. ISO specifications for ceramic (ISO 4824) and acrylic (ISO 3336) teeth adopt different approaches towards ensuring a reasonable bond. ISO 4824 requires only that there is some means of mechanical attachment in the ceramic tooth base, i.e. diatoric holes provided for attachment must be patent. ISO 3336 for synthetic polymer teeth requires a bond test to be performed. When a denture tooth is fractured away from a sample of denture base the fracture path must not occur along the interface between the tooth and denture base, i.e. the fracture must be cohesive.

Table 15.1 lists some of the physical and mechanical properties of artificial teeth.

Acrylic resin teeth are, naturally, more compatible with the denture base than porcelain teeth. There is a serious mismatch in coefficient of thermal expansion and modulus of elasticity between porcelain and acrylic resin. This may lead to crazing and cracking of the denture base in the region around the base of the porcelain teeth. Porcelain has a density value about twice that of acrylic resin and dentures constructed with porcelain teeth are much heavier.

Porcelain is brittle and teeth constructed from this material are more likely to chip and fracture than acrylic teeth.

There is a vast difference in hardness between acrylic resin and porcelain. Acrylic teeth are more likely to suffer abrasion than porcelain teeth, although this does not constitute a serious problem in more than a few rare cases.

When excessive wear is evident on acrylic denture teeth, special environmental factors or patient habits are often responsible. For example, working in a dusty or gritty environment may accelerate wear if particles of grit are ground between teeth of an upper and lower denture. Likewise the use of a very abrasive material, such as pumice, for cleaning dentures may result in marked abrasion.

The extreme hardness of porcelain is a disadvantage when adjustments, requiring grinding of teeth, are necessary. With acrylic teeth, such adjustments are carried out quite simply. For porcelain teeth however, the process is difficult and results in the glaze being removed from the surface of the porcelain.

It is a clinical impression that porcelain teeth transmit higher forces to the supporting soft tissues than acrylic teeth. This is a function of the greater modulus of elasticity of porcelain.

The difficulties of grinding porcelain teeth combined with their tendency to transmit a greater force to the underlying tissues dictates the type of clinical case for which they can be used. They should not be used where there is diminished interocclusal distance or when there is poor ridge support.

One advantage of ceramic materials used in various aspects of medicine and dentistry is their perceived biocompatibility. This is related to their structure and lack of chemical reactivity under normal conditions. One aspect of the biocompatibility of ceramic denture teeth which has been a source of some controversy over the years is the occurrence of radioactive compounds of uranium-238. An amendment to ISO 4824 was introduced to test for the presence of uranium-238 using neutron activation. The upper limit for the concentration of the radioactive isotope in the ceramic teeth is $0.2 \ Bq \ g^{-1}$.

The vast majority of artificial teeth used for denture construction are now of the acrylic type. Acceptable appearance coupled with convenient handling, greater toughness and compatibility with

Table 15.1 Some properties of artificial teeth.

	Acrylic resin	Porcelain
Density (g cm^{-3})	1.2	2.4
Coefficient of thermal expansion (ppm°C^{-1})	80	7
Modulus of elasticity (GPa)	2.5	80
Hardness (VHN)	20	500

the acrylic denture base give the acrylic resins an advantage over the alternative porcelain materials.

The appearance of both porcelain and acrylic teeth can be customized using surface stains. Those for porcelain teeth are similar to the glaze stains used for porcelain crown and bridge materials. Their use necessitates the teeth being placed through a glazing cycle by a ceramic technician. The surface stains for acrylic are applied in the form of a surface lacquer.

Both approaches can produce a dramatic increase in the realism of denture teeth. However, the effect of acrylic surface stains is rather short-lived as the lacquer is soft and hence worn away quite rapidly.

15.5 Suggested further reading

Woodforde J. (1968) *The Strange Story of False Teeth.* Routledge & Kegan Paul, London.

Chapter 16

Impression Materials: Classification and Requirements

16.1 Introduction

Many dental appliances are constructed outside the patient's mouth on models of the hard and/or soft tissues. The accuracy of 'fit' and the functional efficiency of the appliance depends upon how well the model replicates the natural oral tissues. The accuracy of the model depends on the accuracy of the impression in which it was cast.

The impression stage is the first of many stages involved in the production of dentures, crowns, bridges, orthodontic appliances etc. It is of great importance, therefore, that inaccuracies are minimized at this stage, otherwise they will be carried through and possibly compounded later on.

Impression materials are generally transferred to the patient's mouth in an impression 'tray'. The tray is required because the materials are initially quite fluid and require support. Once positioned in the patient's mouth, the materials undergo 'setting' by either a chemical or physical process. After 'setting', the impression is removed from the patient's mouth and the model cast using dental plaster or stone.

16.2 Classification of impression materials

Many criteria may be used to classify impression materials. The most widely used and understood method is to classify them according to chemical type. Hence, we have silicone materials, alginates, etc. Most dentists are able to associate a material from a particular chemical group with a particular set of characteristics or properties which render it suitable for some applications but not for others. Other methods of classification are sometimes used and these may be based upon consideration of the properties of the materials either before or after setting.

Before setting, the property most normally used to characterize materials is viscosity. This may effect the fine detail which can be recorded in impressions of hard tissues and may influence the degree of tissue compression or displacement achieved with soft-tissue impressions. Thus, materials which are initially very fluid are often classified as *mucostatic* impression materials because they are less likely to compress soft tissues, whilst materials which are initially more viscous are classified as *mucocompressive*. It should be remembered however, that viscosity often varies with the applied stress (p. 15). Thus, certain materials which appear fairly viscous whilst under low stress conditions may become more fluid during the recording of the impression, when the material is placed under higher stress. When a substance behaves in this way, it is said to be *pseudoplastic*. Another complicating factor is the spacing of the impression tray. This controls the thickness of the impression material and hence the pressure transmitted to the underlying tissues. A relatively fluid impression material confined in a close-fitting impression tray will compress the soft tissues to a greater extent than the same material used in a loosely-fitting tray. Classification of materials according to viscosity is not, therefore as simple as it may seem. Figure 16.1 gives a simplified classification according to viscosity in which materials with the highest viscosity are shown at the left of the figure and those with the lowest viscosity are shown on the right. There are often significant variations between different brands of the same type of material and these variations can spread across the divisions between different levels of viscosity.

A more widely used classification of materials involves consideration of the properties of the set material. This factor is primarily responsible for governing the principal applications of the materials. The properties which are most important are *rigidity* and *elasticity*, since they determine whether an

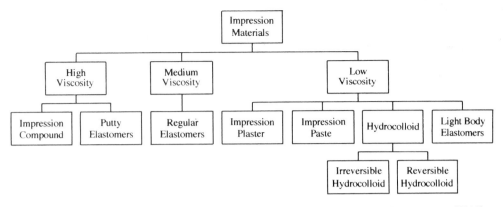

Fig. 16.1 Classification of impression materials by viscosity at a constant shear rate and temperature (23°C).

impression material can be used to record undercuts. When standing teeth are to be recorded, or when the patient has deep soft-tissue undercuts, the set impression material must be flexible enough to be withdrawn past the undercuts and elastic enough to give recovery and an accurate impression. Hence impression materials are classified as being *elastic or non-elastic*. The term elastic as applied to impression materials is fairly unequivocal since the materials which form this group all possess the ability to be stretched or compressed and give a reasonable degree of elastic recovery following strain. They could be described as possessing rubbery characteristics. The term non-elastic however, is not a particularly good term with which to describe a group of products which in some cases are clearly plastic (e.g. impression waxes) and in other cases are very rigid but show little evidence of plastic deformation (e.g. impression plasters). It may be less confusing if the terms rubbery and non-rubbery were used instead of elastic and non-elastic. However, the latter terms have been used for many years and are therefore likely to be familiar to dentists.

Figure 16.2 lists the major groups of impression materials using the classification referred to above.

16.3 Requirements

The requirements of impression materials can be conveniently discussed under four main headings:

(1) Factors which affect the *accuracy* of the impression.
(2) Factors which affect the *dimensional stability* of the impression, that is, the way in which the accuracy varies with time after recording the impression.
(3) Manipulative variables such as ease of handling, setting characteristics, etc.
(4) Additional factors such as cost, taste, colour etc.

Accuracy

In order to record the fine detail of the hard or soft oral tissues, the impression material should be fluid on insertion into the patient's mouth. This requires a low viscosity or a degree of pseudoplasticity.

The way in which the material interacts with saliva is another factor affecting fine-detail reproduction. Some products are hydrophobic and may be repelled by moisture in a critical area of the impression. This

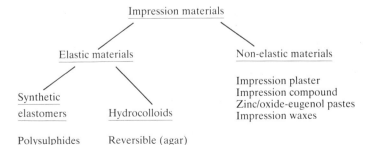

Fig. 16.2 Impression materials. Classification according to elastic properties and chemical type.

normally results in the formation of a 'blow hole' in the impression. For such products, a dry field of operation is essential. Other materials are more compatible with moisture and saliva and no special precautions are necessary.

The fine detail recorded in an impression will only be transferred to the gypsum cast if there is adequate 'wetting' of the impression surface by the freshly mixed dental stone or plaster. In cases where the impression is made from a hydrophobic material the hydrophilic slurry of calcium sulphate hemihydrate in water may not be able to approach closely enough to the surface to the impression (on a microscopic scale). This can result in blow holes and loss of fine detail. The ability of impression materials and gypsum products to reproduce detail in the cast is normally determined by measuring the contact angle which a drop of aqueous calcium sulphate solution makes with the surface of the impression material. A low contact angle is favourable as it indicates good wetting.

The 'setting' of impression materials, whether it involves a chemical reaction or simply a physical change of state, generally results in a dimensional change which, naturally, affects accuracy. For most materials, the dimensional change is a contraction and, providing the impression material is firmly attached to the impression tray, this produces an expansion of the impression 'space' and an oversized die, as illustrated in Fig. 16.3. Materials which expand during setting result in undersized dies or casts. The effect on the accuracy of fit of the resultant restoration depends on the type of restoration and the complexity of shape involved. For the simple crown preparation, illustrated in Fig. 16.3, the oversized die will result in a 'loose-fitting' crown. For greatest accuracy, the dimensional change should be minimal.

On being withdrawn from the patient's mouth, which is typically at a temperature of 32–37°C, into the dental surgery, at a temperature of around 23°C, the impression undergoes approximately 10°C cooling. This results in thermal contraction, the magnitude of which depends on the value of coefficient of thermal expansion of the impression material and impression tray to which it is attached. It is difficult to calculate the precise value of the thermal contraction or to predict accurately the direction in which it operates since the contraction of the tray and that of the material act in opposite directions, providing the impression material remains attached to the tray. This is illustrated in Fig. 16.4. The effects of thermal changes are minimized if the values of coefficient of thermal expansion of the impression material and tray material are small.

It is important that the impression material remains attached to the impression tray during the recording of the impression. Partial detachment may cause gross distortions of the impression which may remain undetected and will almost certainly lead to ill-fitting appliances or restorations. Manufacturers of impression materials often supply tray adhesives which are used to enhance bonding. Additional retention is achieved by using perforated trays.

In addition to the requirements given above, there are two further requirements which apply specifically to materials used for recording undercuts. These materials must have adequate elastic properties and adequate tear resistance, coupled with a rigidity which is low enough to enable the impression to be removed.

Figure 16.5 shows diagramatically the way in which a set material is placed under stress during the withdrawal of the impression. The thickest parts of the impression are compressed against the tray when they pass the widest part of the tooth crown. As the impression is withdrawn it is likely that the material is also subjected to tensile stresses as the trapped material is stretched. If a material is rigid after setting it may not be possible to remove it from undercut areas. This obviously has a negative effect on the ability to achieve an adequate impression, but more seriously may undermine the viability of the remaining teeth as they may be subjected to a considerable stress if an attempt is made to remove the impression.

Figure 16.6 gives a series of diagrams to illustrate what happens when an impression of an undercut tooth is recorded with (a) an elastic material, (b) a plastic material, and (c) a viscoelastic material. The impression recorded with the elastic material accurately records the true shape of the tooth with the

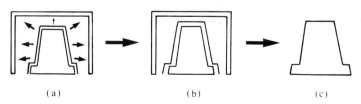

(a)   (b)   (c)

Fig. 16.3 Diagram illustrating the effect of setting contraction. (a) If the impression material is bonded to the tray, contraction occurs towards the tray. (b) Contraction results in an oversized impression space. (c) This results in an oversized die.

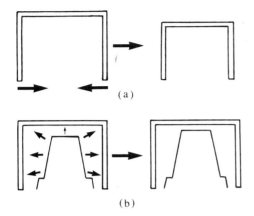

Fig. 16.4 Diagram illustrating the effects of thermal contraction. (a) The tray contracts and reduces the impression space. (b) The impression material contracts towards the tray (providing it is bonded) and increases the impression space.

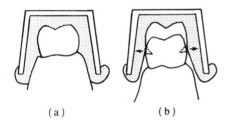

Fig. 16.5 Diagram illustrating how an impression material is placed under stress during removal from an undercut area. (a) Impression in place before removal. (b) During removal – the impression material is subjected to both compressive and tensile stresses.

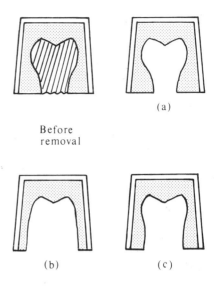

Before removal

After removal

Fig. 16.6 Diagram illustrating attempts to record the impression of an undercut tooth crown with the following: (a) an elastic material; (b) a plastic material: (c) a viscoelastic material.

On removing elastic impression materials from undercut areas they are often put under a considerable tensile stress. The materials should be capable of withstanding such stresses without tearing. One important practical example of when tear resistance is required is shown in Fig. 16.7. For a crown preparation having subgingival shoulders, a thin, undercut region of impression material is formed. In order to obtain a complete impression this must not tear during removal of the impression.

correct degree of undercut. The impression recorded with the plastic material has been grossly distorted during removal and has not recorded any undercut. The impression recorded with the viscoelastic material gives a distorted shape. The degree of distortion depends on the severity of the undercut, the thickness of the impression material and the time for which the impression is maintained in a compressed state (Fig. 16.5b) as well as the viscoelastic properties of the material itself. The behaviour of viscoelastic materials is described on p. 13, where the influence of time as an important parameter is discussed in some detail. Ideally, an impression material used to record undercuts should be perfectly elastic. If a degree of viscoelaticity exists, distortions can be minimized by ensuring that the material is not maintained in the strained position for longer than necessary, by removing the impression quickly.

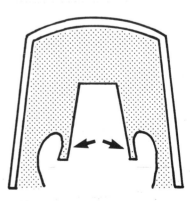

Fig. 16.7 Exaggerated view of a material being used to record an impression of a crown with subgingival shoulders. The thin areas of impression material, which are most prone to fracture, are arrowed.

Dimensional stability

The previous section deals with factors which affect the accuracy of an impression material during the periods of insertion into the patient's mouth, setting, and withdrawal. The next stage is to cast a gypsum model into the impression. This stage is, however, often delayed for one of several reasons. It may not be convenient for the dentist himself to cast the model, in which case the impression is sent to a dental laboratory. If the laboratory is not on the same premises it may be several hours before the model is cast. If the laboratory is a long distance from the surgery it may be necessary to send the impression by post, in which case the delay between recording the impression and constructing the cast may be several days. The way in which the accuracy of the impression changes during this period is a measure of its dimensional stability. An ideal impression material would have perfect dimensional stability, such that the impression would retain its original accuracy indefinitely.

Several factors may contribute towards dimensional changes during storage or transportation of impressions. Continuation of the setting reaction beyond the apparent setting time may cause dimensional changes over a period of time. For viscoelastic materials, slow elastic recovery may continue for some time after withdrawal of the impression, producing a dimensional change. In this case the dimensional change results in a more accurate impression. For some elastic materials it has been suggested that one should allow a rest period after withdrawing the impression, before pouring the gypsum cast, to allow elastic recovery to occur more fully. Some impression materials develop internal stresses on cooling from the temperature at which the impression is recorded to room temperature. This particularly applies to thermoplastic impression materials such as impression compound. On storage of the impression, distortions may occur as the material attempts to relieve the internal stresses. Finally, many impression materials contain volatile substances, either as primary components or as byproducts of the setting reactions. Loss of such volatile materials during storage results in a shrinkage of the impression material with a consequent decrease in accuracy. For the majority of materials, accuracy is best maintained by pouring the gypsum cast soon after recording the impression.

Manipulative variables

Many methods of dispensation are used for impression materials. Some involve the mixing of powder and water, others paste and liquid, others two pastes and some require no mixing at all. The latter materials, generally, require warming in either a water bath or bunsen flame in order to soften them. They record the impression by rehardening at mouth temperature. For materials where mixing is required, the two-paste systems, generally supplied in toothpaste-like tubes, have certain advantages. Proportioning is easy; one simply 'squeezes' out equal lengths of paste from each tube onto a paper mixing pad or a glass plate. The manufacturer normally supplies the two pastes with contrasting colours so that it is easy to see when mixing has been completed satisfactorily – there are no streaks of colour left in the mix. For powder/liquid and paste/liquid systems, it is not possible to define clearly the point at which mixing has been completed satisfactorily. If mixing is incomplete, certain parts of the impression may remain unset.

The setting characteristics of the material have an important effect on the ease of handling and, therefore, often influence the dental surgeon's choice of product. Materials which soften on warming and 'set' on cooling are sometimes difficult to control, particularly in inexperienced hands. The setting characteristics are almost totally under the control of the operator since they depend on the temperature to which the material is heated and the time for which it is maintained at that temperature before recording the impression.

For those materials which set by a chemical reaction, setting begins immediately after mixing unless the manufacturer incorporates a retarder. The *working time* of the material is the time, from start of mix, until the material is no longer suitable for recording an impression. It is normally characterized by the time taken for the viscosity to increase by a given amount above that of the freshly mixed material. Several methods are available for measuring the increase in viscosity as a function of time, including cone and plate viscometers, extrusion rheometers, reciprocating rheometers and simple parallel-plate plastimeters. In each case, the value of working time obtained is somewhat arbitrary, since it depends on a subjective decision as to the degree of increase in viscosity which can be tolerated before the material becomes unworkable. Three typical viscosity – time curves for impression materials are given in Fig. 16.8. Curve A represents a material for which viscosity is high immediately after mixing but increases relatively slowly over the first three minutes. Curve B represents a material, the initial viscosity of which is low but increases rapidly after mixing. Curve C represents a material for which

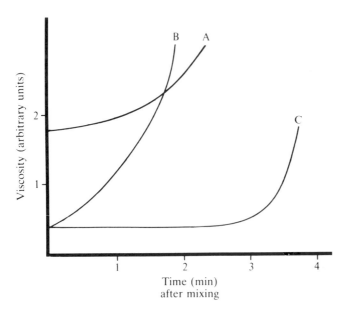

Fig. 16.8 Viscosity versus time curves for three impression materials. Material A is initially quite viscous and its viscosity slowly increases. Material B is initially fluid (low viscosity) but its viscosity increases sharply. Material C is initially fluid and has an induction period during which viscosity is constant. This is followed by a rapid increase in viscosity.

viscosity remains constant for some time due to retardation of the setting reaction. Following the induction period, the viscosity increases rapidly. With materials which do not have an induction period the impression should be recorded as soon as possible after mixing to ensure that the viscosity has not increased unduly.

For elastic impression materials the increase in viscosity during setting may not be the most appropriate way to measure the working time. For these materials the initial onset of some elastic behaviour may be taken as a time beyond which it would be inappropriate to seat the material in the patient's mouth in order to record an impression. The ISO Standard for Elastomeric Impression Materials (ISO 4823) defines working time for these products as follows:

'The period of time beginning with the start of mixing and ending with the loss of plasticity and development of elastic properties such that the material is no longer suitable for making an impression'.

Whereas the working times of materials are determined at room temperature, setting times are generally determined at mouth temperature. The *setting time* of an impression material may be defined in terms of the time required to complete the setting reaction. It is more normal, however, to use a definition which is based on the time to reach a certain degree of rigidity, hardness or elasticity. Setting times measured in this way often gives

values which are significantly shorter than the times required to complete the setting reaction, indicating that setting continues slowly for some time after removal from the mouth. In order to obtain the optimum performance from any impression material, it is wise to leave the material in the patient's mouth for an extra minute or so after setting has apparently been completed. This applies particularly to the elastic materials for which significant improvements in elasticity may occur after the apparent completion of setting.

For the convenience and comfort of both the dental surgeon and patient the most ideal combination of properties for an impression material is a long working time and short setting time. This can be achieved with materials which set by a chemical reaction providing the reaction rate is much quicker at mouth temperature than at room temperature.

16.4 Clinical considerations

Choice of impression material

The fundamental choice for impression materials is between rigid and elastomeric products. As a broad generalization, rigid materials are used when undercuts are not present amongst the surfaces to be recorded. The one exception to this is impression plaster which can be used in some circumstances where undercuts are present. The impression fractures during removal and then needs to be reassembled like a jigsaw before the master cast is prepared. Rigid impression materials can also be used in edentulous subjects where soft tissue (compressible) undercuts are present.

Both rigid and elastomeric materials are available which exhibit a wide range of accuracy and physical properties. The selection of a material for a specific clinical application is usually based on a combination of cost and required accuracy. The more accurate/dimensionally stable materials also tend to be more expensive and hence are used when required rather than routinely.

Impression trays

The purpose of an impression tray is to give rigid support to the impression material and to facilitate its introduction into the mouth. Trays can be either custom made or pre-formed (stock).

Custom trays are produced on study casts of a patient's mouth that have been made using an impression material of lower accuracy/dimensional stability in a stock tray. They are designed to be rigid and to have optimal spacing between the tray and the tissues that are to be recorded to obtain the best results with the impression material to be used in that tray. Custom trays should also have appropriate extensions in all directions to record the oral soft tissues.

Stock trays are produced in a variety of shapes and sizes so that the clinician selects the 'best fit' available for the patient. Such trays are often either too short or too long (under- or overextended) in relation to the extent of the oral soft and hard tissues that need to be recorded for clinical purposes. Modification to the extension of a tray can be achieved by cutting it back (with disposable plastic trays) or by further extending the periphery using a rigid thermoplastic material like 'green stick' tracing compound. It may be possible to provide some support for tray extension into the vestibular sulcus using wax, but this material is too flexible to support adequately distal extension to impression trays. Inevitably, an impression material used in a stock tray will vary in thickness and hence the elastic properties of the material will not necessarily be optimal for that material. The accuracy of an impression in a stock tray depends upon the ability of an elastomeric material to perform adequately under less than optimal conditions.

Tray design must include some method for retaining the impression material attached to the tray. The methods commonly used include mechanical interlocks (holes perforating through the tray, wires attached to the base of the tray or increased bulk at the rim of the tray or 'rim lock') and the use of adhesives. The adhesives tend to be of the *contact adhesive* type, hence it is important that the adhesive layer has had adequate time to dry before the impression material is placed in the tray.

Trays designed for use with reversible hydrocolloids have an in-built water-cooling mechanism to accelerate gelation of this thermally softened material. Whilst it would be technically possible to use reversible hydrocolloids in uncooled trays, the gelation time would be far too long to make them clinically viable.

It has already been stated that trays need to be rigid to support the impression material. This can pose problems with very high viscosity impression *putties* and plastic stock trays.

Tissue management

When impressions are being recorded for fixed or removable prosthodontics it is important not only to record the surfaces of the teeth with the impression but also the relationship between the teeth and the soft tissues surrounding them. For removable prosthodontics this can be achieved by careful impression technique and by smearing or syringing impression material into areas of the mouth which may be recorded badly during conventional placement of a loaded impression tray into the mouth.

With fixed prosthodontics (crown/bridgework) the preparations on the teeth commonly extend up to or beneath the gingival margin. It is necessary, therefore, to displace the gingival tissues away from the preparation prior to syringing in light bodied material around the teeth. This displacement can be achieved either by packing a retraction cord into the gingival crevice or by widening the crevice temporarily using either an electrosurgical unit or a soft tissue laser (this technique is known as troughing).

There are a wide variety of gingival retraction cords available, varying from silk suture material through custom made laid or braided cords to knitted cords. One manufacturer incorporates a thin copper filament in their cord to help it to remain in place within the gingival crevice. All are available in a range of diameters to cope with gingival crevices of varying depth and width.

The objective of placing a retraction cord is to displace the gingival tissue laterally away from the prepared tooth surface rather than apically. Consequently the packing technique needs to be directed to give lateral displacement of the cord, which is introduced in the crevice using a slim, flat-bladed instrument like a 'flat plastic' or using a custom designed cord packer.

There is some dispute about how many retraction cords should be placed within the crevice. Some authorities maintain that a very fine cord should be placed in the base of the crevice to help provide moisture control (the haemostatic cord) with a second layer at the coronal extent to displace the gingiva laterally (the expanding cord). The more superior cord is removed whilst the impression is recorded, whilst the fine cord is left within the crevice. One of the complications of the use of retraction cord is gingival recession exposing a restoration/tooth margin which can give aesthetic problems in the anterior portion of the mouth. The use of a dual cord technique is thought to increase the risk of recession and consequently a single large cord is advocated by other authorities. Whichever approach is adopted, the expanding cord should not be left within the gingival crevice for more than 20 minutes to minimize the risk of recession. Care should be taken when removing cord from the crevice to ensure that the cord is wet. Dry cord will tend to stick to the mucosa lining the crevice and tear this away if it is removed, causing gingival bleeding.

Retraction cords are often used in association with a haemostatic agent to assist with moisture control. Some cords are impregnated with the haemostat whilst others are dipped in a haemostatic solution prior to placement. These agents include adrenaline (epinephrine) and aluminium and ferric chlorides. Adrenaline containing cord must be used with great care as it contains large quantities of drug which can be absorbed through the gingival capillary bed and hence exert a systemic effect. This would be of particular concern in people with compromised cardiological function. They are probably best avoided. Some of the other haemostatic agents have a relatively low pH and can remove the smear layer/dissolve superficial dentine apical to the margins of the preparation. This may induce dentine sensitivity post-operatively in some teeth.

The alternative technique of troughing uses the cutting power of an electrosurgery unit or a soft tissue laser to widen the gingival crevice and produce haemostasis. The key to success with either instrument is to use a careful technique and, with the electrosurgery unit, a fine single wire cutting tip to ensure minimal soft tissue damage. There is no greater likelihood of gingival recession after troughing than in association with the use of conventional retraction cord unless the gingival tissues are particularly thin or there is an absence of attached gingiva. The electrosurgery unit is also particularly useful for removing areas of gingival overgrowth that may be present when replacing previous crowns that have had mar-

ginal deficiencies or where provisional restorations have been poorly contoured.

Impression technique

The specific technique used for each material will vary from product to product. However, there are some broad generalizations that are applicable to all. To obtain greatest accuracy the teeth need to be clean and dry. Salivary contamination is usually prevented using a combination of cotton rolls and absorbent pads – 'dry guards'. It has been suggested that rubber dam can be used to provide isolation, this is only practical when an addition-cured silicone rubber is *not* being used. The plasticizers in the rubber dam will poison the platinum catalyst in the impression material, inhibiting its set.

Material needs to be placed on both the occlusal surfaces of teeth (if present) and within the tray. If this is not done there is a tendency to entrap air within the occlusal surface of the tooth giving bubbles on the impression which will fill subsequently with the material from which the models are formed, producing inaccuracies on the occlusal surface of the prepared model. This is a particular problem when working with teeth with steep cusp angles and tortuous fissure patterns.

Obviously the impression needs to be placed in the mouth whilst the impression material is fluid and left in the mouth until it is set fully. During this time the impression tray needs to be kept as still as possible to avoid distortion of the setting material, producing distorted casts.

All manufacturers give guidance on the working and setting times of their products. These should be adhered to whenever possible to avoid removing an impression whilst it is still partially set. This is particularly important for elastomeric materials which do not fully develop their physical properties until set and hence will distort if removed too early.

Clinically it must be remembered that an impression material that is in direct contact with the lips/tongue will set more rapidly than the bulk of the material in the tray. The material in contact with the lips will be raised fairly rapidly to mouth temperature whilst the bulk of material in the tray will remain closer to room temperature, giving differential setting. This can make a subjective assessment of the quality of set of a material difficult.

After removing the impression from the mouth it is necessary to check to see that the surfaces of the teeth are accurately represented in the impression. It is also wise to ensure that the material remains attached to the supporting impression tray. The forces required to remove the impression from the mouth can disrupt the adhesive bond between material and tray, particularly in the molar region of lower impressions. If this support is disrupted, the accuracy of the impression will be reduced, with the impression material recording the molar being lifted away from the tray, distorting the occlusal plane and potentially giving grossly inaccurate occlusal contacts.

Impression material which extends beyond the tray distally will be unsupported and should be trimmed back to the extent of the impression tray. If this is not done, there may be problems with distortion of this distal extent of the model produced by the weight of the model-making material (commonly dental plaster or stone).

Cross-infection control

It is important that impressions are disinfected prior to their being sent to the laboratory for the manufacture of models and/or prostheses/appliances, to protect the laboratory staff from the transmission of infection from patients. Equally, work leaving the laboratory also ought to be disinfected to prevent transmission of organisms from the laboratory to the patient. The disinfection of impressions poses particular problems as some materials are water based (dental plaster and the hydrocolloids), some are subject to water uptake and/or loss if exposed to inappropriate conditions (hydrocolloids and polyethers) and the quality of the surface of gypsum-based die materials can be affected by the surface disinfectants used to prevent cross-infection.

The first stage in prevention of transmission from the patient to the technician is carefully to rinse the surface of the impression to remove gross contamination with blood or saliva. Current recommendations in the UK would then suggest that all impressions should be further disinfected by immersing them in sodium hypochlorite solution at a concentration of 10 000 parts per million available chlorine for 10 minutes. (Diluted household bleach at either 1:5 or 1:10 will achieve this, depending on whether the original solution was 5% or 10%.) The bleach should be washed off the surface of the casts and then models poured as soon as possible. This immersion time is sufficient to inactivate most oral micro-organisms (including human immunodeficiency virus (HIV) and hepatitis B virus (HBV), whilst at the same time avoiding distortion of impressions. A similar regime can be used for the disinfection of the various trial stages during denture construction after they have been in the mouth. Aerosol-based disinfection processes are not satis-

factory as a result of the potential to miss some areas of the impression with the spray and also the health and safety risk of using powerful disinfectants in an aerosol form. Glutaraldehyde and sodium dichloro-isocyanate solutions have also been advocated, but pose a greater health and safety risk to personnel in use than hypochlorite. The latter solution should be stored in air-tight containers and changed at least daily (more frequently with high rates of use) to maintain its disinfectant properties. Recently developed disinfectants such as sodium peroxy-monosulphate (which is active in a 2% solution against bacteria, fungi and viruses) are likely to overcome many of the handling and storage problems of sodium hypochlorite. This product is effective with a 10 minute immersion period and can be used with the full range of dental impression materials, with the exception of the reversible hydrocolloids.

When managing patients who pose an established risk of spread of infection to laboratory personnel then greater efforts need to be made to sterilize rather than to disinfect impressions. Such patients would include those who have AIDS or those who are sero positive for HIV or HBV. Cold sterilization of impressions involves their immersion in 2% glutaraldehyde under acidic, neutral or alkaline conditions for 10 hours or with a phenolic buffer for 6.75 hours. This sterilization regime determines the impression materials that can be used for this group of subjects as the silicone rubbers are the only group of materials which shows adequate dimensional stability under these conditions. Despite careful rinsing there still tends to be some deleterious effects on the surface finish of gypsum-based model materials, giving softened powdery surfaces. When making dentures for such patients it is necessary to produce multiple copies of the working models as these will become contaminated with oral washings from the surface of the various stages of denture construction at registration and try in. It is not possible to sterilize a gypsum-based model and hence these need to be discarded after each clinical stage with the laboratory work being sterilized before being returned to the laboratory.

16.5 Suggested further reading

Blair, F.M. & Wassell R.W. (1996) A survey of the methods of disinfection of dental impressions used in dental hospitals in the United Kingdom. *Br. Dent. J.* **180**, 369–375.

Craig, R.G. (1988) Review of dental impression materials. *Adv. Dent. Res*, **2**, 51–64.

Wassell, R.W. & Abuasi H.A. (1992) Laboratory assessment of impression accuracy by clinical simulation. *J. Dent*, **20**, 108–14.

Chapter 17
Non-elastic Impression Materials

17.1 Introduction

Four main types of products form the group of impression materials classified as non-elastic materials:

(1) Impression plaster;
(2) Impression compound;
(3) Impression waxes;
(4) Zinc oxide/eugenol impression pastes.

They are classified together for convenience rather than for reasons of similarity in composition or properties. A factor which links the materials is their inability to accurately record undercuts. One of the materials (plaster) is brittle when set and fractures when withdrawn over undercuts. The other products are likely to undergo gross distortions due to plastic flow if used in undercut situations.

17.2 Impression plaster

Impression plaster is similar in composition to the dental plaster used to construct models and dies (Chapter 3). It consists of calcined, β-calcium sulphate hemihydrate which when mixed with water reacts to form calcium sulphate dihydrate.

The material is used at a higher water/powder ratio (approximately 0.60) than is normally used for modelling plasters. The fluid mix is required to enable fine detail to be recorded in the impression and to give the material *mucostatic* properties. The setting expansion of dental plaster is reduced to minimal proportions by using *anti-expansion agents*. Potassium sulphate is the most common of these and has the secondary effect of accelerating the setting reaction, details of which are discussed on p. 33. A retarder, such as borax, is normally incorporated, in order to give a material in which the setting characteristics are controlled. A pigment such as alazarin red is also commonly used, in order to make a clear distinction between the impression and the model

after casting of the model. The anti-expansion agent, retarder and pigment are incorporated into the impression plaster powder by some manufacturers. As an alternative an *anti-expansion solution*, containing potassium sulphate, borax and pigment, may be prepared and used with a standard white plaster.

Freshly mixed plaster is too fluid to be used in a stock impression tray and is normally used in a special tray, constructed using a 1–1.5 mm spacer. The tray may be constructed from acrylic resin or shellac. Another technique is to record the plaster impression as a wash in a preliminary compound impression. The compound is deliberately moved during setting to create space for the plaster wash. The technique for insertion of the impression into the mouth involves 'puddling' the impression into place. With other materials the tray is simply seated home in a single movement. With plaster the tray is gently moved from side to side and antero-posteriorly to best take advantage of the handling characteristics of the material, particularly its fluidity.

Before casting a plaster model in a plaster impression, the impression must be coated with a separating agent, otherwise separation is impossible.

The mixed impression material is initially very fluid and is capable of recording soft tissues in the uncompressed state. In addition, the hemihydrate particles are capable of absorbing moisture from the surface of the oral soft tissues, allowing very intimate contact between the impression material and the tissues. The fluidity of the material, combined with the ability to remove moisture from tissues and a minimal dimensional change on setting, results in a very accurate impression which may be difficult to remove.

The water-absorbing nature of these materials often causes patients to complain about a very dry sensation after having impressions recorded. Disinfection of a plaster impression can be achieved with a 10 minute soak in sodium hypochlorite solution as described previously.

Following setting, the plaster impression material is very brittle. It can undergo virtually no compressive or tensile strain without fracturing. The material is, therefore, not suitable for use in any undercut situations.

One technique for recording impressions of undercut areas, commonly used before the advent of elastic materials, was to allow the impression plaster to 'set' and then to fracture it in order to facilitate removal from the mouth. The material is weak and easily fractured due to its high water/powder ratio. The fragments are then reconstructed in order to form the completed impression.

The properties of impression plasters can be compared with those of model plasters and stones by reference to Table 3.2. The main differences between impression plaster and model plaster are: more rapid setting in order to avoid inconvenience/discomfort to both the patient and dentist; smaller setting expansion for greater accuracy – the expansion is actually equivalent to that observed for a low expansion die stone (type 4) and much lower strength so that fracture can occur easily if the material engages an undercut.

Dental impression plaster remains a useful material, particularly when recording impressions of patients with excessively mobile soft tissues overlying the residual alveolar bone (a 'flabby' ridge). It is important to capture such tissue at rest rather than risk an abnormal pattern of displacement with a more viscous impression material. A two-stage technique is commonly used in which a special tray is made with appropriate spacing for zinc oxide/eugenol paste where the mucosa is well supported and having a window overlying the 'flabby' area. An impression of the bulk of the ridge is recorded in zinc oxide/eugenol paste. Any excess material is removed from the window and the impression re-seated in the mouth. The shape of the flabby ridge at rest is then recorded by painting plaster into its surface with a brush and keying this impression into the impression tray.

17.3 Impression compound

Impression compound is a thermoplastic material, having properties which in many ways are similar to those of the dental waxes discussed in Chapter 4. The composition varies from one product to another but an indication of typical composition is given in Table 17.1. Two types of impression compound are available. These are usually classified as type I (lower fusing) and type II (higher fusing). The type I materials are impression materials whereas the type II materials are used for constructing impression trays. The difference in fusing temperature between type I and type II materials naturally reflects a difference in the composition of the thermoplastic components of each.

The lower fusing, type I impression materials may be supplied in either sheet or stick form. The sheet material is used for recording impressions of edentulous ridges, normally using stock trays. The stick material is used for border extensions on impression trays or for recording impressions of single crowns using the *copper ring* technique.

The sheet material is normally softened using a water bath. Both the temperature and time of conditioning in the water bath affect the performance of the material. If the conditioning temperature is too low the material does not soften properly, and if too high, it becomes sticky and unmanageable. A temperature in the range 55–60°C is normally found to be ideal.

The conditioning time must also be carefully monitored. It should not be so long that important constituents, such as stearic acid, can be leached out, nor should it be so short that the material is not thoroughly softened. The materials are poor conductors of heat and it may take several minutes for the centre of the material to become softened. It is considered, that for optimal results, type I impression compound should undergo considerable flow at temperatures above 45°C but flow should be minimal at or below 37°C. The stick material is generally

Table 17.1 Composition of a typical impression compound material.

Component	Example	Function
Thermoplastic material (47%)	Natural or synthetic resins and waxes	Characterizes the softening temperature
Filler (50%)	Talc	Gives 'body' by increasing viscosity of the softened material; reduces thermal contraction
Lubricant (3%)	Stearic acid	Improves flow properties

softened using a bunsen burner. A measure of skill and experience is required in order to soften the material sufficiently without causing it to become too fluid or to ignite. The material is tempered in a water bath before placing in the patient's mouth.

The copper ring technique involves the recording of single crown preparations in stick compound employing a hollow, open-ended copper tube as a type of 'tray'. The principle is illustrated in Fig. 17.1. The surface of the compound is copper plated in an electroplating bath and an epoxy resin/metal die made. A separate locating impression is also recorded of the prepared tooth. The die is inserted into this impression and then a stone working model is made by pouring stone into the impression. This technique has largely been superseded by the use of silicone rubbers for crown and bridgework. However, it can be of value, particularly in areas where moisture control is a problem.

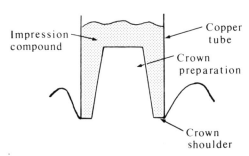

Fig. 17.1 Diagram illustrating the principle of the copper ring technique for obtaining impressions of crown preparations.

One of the main requirements for impression compound, set out in American and British Standards, is for the value of flow at mouth temperature (37°C) and 45°C (Table 17.2). It is this test which primarily distinguishes the type I and type II materials. The type I material should flow readily at just above mouth temperature, whilst the type II

Table 17.2 Flow of impression compound as required by ADA, specification no 3, and BS 3886.

Flow	at 37°C	at 45°C
Type I	20% or less[†] 6% or less[*]	85% or more
Type II	2% or less	between 70 and 85%

[*] ADA specification no 3.
[†] BS 3886.

material should ideally not distort at mouth temperature. The flow is measured at the stated temperature by applying a load of 2 kg to the flat ends of a cylindrical specimen 6 mm high by 10 mm diameter for 10 minutes.

The other main requirement of standards is for impression taking properties. This applies to type I materials only. The material should be capable of recording sharp grooves 0.2–4 mm wide cut into the surface of a metal test block.

Impression compound is the most viscous of the impression materials in common use. Table 17.3 gives typical values of viscosity for some materials, measured at a given shear rate. It can be seen that under these conditions the viscosity is some 70 times greater than that for impression plaster and more than 100 times greater than values for some of the light-bodied elastomers. The very high viscosity of impression compound is significant in two ways. Firstly, it limits the degree of fine detail which can be recorded in an impression. Secondly, it characterizes compound as a mucocompressive impression material. In certain circumstances, the high viscosity is used to advantage. For example, when recording impressions of some edentulous patients it is necessary to record the full depth of the sulcus so that a denture with adequate retention can be designed. Only a viscous material, such as compound, is able to displace the lingual and buccal soft tissues sufficiently.

Table 17.3 Viscosity values for some impression materials.*

Material	Viscosity (Pas)
Impression compound	4000
Impression plaster	60
Zinc oxide/eugenol paste	60
Alginate	50
Light-bodied elastomer	30
'Putty' elastomer	800

* Measured at $50\,s^{-1}$ shear rate at 23°C and 1 minute after mixing – for materials which require mixing.

Compound is fairly rigid after setting and has poor elastic properties. A large stress would be required to remove an impression from undercut areas and the resultant impression would be grossly distorted. The materials have large values of coefficient of thermal expansion and undergo considerable shrinkage on removal from the mouth. This can be partially overcome by resoftening the surface of the impression with a bunsen flame and reseating the impression.

Three factors combine to produce significant internal stresses within the compound impression.

(1) The high value of coefficient of thermal expansion.
(2) The poor thermal conductivity.
(3) The relatively large temperature drop from the softening temperature to room temperature.

The gradual relief of internal stresses may cause distortion of the impression. For the most accurate results, the model should be poured as soon as possible after recording the impression.

Impression compound is most widely used for recording preliminary impressions of edentulous arches. The high viscosity of the material enables the full depth of the sulcus to be recorded. This gives a model on which a special tray can be constructed. A major impression is recorded in the special tray using a less viscous material, such as zinc oxide/eugenol impression paste.

The use of impression compound has declined markedly over recent years as newer materials and techniques have become available. The declining use of impression compound is reflected in the lack of any development of an international standard (ISO) for these materials. Impression compound is still used widely in stick form to modify/refine the peripheral extent of a special tray, particularly for complete dentures or in the edentulous regions for partial dentures. Denture retention relies on a number of factors including developing an adequate border seal around the denture against the soft tissues. This is achieved by extending the denture so that it just begins to displace the movable soft tissues at the periphery of the denture. Obviously such extensions cannot impinge on areas of muscle activity or the denture will be displaced in function. Thus, there is a need to record a dynamic shape of the oral soft tissues. This is achieved by trimming back the special tray until it is just short of the lines of movement of the mucosa. The periphery of the tray is then coated in softened 'green stick' tracing compound and the tray replaced in the mouth. The cheeks are then manipulated by the dentist to simulate functional movement to produce a dynamically generated shape in the softened thermoplastic material. Care must be taken to ensure that the patient is not burnt during this process.

Green stick compound is also used to provide localized mucocompression at the distal extent of the palatal coverage for an upper denture. This is necessary to give border seal in this area (the post

dam) when using an otherwise mucostatic impression technique.

17.4 Impression waxes

Impression waxes are rarely used to record complete impressions but are normally used to correct small imperfections in other impressions, particularly those of the zinc oxide/eugenol type. They are thermoplastic materials which flow readily at mouth temperature and are relatively soft even at room temperature. They are applied with a brush in small quantities to 'fill in' areas of impressions in which insufficient material has been used or in which an 'air blow' or crease has caused a defect.

Waxes can also be used to produce a mucocompressive impression of the edentulous saddles for a lower, free-end saddle partial denture – the so-called Applegate technique. The wax is first melted before being applied to the area of the impression that is faulty or to the impression tray. The impression tray is then returned to the mouth and should be reseated with firm finger pressure. It is important to leave the impression in the mouth for sufficient time to raise the wax to oral temperature so it will undergo plastic flow under pressure to record accurately the denture bearing area.

These materials consist, typically, of a mixture of a low melting paraffin wax and beeswax in a ratio of about 3:1. This composition ensures a very high degree of flow at mouth temperature.

17.5 Zinc oxide/eugenol impression pastes

These materials are normally supplied as two pastes which are mixed together on a paper pad or glass slab. Typical compositions of the two pastes are given in Table 17.4. There is normally a good colour contrast between the two pastes, the zinc oxide paste, typically, being white and the eugenol paste, a reddish brown colour. This enables thorough mixing to be achieved as indicated by a homogeneous colour, free of streaks, in the mixed material.

The pastes are normally dispensed from toothpaste-like tubes and are mixed in equal volumes. The proportioning is achieved, simply, by expression equal lengths of each paste onto the mixing pad or slab. The manufacturers normally label one of the tubes as the catalyst paste and the other the base paste. Some manufacturers refer to the zinc oxide paste as the catalyst paste, whilst others refer to it as the base paste.

On mixing the two pastes, a reaction between zinc oxide and eugenol begins. Figure 17.2 gives the

Table 17.4 Composition of impression pastes.

	Component	Function
Paste 1	Zinc oxide	Reactive ingredient which takes part in setting reaction
	Olive oil, linseed oil or equivalent	Inert component used to form paste with zinc oxide
	Zinc acetate or equivalent (in small quantities)	To accelerate setting
	Water (trace) in some products	To accelerate setting
Paste 2	Eugenol (oil of cloves)	Reactive ingredient – takes part in setting reaction
	Kaolin, talc or equivalent	Inert filler used to form a paste with eugenol

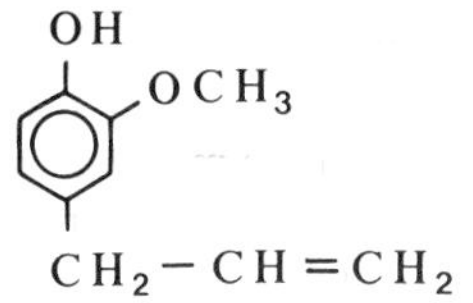

Fig. 17.2 Structural formula of eugenol.

structural formula of eugenol. The basis of the reaction is that the phenolic – OH of the eugenol acts as a weak acid and undergoes an acid – base reaction with zinc oxide to form a salt, zinc eugenolate, as follows:

$$2C_{10}H_{12}O_2 + ZnO \rightarrow Zn(C_{10}H_{11}O_2)_2 + H_2O$$

Two molecules of eugenol react with zinc oxide to form the salt. The structural formula of zinc euge-nolate is given in Fig. 17.3. It can be seen that the ionic salt bonds are formed between zinc and the phenolic oxygens of each molecule of eugenol. Two further co-ordinate bonds are formed by donation of pairs of electrons from the methoxy oxygens to zinc. These bonds are indicated by the arrows in Fig. 17.3. Although the structural formula shows the two aromatic rings lying in the plane of the paper, in fact,

they occupy perpendicular planes, such that one ring is in the plane of the paper whilst the other is in a plane at 90° to the plane of the paper. The structure can, therefore, be visualized as a central zinc atom held by two eugenol 'claws'. Compounds with this type of structure are normally referred to as *chelate compounds*.

The setting reaction is ionic in nature and requires an ionic medium in which to proceed at any pace. The ionic nature is increased by the presence of water and certain ionizable salts which act as accel-erators. Some manufacturers do not incorporate water into the pastes and for these materials setting is retarded until the mixed paste contacts moisture in the patient's mouth. Water is then absorbed and setting is accelerated. Other manufacturers include water as a component of at least one of the pastes, in order that setting can commence immediately after mixing.

These materials are normally used to record the major impressions of edentulous arches. The impression is normally recorded in a close-fitting special tray, constructed on the model obtained from the primary impression, or inside the patient's existing denture. The periphery of the special tray or denture needs to be modified with tracing compound to ensure appropriate contour of the impression and to give support to the paste in these critical areas.

The thickness of paste used is normally around 1 mm. This thin section of material results in an insignificant dimensional change on setting and subsequent storage of the impression. The relatively low initial viscosity of the mixed paste, coupled with its pseudoplastic nature, allows fine detail to be recorded in the impression. Defects sometimes arise on the surface of the impression but these can be corrected using an impression wax.

The major restriction on the use of these materials is their lack of elasticity. The set material may distort or fracture when removed over undercuts. The materials are sometimes used to record small undercuts in soft tissues but the tendency of some pastes to flow under relatively small pressures should be remembered. There is some variation in the properties of set impression pastes. Some are rela-tively hard and brittle when set, resembling impres-

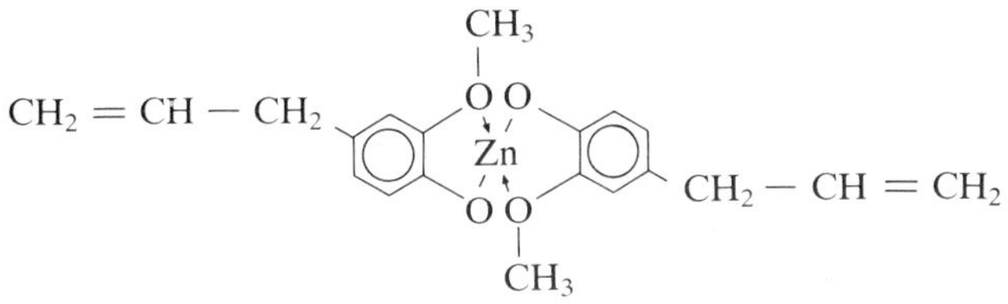

Fig. 17.3 Structural formula of zinc eugenolate.

sion plaster in this respect. Others show a less precise set point appearing to only increase in viscosity during setting, remaining relatively soft after several minutes. Naturally there is a greater tendency for the soft materials to undergo flow during the removal of the impression. Use of either the soft or hard type impression pastes depends more on operator preference than on any logical scientific argument.

For the vast majority of patients the zinc oxide eugenol impression pastes may be considered non-irritant. Occasionally, however, eugenol may promote an allergic response in some patients. To cater for this type of patient, eugenol-free zinc oxide impression pastes are available. The eugenol is replaced by an alternative organic acid.

The properties of impression pastes which are embodied as requirements of standards vary from one national standard to another. The fact that there is no International Standard (ISO) for these products is probably indicative of the declining use of these materials. ADA specification no 16 sets out requirements for consistency and hardness which are used to categorize impression pastes as either type 1 (hard) or type II (soft) as well as limiting the values of initial and final setting times. BS specification 4284 includes a test for consistency but materials are not classified as 'hard' or 'soft' in this standard.

Also within BS4284 are requirements for working time and setting time as determined by a rheometer, strain in compression, dimensional stability, impression taking properties and compatibility with gypsum. For strain in compression a cylindrical sample 20 mm high by 12.5 mm diameter is subjected to a load of 500 g across the flat ends of the cylinder. A maximum strain of 12% is allowed. However, a weakness of this test is that no attempt is made to differentiate between elastic and plastic strain. It is probably safe to assume that for these materials the strain will be primarily plastic in nature. The impression taking properties are determined from the ability to reproduce fine engraved lines on a metal block. The finest line is only 0.025 mm wide. The dimensional stability is determined by measuring the extent to which the distance between two fixed points on the surface of a sample of set material changes between 15 minutes and 6 hours. The maximum allowed change is only 0.02%. These requirements confirm the ability of the materials to record fine detail and their good dimensional stability. In addition to recording conventional non-undercut impressions the materials described in this chapter have also traditionally been used for recording interocclusal relationships, although there is now increased use of elastomeric materials for this purpose.

Chapter 18
Elastic Impression Materials: Hydrocolloids

18.1 Introduction

Hydrocolloid impression materials used in dentistry are based on colloidal suspensions of polysaccharides in water. A colloidal suspension is characterized by the fact that it behaves neither as a solution, in which the solute is dissolved in the solvent, nor as a true suspension, in which a heterogeneous structure exists with solid particles being suspended in a liquid. The colloidal suspension lies somewhere between these two extremes; no solid particles can be detected and yet the mixture does not behave as a simple solution. The molecules of the colloid remain dispersed by nature of the fact that they carry small electrical charges and repel one another within the dispersing medium. When the fluid medium of the colloid is water it is normally referred to as a hydrocolloid.

Dental hydrocolloid impression materials exist in two forms: sol or gel form. In the sol form, they are fluid with low viscosity and there is a random arrangement of the polysaccharide chains. In the gel form, the materials are more viscous and may develop elastic properties if the long polysaccharide chains become aligned. Alignment of the polysaccharide chains as *fibrils* which enclose the fluid phase normally causes the gel to develop a consistency similar to that of jelly. The greater the concentration of fibrils within the gel the stronger the jelly structure will be. This point is best illustrated by consideration of the properties of commercial, flavoured gelatin (jelly). The material which is initially purchased is a fairly strong gel but after dilution with water the resulting gel is much weaker. This is relevant to dental hydrocolloids since the strength of the gel is important and depends on the concentration of polysaccharide material dispersed in the aqueous phase.

The conversion from sol to gel forms the basis of the setting of the hydrocolloid impression materials. The products are introduced into the patient's mouth while in the fluid, sol form. When conversion to gel is complete, and elastic properties have been developed, the impression is removed and the model cast.

The formation of gel and development of elastic properties through alignment of polysaccharide chains may take place by one of two mechanisms. For some materials, gel formation is induced by cooling the sol. Chains become aligned and are mutually attracted by Van der Waals forces. Intermolecular hydrogen bonds may be formed between adjacent chains, enhancing the elasticity of the gel. On reheating the gel, these bonds are readily destroyed and the material reverts to the sol form. These materials are the *reversible hydrocolloids* (agar). The principle of gel formation is given in Fig. 18.1.

For other materials, gel formation involves the production of strong intermolecular cross-links between polysaccharide chains. These materials do not require cooling in order to encourage gel formation and once formed the gel does not readily revert to the sol form. These materials are the *irreversible hydrocolloids* (alginates).

18.2 Reversible hydrocolloids (agar)

These materials are normally supplied as a gel in a flexible, toothpaste-like tube or syringe. The gel consists primarily of a 15% colloidal suspension of agar in water. Agar is a complex polysaccharide which is extracted from seaweed. Figure 18.2 gives a very simplified indication of the type of molecular structure. The high molecular weight, coupled with the large concentration of free hydroxyl groups, renders the material suitable for hydrocolloid formation.

Small quantities of borax and potassium sulphate are normally present in the gel. Borax is added to

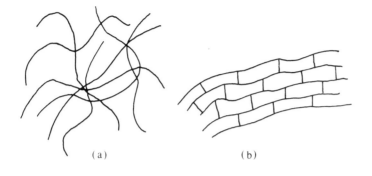

Fig. 18.1 Diagram illustrating the formation of an aqueous polysaccharide gel by ordering of the polymer chains. (a) Disordered chains (present in sol). (b) Ordered chains (present in gel). Chemical cross-links are formed in irreversible materials.

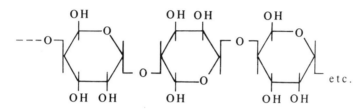

Fig. 18.2 Simplified structural formula of a polysaccharide chain similar to that used in agar.

give more 'body' to the gel, although the mechanism by which this is achieved is unclear. Unfortunately, borax retards the setting of gypsum model and die materials and models formed in agar impressions may have surfaces of poor quality. The presence of potassium sulphate in the agar gel counteracts this effect of the borax, since it accelerates the setting of gypsum products (see p. 33). Alternatively, the impression may be dipped in a solution of accelerator.

Manipulation: Reversible hydrocolloids are normally conditioned, prior to use, using a specially designed conditioning bath. This consists of three compartments each containing water (Fig. 18.3).

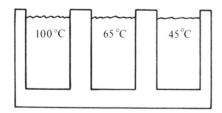

Fig. 18.3 A specialized water bath used for conditioning agar impression material.

The tube or syringe of gel is first placed in the 100°C bath. This rapidly converts the gel to sol and the contents of the tube become very fluid. The tube is then transferred to the 65°C bath where it is stored until required for use. This temperature is high enough to maintain the material in the sol form. At this stage, the material is mixed by squeezing the tube, thus ensuring an even distribution of components. A few minutes before the impression is recorded, the contents are cooled to 45°C. If the material is maintained at this temperature for long, it slowly begins to revert to the gel form. When the impression is recorded, the sol is expressed from the tube into an impression tray and seated in the patient's mouth. Reversible hydrocolloids are available in a variety of viscosities to help us achieve high levels of accuracy for use in crown and bridgework. A high viscosity sol is transferred from the tempering bath into a stock tray and a low viscosity material can be syringed directly onto the prepared teeth. The tray is then inserted into the mouth over the teeth concerned. There is a temperature hysteresis effect on the gel to sol and sol to gel transition in that the latter process occurs at a lower temperature than the gel to sol transition. The conversion from sol to gel takes place slowly at mouth temperature and it may be many minutes before the material develops sufficient elasticity to permit removal of the impression. The rate of conversion of sol to gel may be accelerated by spraying cold water onto the impression tray whilst it is in the mouth, or by using water-cooled impression trays. The latter are metal stock trays with a narrow-bore metal tube attached to the outer surface. The tube is connected to a cold water supply and the circulating water reduces the temperature of the tray. The coolest areas of the sol are converted to gel more rapidly, so the material in contact with the tray sets more rapidly than that in contact with the oral tissues. It is argued that this arrangement may be advantageous. If slight movements of the impression tray take place during setting, the material adjacent to the oral tissues can flow to compensate, thus reducing inaccuracies.

Removal from the mouth is accomplished with a snapping action. The reversible hydrocolloids are very susceptible to water uptake and loss (syneresis and imbibition). After recording an impression it should be rinsed to remove debris and then stored covered in a damp gauze. The model should be poured within 30 minutes of the impression being recorded. It is not possible to use a hydrocolloid impression to make metal coated or epoxy resin dies.

One clinical advantage of the reversible hydrocolloids relates to their ability to take up moisture. A poorly fitting provisional crown can result in gingival inflammation and an increased rate of crevicular fluid flow. In turn this makes the recording of an accurate impression of the crown margins more difficult. When a reversible hydrocolloid is used in such patients it tends to 'draw' moisture from the marginal gingival tissues. This has the effect of producing a relatively poor first impression but a greater chance of success with the second as the levels of fluid flow will be decreased. It is possible to re-use reversible hydrocolloids. However, concerns about cross-infection control and alteration to the material's physical properties by altered water content and the incorporation of small chips of dental stone into the material during repeated use make this approach unacceptable.

Properties: Many of the important properties of agar impression materials are embodied in the ISO Standard for dental aqueous impression materials based on agar, ISO 1564. This standard classifies materials according to consistency as:

Type 1   high consistency
Type 2   medium consistency
Type 3   low consistency

Some of these products can be used alone to record impressions whilst others are designed to be used in techniques requiring two materials of different consistency. For example, the type 1 material can be used for making impressions of complete or partial dental arches with or without the use of syringe-extruded increments of type 2 or 3 material. When type 1 is used in combination with types 2 or 3 the type 1 material is softened and extruded into the impression tray whilst the type 2 or 3 material is extruded from a syringe into the mouth to cover the area which is to be recorded.

The type 2 materials are multi-purpose in appli-

cation as they can also be used for making impressions of complete and partial dental arches with or without the use of a syringe-extruded increment, but these products can also themselves be syringe-extruded for use in the *combination* technique. The type 3 materials are designed specifically for syringe use and are used with a type 1 or type 2 material in the combination technique. Table 18.1 gives some of the requirements of type 1 and type 2 materials compared with alginate materials. In the sol form, agar is sufficiently fluid to allow detailed reproduction of hard and soft oral tissues. Its low viscosity classifies it as a mucostatic material, as it does not compress or displace soft tissues. The requirement for detail reproduction in ISO 1564 is tested through confirming that the material is able to reproduce a 0.02 mm line on a metal test block. In order to demonstrate compatibility with gypsum a line 0.05 mm thick must be reproduced when a gypsum cast is prepared from an agar impression.

Table 18.1 Comparison of the requirements of reversible and irreversible hydrocolloid impression materials (ISO 1564 and ISO 1563).

	Reversible (agar)	Irreversible (alginate)
Strain in compression (%)	4 min, 15 max	5 min 20 max
Recovery from deformation (%)	96.5 min	95 min
Detail reproduction (mm)	0.02	0.05
Compatibility with gypsum (mm)	0.05	0.05
Resistance to tearing (N/mm)	0.75	—
Compressive strength (MPa)	—	0.35

In the gel form, agar is sufficiently flexible to be withdrawn past undercuts. In the standard test for agar materials (ISO 1564) this requirement is tested using a cylinder of material 20 mm long and 12.5 mm diameter. The height of the cylinder is measured under a minor load of 125 g and then under a major load of 1.25 kg. The resulting strain in compression produced by changing from the minor to the major load is required to be between 4% and 15%. This is great enough to ensure that the set material can be readily removed from undercuts, but not so great that the material undergoes deformation under the load of the gypsum model material.

The materials are viscoelastic and the elastic recovery can be optimized by using correct technique. A suitable model used to explain the nature of viscoelastic materials is described on p. 13 (see Fig. 2.15). The amount of permanent deformation exhibited by a viscoelastic impression material is a function of the severity of the undercuts and the time for which the material is under stress during the removal of the impression. The elastic recovery is enhanced and permanent deformation reduced if the impression is removed in one quick movement, ensuring that the impression material is under stress only momentarily. Elastic recovery or recovery from deformation is another requirement of the international standard for agar impression materials (ISO 1564). A cylindrical specimen 20 mm high and 12.5 mm diameter is compressed by 4 mm (i.e. 20% of its height) for one second. Following this compression the material is required to exhibit at least 96.5% recovery – expressed as a percentage of the original specimen length.

Agar gel has very poor mechanical properties and tears at very low levels of stress. Interproximal and subgingival areas are very difficult to record with this type of impression material. Tear resistance is determined (ISO 1564) using a specimen of the type shown in Fig. 18.4. The specimen is gripped at each end and then stretched and the force required to propagate a tear from the notch tip is determined. The tear resistance (T_s) is calculated as:

$$T_s = F/d \text{ N/mm}$$

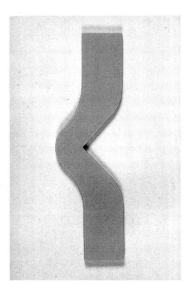

Fig. 18.4 Specimen used for determination of tear resistance of impression materials based on agar.

where F is the maximum force and d is the thickness of the specimen. The standard requires that T_s should be at least 0.75 N/mm for type 1 and type 2 materials and 0.5 N/mm for type 3 materials.

The material has very poor dimensional stability – a function of the very high water content of the gel. On standing, water is readily lost by a combination of syneresis and evaporation. The process of *syneresis* may be envisaged as a squeezing out of water from between polysaccharide chains. As a result, one can often observe small droplets of water on the surface of an agar impression. The water may be lost by evaporation, causing shrinkage of the impression and seriously affecting accuracy.

In the presence of excess water, agar gel may absorb water by a process which is, effectively, the reverse of syneresis. This process is referred to as *imbibition*. When water is imbibed it causes a separation of the aligned polysaccharide chains and a swelling of the impression. In order to assure optimum accuracy the model should be cast as soon as possible.

The primary uses of agar impressions are for partial denture and crown and bridge patients. For these applications, the poor tear resistance is considered to be their major disadvantage.

The materials are widely used as laboratory duplicating materials. For this application their main advantage is that the material can be re-used, a significant factor in this application where the products are used in relatively large bulk. In the construction of partial dentures and orthodontic appliances it is often necessary to produce more than one cast. It is not always possible or advisable to pour two or more casts from one impression and in such cases the first cast is duplicated using a reversible hydrocolloid duplicating material.

The technique for duplication involves standing the cast on a glass slab surrounded by a metal duplicating flask which is designed to allow an even thickness of material all round. The duplicating hydrocolloid, which is normally thinner in consistency than the impression hydrocolloids, is heated to cause conversion to the sol state and then allowed to cool to about 50°C before use. The fluid material is then poured through a hole in the top of the duplicating flask until the flask is full and excess material spills from an overflow vent in the flask. The material is best poured at as low a temperature as possible, whilst maintaining the sol state, in order to minimize contractions which occur during gelation.

A further means of reducing contraction effects is to cool the flask from the base to prevent the colloid from shrinking away from the cast. When gelation is complete the master cast is removed with a rapid movement rather than by easing it away, in order to optimize elastic recovery within the gel.

Reversible hydrocolloids are viscoelastic materials and are likely to undergo permanent deformation if subjected to stresses for more than a few seconds. The duplicate cast should be poured straight away after removal of the master cast in order to avoid dimensional changes in the hydrocolloid caused by syneresis. Setting of gypsum casts in contact with hydrocolloids may be inhibited by the presence of Borax in the latter. This potential problem can normally be avoided by treating the surface of the hydrocolloid with an accelerator for gypsum, such as potassium sulphate.

18.3 Irreversible hydrocolloids (alginates)

Alginate impression materials are supplied as powders which are mixed with water. The typical composition of an alginate powder is given in Table 18.2. The relative concentration of each ingredient varies from one product to another. Some alginates are more fluid than others because they contain less filler, while some products are faster setting than others because they contain less trisodium phosphate.

Manipulation: The normal method of dispensing the materials is in large tubs. Scoops are provided for measuring the powder whilst plastic measuring cylinders are generally used to meter the correct volume of water. An alternative method of dispensation is to supply the alginate powder in small sachets. The contents of one sachet are sufficient for one impression. The operator simply adds the correct volume of water. This ensures a correct concentration of ingredients in each impression. Materials supplied in tubs have a tendency to undergo separation as the dense ingredients fall to the bottom of the container. This must be overcome by inverting the container before use. It also prevents compaction of the powder and ensures that a reproducible volume of material is used in each mix. After proportioning, the powder and water are mixed together in a plastic mixing bowl using a wide-bladed spatula. Rapid spatulation is required to give thorough mixing and an alginate sol of 'creamy' consistency. The material is used in either stock trays or special trays and an adhesive is used to aid retention of the impression material to the tray.

Setting reaction: On mixing and spatulating the powder and water, an alginate sol is formed. The sodium phosphate, present in the powder, dissolves readily in the water whilst the gypsum is only sparingly soluble (solubility about 0.2%).

The structural formula of sodium alginate is given in Fig. 18.5a. This may be represented by the simplified structure given in Fig. 18.5b for the purpose of clarifying the setting reaction.

Sodium alginate readily reacts with calcium ions derived from the dissolved gypsum to form calcium alginate, as shown in Fig. 18.6. The replacement of monovalent sodium with divalent calcium results in the cross-linking of the alginate chains and the conversion of the material from the sol to gel form. As the setting reaction proceeds, and the degree of cross-linking increases, the gel develops elastic properties.

Sodium phosphate plays an important role in controlling the setting characteristics of alginate materials. It reacts rapidly with calcium ions as they are formed giving insoluble calcium phosphate:

$$3Ca^{2+} + 2Na_3PO_4 \rightarrow Ca_3(PO_4)_2 + 6Na^+$$

This reaction denies the supply of calcium ions required to complete the cross-linking of alginate chains and thus extends the working time of the

Table 18.2 Composition of alginate impression material powders.

Material	Amount (%)	Function
Sodium or potassium salt of alginic acid	11–16	Main reactive ingredient; forms sol with water and becomes cross-linked to form gel
$CaSO_4 . 2H_2O$ (gypsum)	11–17	Source of Ca^{2+} ions which cause cross-linking of the alginate chains
Na_3PO_4	1–3	Used to control the working time
Inert filler – such as diatomaceous earth	65–75	Gives 'body' and enables easy manipulation
Reaction indicator (present in some products)		Gives a colour change when setting is complete

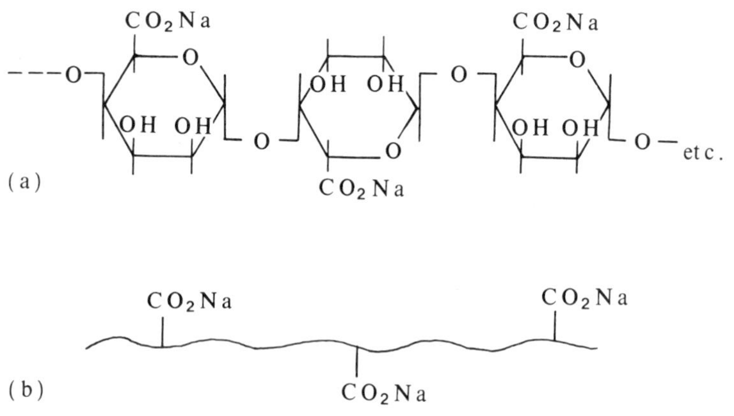

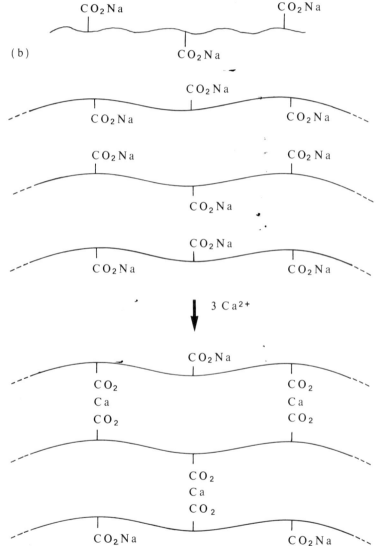

(a)

(b)

Fig. 18.5 The structural formula of sodium alginate. (a) Actual formula. (b) Simplified formula.

$3 \, Ca^{2+}$

Fig. 18.6 Schematic representation of the cross-linking of alginate chains by replacement of sodium ions with calcium ions.

material. When all the sodium phosphate has reacted, calcium ions become available for reaction with sodium alginate, the setting reaction is initiated and the viscosity of the material increases rapidly.

Properties: The freshly spatulated material has low viscosity (see Table 17.3), although this can be varied to some extent by alterations in the amount of inert filler incorporated by the manufacturer. The low viscosity, coupled with a degree of pseudoplasticity, classifies alginates as mucostatic impression materials. They are able to record soft tissues in the uncompressed state. For some applications low viscosity may be a disadvantage, for example, when trying to record the depth of the lingual sulcus. A higher viscosity is required to displace the lingual soft tissues in order that the full depth can be recorded.

It follows from the description of the setting reaction that these products go through an induction period following mixing, during which the viscosity remains almost unaltered. This is followed by rapid setting. The setting characteristics of these materials, therefore, approach the ideal requirement of adequate working time followed by rapid setting. They are almost unique from this point of view. The setting characteristics can be further controlled by the operator by fixing the temperature of the water used. The use of warm water reduces the working time and setting time both by accelerating the rate at which sodium phosphate is consumed and by subsequently increasing the rate of the cross-linking reaction. The use of cold water, naturally, has the reverse effect.

In contrast to the reversible hydrocolloids, alginate material adjacent to the oral tissues sets more rapidly, while that adjacent to the cooler tray wall sets more slowly. Hence, the operator must ensure that the impression tray is not moved during setting, otherwise distortions occur.

Some of the properties of dental alginate impression materials are outlined in the requirements of ISO 1564. These are outlined in Table 18.2 where a comparison with the agar products can be made. Alginate is commonly used in bulk within a stock or an appropriately spaced special tray. Greater levels of accuracy of occlusal and interproximal area are achieved if the surfaces of the teeth are dried and excess alginate is smeared onto the tooth surfaces using a finger. This helps to prevent the incorporation of air bubbles in the surface of the impression, which would be manifest as 'pimples' on the surface of the models of the teeth.

Following setting, the material is flexible and elastic enough to be withdrawn past undercuts, although it should be remembered that, as for agar, the alginate materials are viscoelastic and due regard to this should be made when withdrawing the impression from the patient's mouth (see Section 18.2). The degree of cross-linking continues to increase after the material has apparently set. Waiting a further minute or two before removing the impression enhances the elastic nature of the materials.

Reference to Table 18.2 indicates that typically alginate and agar materials are equally flexible and the range of strain in compression values allowed is similar for the two materials. Some alginate products are more flexible as indicated by the higher maximum value of strain in compression. Elastic recovery is similar for the two materials, although the standards require agar materials to have a slightly higher recovery from deformation. Alginate gels have poor mechanical properties and are liable to tear when removed from deep undercuts, particularly in interproximal and subgingival areas. Curiously the ISO Standard for alginate materials does not specify a requirement for resistance to tearing but instead specifies a minimum compressive strength (Table 18.2). Since these materials are more likely to fracture by tearing in tension than through crushing in compression it is likely that this shortcoming will be addressed in future editions of the standard.

Permanent distortions due to viscoelastic effects and tearing are reduced slightly by using a large bulk of material. It is normal to have approximately 3–5 mm of material between the tissues and the tray.

The model should be cast as soon as possible, in order to prevent inaccuracies due to dimensional changes, because alginate impressions undergo syneresis and imbibition by the same mechanisms described for agar (see Section 18.2). The impressions may be stored for a short time if covered with a damp napkin.

Alginate impression materials are widely used for a variety of applications. In prosthodontics, they are used for recording impressions of edentulous and partially dentate arches. In orthodontics, they are used for recording impressions prior to appliance construction and they are used extensively for recording impressions for study model construction. They are only rarely used for crown and bridge work because their poor tear resistance is a serious disadvantage when considering this application.

Decontamination: Over recent years the need for strict cross-infection control in dentistry has taken on a new significance, as stated earlier. The need for a simple and effective means for the decontamination of impressions has been identified. Most such procedures involve treatment in aqueous solutions of hypochlorite or aldehyde (formaldehyde or glutaraldehyde). For both agar and alginate type materials soaking in aqueous media presents a potential problem because of the previously mentioned process of imbition which causes dimensional change and distortion. Evidence is emerging that for alginates a relatively short term treatment (approximately 10 minutes) can be effective without causing undue dimensional change. Alternatively, the use of rinsing combined with short 'dips' in glutaraldehyde solution or the use of a hypochlorite spray has been suggested. An alternative is to disinfect the poured stone cast by immersing it in sodium hypochlorite, again for 10 minutes.

18.4 Combined reversible/irreversible techniques

Techniques involving the combined use of reversible and irreversible hydrocolloids have been advocated in recent years. The technique involves loading a conventional impression tray with alginate material and syringing reversible hydrocolloid around the region of the mouth to be recorded. The bulk of the final impression therefore consists of alginate whilst the surface close to the hard and soft oral tissues consists of reversible hydrocolloid.

The technique is claimed to give the good surface detail reproduction of a reversible hydrocolloid impression whilst overcoming some of the problems of using this material alone. The thin layer of reversible material sets relatively quickly without the need to use special water-cooled trays. The combined materials suffer many of the disadvantages of their parent materials however, such as poor dimensional stability and poor strength.

The ISO Standard for dental reversible/irreversible hydrocolloid impression material system requires that the two materials used together in the system should each satisfy the requirements of the relevant standards for reversible (agar) and irreversible (alginate) materials. They should also be able to bond together adequately as demonstrated by a tensile bond strength in excess of 50 kPa between the two materials. A further requirement is that the dimensional change in the impression after 20 minutes, recorded with the combined materials, should be no greater than 1% when the impression is stored at 23°C and 95% relative humidity.

18.5 Modified alginates

Alginates modified by the incorporation of silicone polymers have been developed. These are supplied as two pastes which are mixed together. A colour contrast between the pastes enables thorough mixing to be achieved although this can be difficult because the pastes are of widely differing viscosity in some products.

The setting characteristics of the modified alginate materials are similar to those of the conventional products. They show marginally better fine-detail reproduction and tear resistance but have poor dimensional stability. They lose water at about the same rate as a conventional alginate if allowed to stand. Casts should be poured soon after recording impression if accuracy is to be maintained.

The materials are considered as hybrids of alginates and silicone elastomers but their properties are closely related to those of the alginates.

18.6 Suggested further reading

Owen, C.P. & Goolam, R. (1993) Disinfection of impression materials to prevent viral cross contamination: A review and a protocol. *Int. J. Pros*, **6**, 480.

ISO 1563 Dental alginate impression material.

ISO 1564 Dental aqueous impression materials based on agar.

ISO 13716 Dental reversible/irreversible hydrocolloid impression material systems.

Chapter 19
Elastic Impression Materials: Synthetic Elastomers

19.1 Introduction

Synthetic elastomers were developed mainly for industrial applications but their potential in medicine and dentistry was quickly realized and they are now widely used as impression materials. They were quick to gain acceptance in dentistry because they offered potential solutions to the two main problems associated with hydrocolloids – poor tear resistance and poor dimensional stability.

Four types of elastomers are in general use:

- Polysulphides;
- Silicone rubbers (condensation curing type);
- Silicone rubbers (addition curing type);
- Polyethers.

A classification and some properties of these materials is given in the ISO Standard for Dental Elastomeric Impression Materials (ISO 4823). Apart from the chemical nature of the material, the primary method of classification is according to consistency. This is measured by pressing 0.5 ml of mixed material between two flat plates using a force of 1.5 N. The consistency, defined by the average diameter of the resulting disc of the material, is related to the viscosity of the material at the time when the force is applied. Materials are categorized as types 0–3, as shown in Table 19.1.

The specification limits defining consistency overlap significantly between types. Hence, a material producing a disc of 31–34 mm diameter could be classified as type 0, 1 or 2. It is the manufacturer who makes the choice in this situation. The situation is further complicated by the use of terms such as 'soft putty', which generally indicates a type 0 material, with a relatively low viscosity (high consistency disc diameter). The situation is clarified somewhat by consideration of the manner in which the materials are used. Types 0 and 1 are normally

Table 19.1 Classification of elastomeric impression materials according to consistency.

Type	Description	Consistency test disc diameter (mm)	
		Min	Max
0	Very high consistency (putty like)	—	35
1	High consistency (heavy bodied)	—	35
2	Medium consistency (medium bodied)	31	41
3	Low consistency (light bodied)	36	—

used in combination with a type 3 material whilst type 2 materials are normally used alone and are sometimes referred to as monophase elastomeric materials. Manufacturers often package their materials in a manner which reflects their preferred combination of high viscosity (type 0 or 1) and low viscosity (type 3) product. The techniques for using the combined high and low viscosity materials are described later in this chapter.

19.2 Polysulphides

Composition: These materials are generally supplied as two pastes which are dispensed from tubes. One paste is normally labelled base paste whilst the other is labelled catalyst paste. The composition of a typical material is given in Table 19.2.

The liquid polysulphide prepolymer in the base paste can be represented by the formula:

$$HS(C_2H_4 - OCH_2 - OC_2H_4 - SS)_{23} - C_2H_4 - OCH_2 - OC_2H_4 - SH$$

Table 19.2 Composition of polysulphide impression materials.

	Component	Function
Base paste	Polysulphide prepolymer with terminal and pendant thiol (–SH) groups	This is further polymerized and cross-linked to form rubber
	Plasticizer–di-*n*-butyl phthalate	To control viscosity
	Inert filler – possibly chalk or titanium dioxide	To give 'body', control viscosity and modify physical properties
Catalyst paste	Lead dioxide or other alternative oxidizing agent	To react with thiol groups – causing setting
	Sulphur	Involved in setting reaction
	Inert oil – normally paraffinic type or di-*n*-butyl phthalate	To form a paste with PbO_2 and sulphur

although the actual structure is known to be slightly more complex than this and contains pendant thiol groups (– SH) in addition to the terminal groups shown in the structural formula. For mechanistic purposes the structure of the prepolymer is conveniently represented by the simplified structure given in Fig. 19.1. The viscosity of the paste is governed by the quantity of filler incorporated by the manufacturer. Three grades of paste are normally available to the practitioner – 'light-bodied', 'regular-bodied' and 'heavy-bodied', having increasing filler contents and viscosity values.

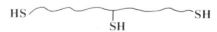

Fig. 19.1 Simplified structural formula of the polysulphide prepolymer showing terminal and pendant – SH groups.

The base paste is normally white, due to the filler, and has an unpleasant odour caused by the high concentration of thiol groups. The colour of the catalyst paste is governed by the nature of the oxidizing agent used; materials containing lead dioxide are normally dark brown. The colour contrast between the two pastes is an aid to efficient mixing, which is continued until a homogeneous colour, with no streaks, is achieved. An adhesive is used to promote adhesion between the impression material and tray.

Setting reaction: On mixing the two pastes, terminal and pendant thiol groups of the prepolymer chains undergo a reaction with lead dioxide. Some of these reactions result in chain extension and cross-linking as shown in Fig. 19.2. The reaction is of the *condensation polymerization* type since one molecule of water is produced as a byproduct of each reaction stage. As chain extension proceeds, the viscosity increases. When the degree of cross-linking reaches a certain level the material develops elastic properties.

Properties: The setting characteristics of the polysulphides differ considerably from those of the alginates (Section 18.3). Setting commences immediately on mixing of the two pastes and is characterized by a gradual increase in viscosity and a rather slow development of elasticity. Setting times of 10 minutes or more are not uncommon, particularly for light-bodied materials. The polysulphide elastomers have very good tear resistance. They can, typically, withstand about 700% tensile strain before tearing. Some of this strain is non-recoverable, since the elastic properties of these materials are far from ideal. They are considered as viscoelastic and recover only slowly and not completely after being compressed or stretched. The time required for recovery and the degree of permanent deformation are functions of the severity of the undercuts and the time for which the material is under strain. In order to optimize elastic recovery the impression should be removed with a single, swift pull.

Many of the properties of these products are directly related to the amount of filler incorporated in the pastes. This particularly applies to viscosity, setting contraction, thermal contraction after removal of the impression from the mouth and dimensional stability (Table 19.3). It can be seen that the heavy-bodied materials are potentially more accurate, since they exhibit less setting and thermal contraction and have better dimensional stability. Their high viscosity means that they are unable to record the same level of fine detail as the more fluid, light-bodied materials.

Dimensional changes occurring after apparent setting of polysulphides are due to two major factors. Firstly, continued reaction occurs for some time after the apparent setting time, causing further shrinkage. Secondly, water produced as a byproduct of the setting reaction may be lost by evaporation from the surface. In this case the dimensional change is also

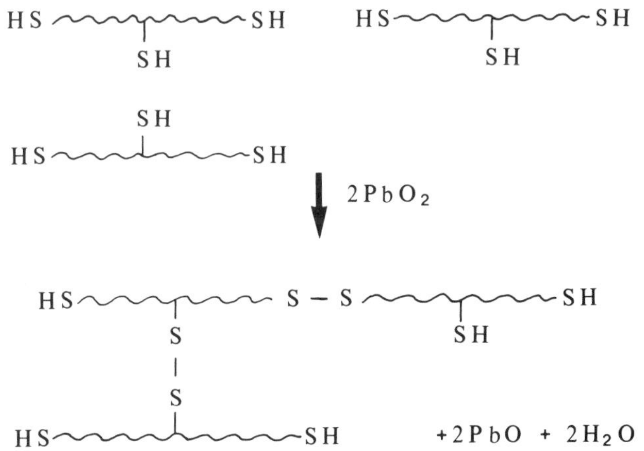

$$HS \sim\!\!\!\sim\!\!\!\sim\!\!\!\sim SH \qquad HS \sim\!\!\!\sim\!\!\!\sim\!\!\!\sim SH$$
$$\qquad\quad SH \qquad\qquad\qquad SH$$

$$SH$$
$$HS \sim\!\!\!\sim\!\!\!\sim SH$$

$$\downarrow 2\,PbO_2$$

$$HS \sim\!\!\!\sim\!\!\!\sim S - S \sim\!\!\!\sim\!\!\!\sim SH$$
$$\qquad\quad S \qquad\qquad\quad SH$$
$$\qquad\quad |$$
$$\qquad\quad S$$
$$HS \sim\!\!\!\sim\!\!\!\sim SH \qquad +2\,PbO + 2\,H_2O$$

Fig. 19.2 Schematic representation of the chain lengthening and cross-linking of the polysulphide prepolymer through oxidation of the –SH groups forming disulphide links. Water is liberated as a byproduct.

Table 19.3 Influence of filler content on some properties of polysulphides.

Filler content	Light-bodied	Viscosity	Setting contraction	Thermal contraction	Dimensional stability
|		|			|
Increasing	Regular-bodied	Increasing	|	|	|
↓		↓	Decreasing	Decreasing	Increasing
	Heavy-bodied		↓	↓	↓

associated with a change in weight of the material. The better dimensional stability of the heavy-bodied materials is due to the fact that they contain a lower concentration of reactive groups and therefore produce fewer byproducts. Although the polysulphides do not have perfect dimensional stability they perform far better than hydrocolloids in this respect.

The use of lead compounds in polysulphide materials has been questioned because of the known toxic effects of lead. It is unlikely that the lead contained in these products is able to exert a harmful effect as the material is in the patient's mouth for only a few minutes and is hydrophobic, reducing the chances of 'washing out' of lead compounds by saliva. The use of lead-free polysulphides is likely to increase, however, as a wider range of alternative materials becomes available.

Clinical Use: These materials are most commonly used in two viscosities, high and low, and must be used in a special tray. They have a number of advantages clinically, including reasonable tear strength and good elastic properties. They have an unpleasant odour and taste. They are moderately hydrophilic and hence can work well in the presence of some moisture. They are commonly used for crown and bridge impressions and only infrequently for other applications. The clinical technique usually adopted for polysulphides is a one-stage procedure.

Freshly mixed low viscosity material is loaded into an impression syringe and the high viscosity material is loaded into the special tray. The light-bodied material is injected around those teeth on which cavities have been cut or crown cores prepared. The tray, containing heavy-bodied material, is then seated so that the two materials can set simultaneously. Figure 19.3 is a line diagram which gives the appearance of the impression viewed in cross-section. It can be seen that the bulk of the impression is recorded in heavy-bodied material – assuring optimum accuracy and dimensional stability. The thin

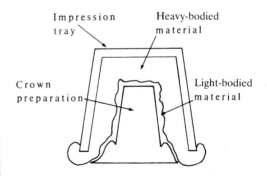

Fig. 19.3 Line diagram showing section of an impression in which heavy-bodied and light-bodied materials have been used to obtain optimal accuracy and dimensional stability.

layer of the impression adjacent to the oral tissues is recorded in light-bodied material – assuring optimum fine-detail reproduction.

Once set the casts can be disinfected with the regime already described and can be poured after a short period to allow for full elastic recoil of the material. The casts should be poured within 24 hours of mixing if possible. Whilst the materials have good short term dimensional accuracy, they will undergo plastic flow after setting. One great benefit is that the surface of the impression can be electroplated using a copper sulphate electroplating bath. An epoxy resin die material can then be used to form the bulk of the working cast. Such metal/plastic dies, whilst expensive to produce, are very hard and are not prone to damage in the laboratory when the crown and bridgework is being made.

This approach can be used when multiple operations are being undertaken on the same die. One example of this would be when a clinician wants to make multiple crowns or a combination of crowns and bridges for a patient on the working cast. It can then be difficult to record accurate impressions of many teeth in one impression. In this circumstance, multiple impressions are used to produce accurate individual metal/resin dies for each of the teeth concerned. A plastic transfer coping is then made for each die. This is a small thimble of plastic which is made without spacing to fit over each die. The transfer copings are then taken back to the patient and placed over each of the prepared teeth. A locating impression is then recorded, capturing all of the copings in the impression. The individual dies are then placed in their respective copings and a working model is produced by pouring a base around the dies, usually from dental stone. This master model is then used by the technician to produce the metal or porcelain crowns and bridges. If this approach is attempted with conventional gypsum-based dies there is a high chance of their margins being damaged during the manufacture of the transfer copings, thus diminishing the chances of achieving an accurate fit with the definitive crown and bridge work.

There have been some limited reports of allergic responses to these materials, from people with an allergy to latex products.

19.3 Silicone rubbers (condensation curing)

Composition: These materials may be supplied as two pastes or as a paste and liquid. Whichever method of dispensation is used the principle of the setting reaction is similar and depends on the cross-linking of hydroxyl-terminated polydimethylsiloxane chains, brought about by an alkyl silicate cross-linking agent and a tin compound as catalyst. The ingredients required for this reaction to occur are reflected in the composition of a typical paste/liquid material, given in Table 19.4. These materials are very similar to the room temperature polymerizing silicones used as denture soft liners. Figure 19.4 gives the structural formula of the silicone prepolymer. The viscosity of the paste is controlled by the amount of inert filler, as in the case of the polysulphides. Light-bodied, regular-bodied, heavy-bodied and 'putty' materials are available. The latter is a paste of a very high viscosity and its availability denotes an important difference between the silicones and polysulphides.

Table 19.4 Composition of a paste–liquid silicone rubber impression material (condensation curing).

	Component	Function
Paste	Hydroxyl-terminated polydimethylsiloxane (liquid silicone prepolymer)	Undergoes cross-linking to form rubber
	Insert filler such as silica	Gives 'body', controls viscosity and modifies physical properties
Liquid	Alkyl silicate such as tetraethylsilicate	Acts as cross-linking agent
	Tin compound such as dibutyl tin dilaurate	Acts as reaction catalyst

Proportioning of the paste/liquid materials is by mixing a given volume of paste with a fixed number of drops of liquid. For paste/paste materials equal lengths of pastes are mixed together. A colour contrast between the pastes enables the operator to see when proper mixing has been achieved.

Setting reaction: On mixing the two components, either two pastes or paste and liquid, a reaction begins immediately in which the terminal hydroxyl groups of prepolymer chains react with the cross-linking agent under the influence of the catalyst (see Fig. 19.4). Each molecule of cross-linking agent may, potentially, react with up to four prepolymer chains causing extensive cross-linking. Each reaction stage also produces one molecule of ethyl alcohol as a

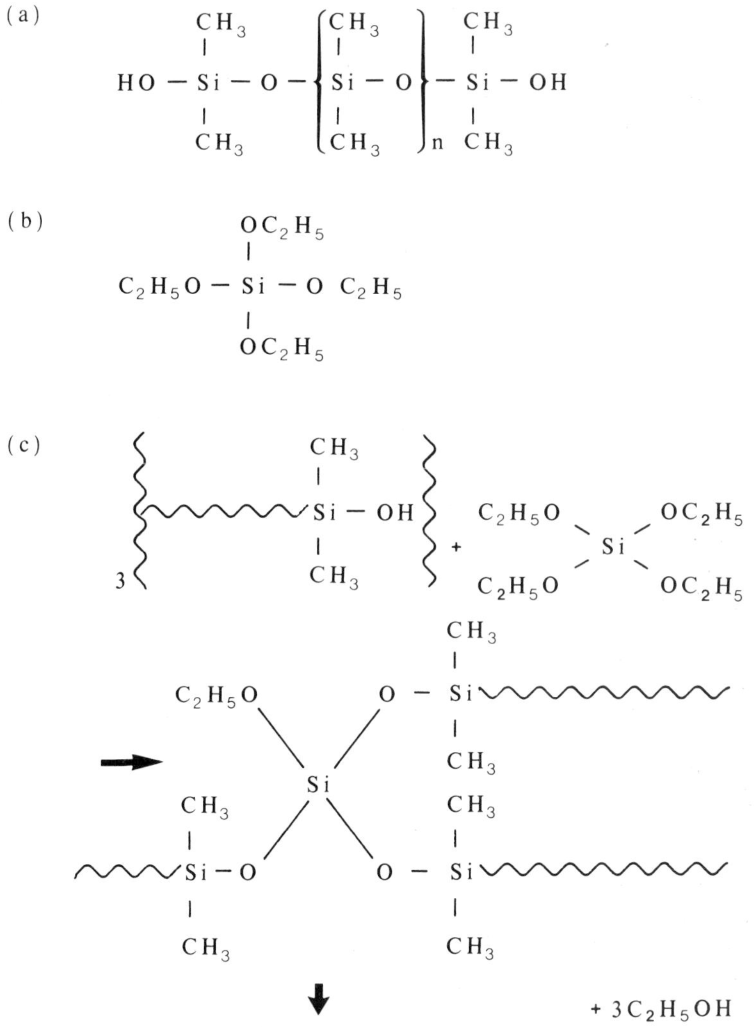

(a)

$$HO - \underset{\underset{CH_3}{|}}{\overset{\overset{CH_3}{|}}{Si}} - O - \left[\underset{\underset{CH_3}{|}}{\overset{\overset{CH_3}{|}}{Si}} - O \right]_n - \underset{\underset{CH_3}{|}}{\overset{\overset{CH_3}{|}}{Si}} - OH$$

(b)

$$C_2H_5O - \underset{\underset{OC_2H_5}{|}}{\overset{\overset{OC_2H_5}{|}}{Si}} - O\,C_2H_5$$

(c)

$$3 \left\{ \mathord{\sim\!\!\sim} \underset{\underset{CH_3}{|}}{\overset{\overset{CH_3}{|}}{Si}} - OH \right\} + \underset{C_2H_5O}{\overset{C_2H_5O}{}} Si \underset{OC_2H_5}{\overset{OC_2H_5}{}}$$

$$\longrightarrow$$

Si central unit cross-linked:

C₂H₅O — O — Si (CH₃)(CH₃) ⌁⌁⌁

CH₃—Si(CH₃)—O — Si — O — Si(CH₃)(CH₃) ⌁⌁⌁

$$+ \, 3\,C_2H_5OH$$

Fig. 19.4 Condensation type silicone elastomer. (a) Hydroxyl-terminated polydimethylsiloxane prepolymer (mixed with inert filler to form paste). (b) Tetraethyl silicate (cross-linking agent). (c) Cross-linking reaction, catalysed by a tin compound. Ethyl alcohol is liberated as a byproduct.

byproduct. Cross-linking produces an increase in viscosity and the rapid development of elastic properties.

Properties: The setting characteristics of the silicone materials tend to be more favourable than those of the polysulphides. Setting times are generally shorter and elasticity is developed earlier.

The silicone impression materials are very hydrophobic and are readily repelled by water or saliva. As a result, it is necessary to dry areas of the mouth for which an accurate impression is required. If a dry field is not secured 'blow holes' are likely to occur in the impression as the material will fail to drive away the residual moisture.

The set material has adequate tear resistance for most purposes. A regular-bodied silicone material can undergo only about 300% extension before fracturing, (compared to 700% for polysulphides) but most of this strain is recoverable. The silicones have elastic properties which most closely approach the ideal of complete and instantaneous recovery following stretching or compression.

Many of the properties are related to the filler content of the pastes. The trends are identical to those given in Table 19.3 for polysulphides. In the case of the silicones an additional, very high viscosity or 'putty' paste exists which has even lower setting and thermal contraction values than the conventional heavy-bodied materials. It also has better dimensional stability.

Dimensional changes after setting, for condensation curing silicones, may be due to continued slow setting or due to loss of alcohol produced as a byproduct of the setting reaction. The latter effect produces a measurable weight loss which is accompanied by a shrinkage of the impression material. Dimensional changes of regular-bodied condensation silicones are slightly greater than those of regular-bodied polysulphides but are small compared to the changes which occur with alginates. In order to obtain optimum accuracy, the models should be case as soon as possible after recording the impression.

Silicone elastomers may be considered essentially non-toxic, despite the fact that they contain a heavy metal catalyst. The materials are extremely hydrophobic and are in the patient's mouth for only a few minutes. The liquid component of the paste/liquid materials may be hazardous if not handled carefully. Accidental splashes may cause considerable irritation and blistering of the eyes.

Applications: For clinical applications of these materials see the end of Section 19.4.

The increased usage of additional curing materials (next section) has led to a gradual decline in the use of the more traditional condensation curing materials.

19.4 Silicone rubbers (addition curing)

Composition: These materials are supplied as two pastes. Each paste contains a liquid silicone prepolymer and filler and one of the pastes contains a catalyst. One paste contains a polydimethylsiloxane prepolymer in which some of the methyl groups are replaced by hydrogen (Fig. 19.5a). The other paste contains a prepolymer in which some methyl groups are replaced by vinyl groups (Fig. 19.5b). One of the pastes contains a catalyst which is normally a platinum-containing compound such as chloroplatinic acid. Four viscosities are available depending on the amount of filler incorporated by the manufacturer.

Proportioning is carried out by extruding equal lengths of each paste onto the mixing pad. A good colour contrast between the pastes enables thorough mixing to be achieved.

A significant advance in recent years has been the availability of addition curing silicones in an auto mixed, cartridge format (Fig. 19.6). The two pastes are housed in separate compartments of the cartridge and are brought together and mixed in the nozzle during extrusion. The mixed material can be extruded into an impression tray or, for light-bodied material, into an impression syringe or directly into the mouth. Light-bodied and regular-bodied materials lend themselves readily to the cartridge extrusion system. Some manufacturers have also managed to package heavy-bodied and even 'soft putty' materials in this way. At least one manufacturer has taken automixing a stage further by producing an electrically driven mixing device which is loaded with bulk quantities of material (sufficient for about *20* impressions). When required, mixed material is produced at the touch of a button.

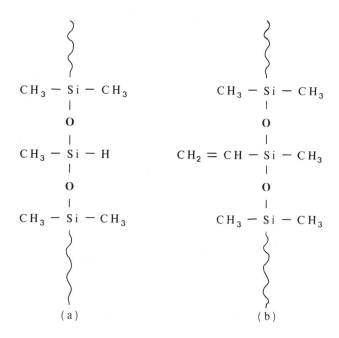

Fig. 19.5 Structural formulae of the silicone prepolymers used in the two pastes of addition curing silicone impression materials. (a) One paste contains some Si–H groups. (b) The other paste contains some Si–CH=CH$_2$ groups.

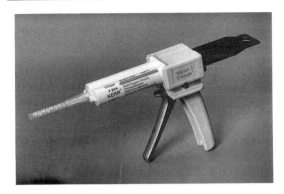

Fig. 19.6 Cartridge mixing and delivery system used for some addition curing silicones.

Setting reaction: On mixing the two pastes a platinum-catalysed addition reaction occurs, causing cross-linking between the two types of siloxane prepolymer (Fig. 19.7). It is noteworthy that the reaction does not involve the production of byproducts although it has been reported that these materials occasionally evolve hydrogen. Some manufacturers recommend that pouring of the cast is delayed until the evolution of hydrogen is complete in order that the cast surface does not become pitted. The mechanism of hydrogen release is unclear but may involve reaction of the platinum catalyst with moisture. Cross-linking produces an increase in viscosity coupled with the development of elastic properties.

As previously stated, one important observation which has been reported over recent years concerns the ability of certain types of latex gloves to retard the setting of addition curing silicones. Dithiocarbamate compounds present in some gloves are thought to be the cause of the observed effect. The use of dithiocarbamate-free gloves is therefore recommended when handling these materials.

Properties: In most respects, the addition curing silicone rubbers have properties similar to those of the condensation type. They have adequate setting characteristics and tear resistance coupled with near ideal elasticity. The combined use of putty and light-bodied materials enables accurate impressions to be recorded. The most significant difference between the addition curing and the condensation curing materials is in their relative dimensional stability. The production of the little or no byproduct in the cross-linking reaction of the addition curing material results in a very stable impression.

Silicone elastomers are inherently hydrophobic in nature – a characteristic which can cause imperfections in impressions if the area to be recorded cannot be thoroughly dried. The mixed silicone material is repelled by moisture and this can result in blow holes in the impression. Attempts have been made to overcome this problem by the incorporation of surface-active agents into the materials in order to make the materials more hydrophilic. The newer materials, which are described as hydrophilic addition silicones, should strictly be described as 'less hydrophobic'. Nevertheless, the improvement in surface characteristics can result in an impression with better fine detail reproduction and fewer blow holes. An alternative approach to solving this problem has been through the use of a surface-active spray which is used to coat the surface of the hard and/or soft tissues prior to recording an impression.

The use of hydrophilic materials or surface-active sprays helps not only to improve the affinity between the impression materials and the oral tissues during recording of the impression, but also in the compatibility with the water-based gypsum model material. This ensures that detail recorded in the impression is transferred through to the model.

Clinical applications: There is virtually no difference between the addition and condensation cured material in terms of their handling characteristics.

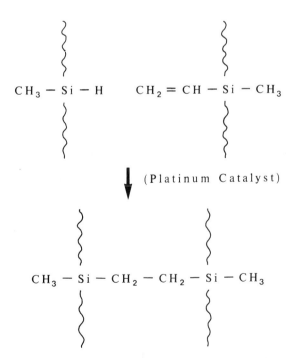

$$CH_3 - Si - H \qquad CH_2 = CH - Si - CH_3$$

$$\downarrow \ (Platinum\ Catalyst)$$

$$CH_3 - Si - CH_2 - CH_2 - Si - CH_3$$

Fig. 19.7 Platinum-catalysed addition reaction which causes cross-linking of prepolymer chains.

The addition cured materials are preferred on the basis of their greater dimensional stability. Both are available in a range of viscosities from light-bodied materials used to record accurate surface detail on prepared tooth surfaces, through medium viscosities, commonly used as a monophase material during either crown and bridgework or denture manufacture, and heavy-bodied materials used to support light body in stock trays for crown and bridge impressions, to putties which are now available in both soft and hard format.

The light-bodied materials can record very accurately the surface detail of tooth preparation but have inadequate dimensional stability to maintain their shape during the production of working casts. They are syringed into place onto the prepared tooth to provide a surface wash giving high quality detail. A more lightly filled material is then used to support the wash, either a heavy body or a putty.

Heavy body and wash or putty and wash impressions can be performed as a one-stage procedure during which both viscosities of material are mixed simultaneously. The clinician then syringes the light-bodied material around the preparation/teeth whilst an assistant places the heavier material into a stock tray. The loaded tray is then inserted into the mouth and the two viscosities blend together and set. Obviously this approach is ergonomically attractive. There are, however, concerns about the accuracy of the one-stage putty wash impressions recorded in some plastic stock trays. The viscosity of the putties is such that on seating the impression tray into the mouth the sides of the tray flex outward. When the impression is removed from the mouth they then rebound inwards, distorting the impression. Unfortunately the distortion is not uniform, as an impression of a circular object when taken in this way results in a die which is ovoid in shape with narrowing bucco-lingually. This occurs with both soft and hard putties but does not occur when the heavy/light body technique is used.

There are two solutions to this problem. Firstly, rigid metal stock trays can be used which do not flex under seating loads. The disadvantage of metal trays is that they are not disposable and hence need to be cleaned and sterilized before re-use which is a laborious task. Alternatively an initial putty impression can be recorded with a polythene spacing sheet between the putty and the teeth. This is allowed to set fully and then the light-body impression is recorded as a second stage. The spacing sheet is required to avoid the large hydraulic pressures which would develop if a light wash was placed inside a well fitting putty impression. These pressures would cause distortion in their own right.

Medium viscosity materials can be used in a similar way to the monophase polyethers, but their dimensional accuracy in stock trays is not quite as good as when using a two-viscosity technique.

There are two problems with the addition cured silicone rubbers. First they are markedly hydrophobic. As a consequence tooth surfaces into which the light body material is being syringed have to be dry. Any moisture contamination will simply result in a failure to record accurately the surface of the prepared tooth. Furthermore, if the tooth is in the upper arch the light body will tend to drip off the preparation under the influence of gravity which is very frustrating. As previously stated the more recently developed materials incorporate wetting agents to lower the surface tension between the impression material and the tooth. One manufacturer has gone so far as to provide a separate aerosol containing the wetting agent to be sprayed on the tooth after drying prior to placement of the light-body material. These developments have improved matters somewhat, but the material remains hydrophobic.

Second, the platinum catalyst system in the addition cured materials is relatively easy to poison, inhibiting the set of the material. Problems can be encountered with the plasticizers in rubber, from gloves or rubber dam, glove powders, some haemostatic agents, particularly those based on ferric salts and freshly placed methacrylate-based materials, including composites, compomers and light-cured glass ionomer cements. These latter products can be used to *patch up* a crown preparation if there is some caries present or an existing restoration falls out during preparation. However, if this is done then the impression should not be recorded in the same visit, as the surface of the impression material adjacent to the patch will not set. The other agents can usually be either avoided or washed/cleaned off the prepared tooth surface prior to recording the impression. Obviously rubber gloves should not be used to protect the hands of somebody mixing a putty impression; vinyl gloves are a viable alternative.

There are no reports in the literature of patients suffering an allergic response to these materials although they can induce a contact dermatitis in dental nurses who mix impression putties without wearing suitable gloves.

The standard disinfection regime of a 10 minute immersion in sodium hypochlorite will have no effect on the dimensional stability of these materials. They are also sufficiently stable that the more rigorous processes associated with managing patients with an established cross-infection risk (i.e. prolonged immersion in glutaraldehyde solution) can be undertaken without a marked effect on their accuracy.

19.5 Polyethers

Composition: These materials are normally supplied as two pastes. The 'base' paste, containing the prepolymer and inert filler is supplied in a large tube. The 'catalyst' paste, containing a reaction initiator together with paste-forming oils and fillers, is supplied in a second, but much smaller tube. The composition is summarized in Table 19.5. Simplified structural formulae for the imine-terminated, ether initiator are given in Fig. 19.8. The group X shown in the structural formula of the polyether prepolymer (Fig. 19.8) has the structure:

$$-CO_2-[CH-(CH_2)_n-O]_m-CH(CH_2)_n-CO_2-$$

with R above each of the two CH groups.

where R represents a hydrogen atom or alkly group. The values of m and n are such that the molecular weight of the difunctional imino molecule is about 4000. The polyester unit (shown in the square brackets) is typically produced by copolymerization of ethylene oxide and tetrahydrofuran. The materials are generally supplied in only one viscosity, equivalent to the regular-bodied materials of other elastomers. The manufacturers do supply a diluent oil, however, which can be used to produce a paste with viscosity akin to that of a light-bodied material.

Table 19.5 Composition of polyether impression materials.

	Component	Function
Base paste (large tube)	Imine-terminated prepolymer	Becomes cross-linked to form rubber
	Inert filler – silica	To give 'body' control viscosity and physical properties
	Plasticizer – e.g. phthalate	To aid mixing
Catalyst paste (small tube)	Ester derivative of aromatic sulphonic acid	Initiates cross-linking
	Inert filler – silica	To form paste
	Plasticizer – phthalate	

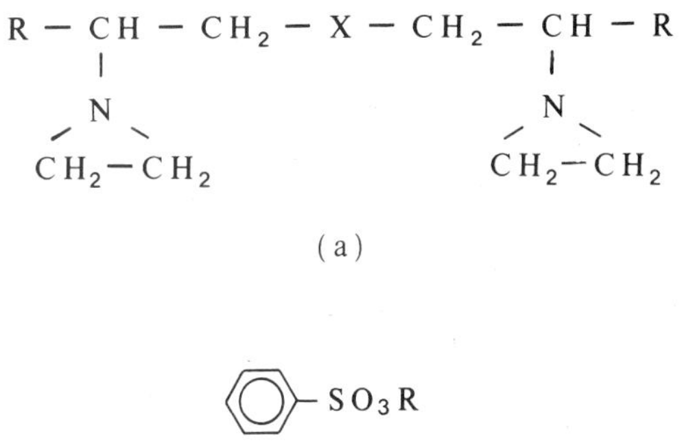

(a)

(b)

Fig. 19.8 (a) Simplified structural formula of the imine-terminated ether prepolymer present in the base paste of a polyether impression material. X represents repeating units of ethers. (b) Structural formula of an aromatic sulphonic acid ester. This is the main active ingredient of the catalyst paste of a polyether impression material. Group R is an alkyl group, for example, butyl.

The two pastes are proportioned by volume. Equal lengths of paste are extruded onto a mixing pad giving a base paste/catalyst paste volume ratio of about 8 : 1. The good colour contrast between the pastes aids mixing.

Setting reaction: When the two pastes are mixed together a cationic, ring opening addition polymerization occurs. The ionized form of the sulphonic acid ester provides the initial source of cations and each stage of the reaction involves the opening of an epimine ring and the production of a fresh cation, as illustrated in Fig. 19.9.

Distinct activation, initiation and propagation stages may be identified in the reaction as shown. The reaction is of the addition type with no byproduct being produced. Since each prepolymer molecule has two reactive epimine groups, individual propagation reactions may produce simple chain lengthening or cross-linking. As the reaction proceeds, the viscosity increases and eventually a relatively rigid cross-linked rubber is produced.

Properties: The polyether materials have adequate tear resistance and elastic properties approaching those of the silicones. They are relatively rigid when set and considerable force may be required to remove the impression after setting, particularly when the undercuts are severe.

The accuracy of polyether impressions compares favourably with other regular-bodied elastomers. The lack of heavy-bodied and putty pastes, however,

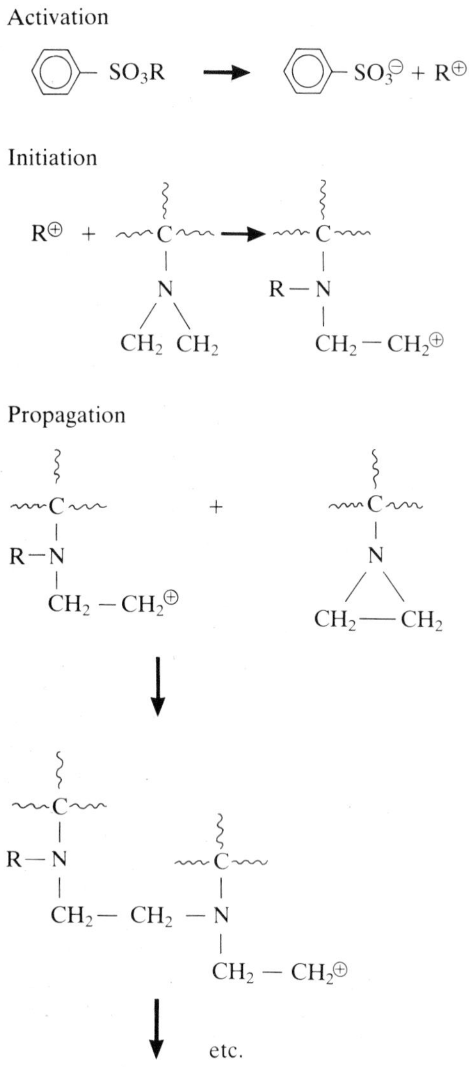

Activation

$$\bigcirc\!\!-\text{SO}_3\text{R} \longrightarrow \bigcirc\!\!-\text{SO}_3^{\ominus} + \text{R}^{\oplus}$$

Initiation

$$\text{R}^{\oplus} + \text{~C~} \longrightarrow \text{~C~}$$

Propagation

etc.

Fig. 19.9 Schematic representation of the cationic, ring opening polymerization involved in the setting of polyether impression materials.

precluded the use of techniques using combined viscous/fluid pastes which are commonly used with other elastomers to optimize accuracy.

The manufacturers of polyether materials have recently introduced products having a range of viscosities. These enable the use of combined heavy- and light-bodied techniques described for poly-sulphides and silicones. This enables precise impressions to be recorded using stock impression trays.

Under conditions of low relative humidity, the polyether materials have very good dimensional stability. This is related, primarily, to the fact that the material contains no volatile constituents and sets by an addition reaction which produces no volatile byproducts. The set material is relatively hydrophilic and absorbs water under conditions of high humidity. This causes the impression material to swell and distort. The use of polyether materials should therefore be avoided in climates where humidity is high and where efficient air conditioning is not available.

Clinical applications: Commonly these materials are used as a *monophase* where a single viscosity of material is used for both the bulk of the impression in the tray and to be syringed around the prepared teeth in the mouth. The polyethers are sufficiently dimensionally stable on setting to allow this approach when using a stock impression tray.

Polyether materials are hydrophilic, consequently they can record an accurate impression when it is difficult to achieve perfect moisture control.

The greatest disadvantage from a clinical standpoint is the rigidity of these materials when set. This can make removal of impressions very difficult in dentate patients when there are marked undercuts present around the teeth, for example when there has been gingival recession exposing root surfaces with open embrasure spaces between the teeth or where bridgework is present elsewhere in the mouth. It is sensible to block out such undercut areas with wax prior to recording the impression if the operator is not to risk being unable to remove the impression or, in extreme cases, removing existing bridgework or even extracting teeth when the impression is removed.

The rigidity of these materials is used to good effect when recording impressions for dental implants. Whilst clinicians attempt to place implants parallel to each other this is not always possible. The transmucosal elements of some implants have a keyway on their upper surface over which a precision machined collar should fit and then be screwed to the implant. The impression process for this style of implant involves attaching brass dummies of the collar to the surface of the implant with long screws. The brass dummies have undercut areas within their superstructure which allows them to be engaged by an overlay impression. However, this impression must exhibit high levels of rigidity to ensure that the brass analogues do not move within the impression once removed from the mouth. The implants are rigid within the base of the jaws so there is no leeway for movement of the analogues in the impression. If the implants are parallel to each other then impression plaster can be used for this purpose. However, when the fixtures are not parallel to each other a polyether is the material of choice for these locating impressions.

Allergic reactions have also been associated with the use of polyether impression materials, usually to the sulphonic acid catalyst system.

A 'standard' disinfection routine of 10 minutes immersion in sodium hypochlorite is unlikely to have a deleterious effect on the accuracy of these materials, although longer periods of immersion in water will result in water uptake and associated dimensional change.

19.6 Comparison of the properties of elastomers

Many of the clinically important properties of elastomeric impression materials are included as requirements in the International Standard (ISO 4823). These requirements are reproduced in Table 19.6. The initial accuracy of any material is related in part to its ability to reproduce fine lines on a test block. This is more closely related to the viscosity of the material than to chemical nature (assuming the area to be recorded is dry). It is seen that type 0 materials (putty type) must be able to reproduce a line 0.075 mm wide whereas a type 3 material (light-bodied) must be able to reproduce a line only 0.020 mm wide. In addition to the ability to reproduce fine detail accuracy also depends on dimensional changes which occur during or immediately after setting. Polymerization shrinkage varies within the range 0.4–1.0% for regular viscosity materials. These values are greater for light-bodied products, and lower for heavy-bodied or putty products. A further dimensional change occurs when the impression cools from mouth temperature to room temperature. Values of the coefficient of thermal expansion are quite large for elastomers ($190–300 \times 10^{-6}\,°C^{-1}$ for

regular-bodied materials) and this can result in a dimensional change of 0.1–0.3%. These values are greater for light-bodied materials and smaller for heavy-bodied and putty materials.

The value of strain in compression gives an indication of the stiffness of the set material. It is determined by measuring compression under a stress of 0.1 MPa. The higher viscosity materials (types 0 and 1) tend to be stiffer than fluid materials (types 2 and 3), although it is clear from Table 19.6 that there are significant differences in stiffness within the type 0–3 categories (i.e. 2–20% for type 2). This reflects significant differences for the different types of material. In general, the polyether materials tend to be much stiffer than the other products whilst the polysulphides tend to be less stiff than the other products. The values of the limits of strain in compression required by the ISO Standard illustrate the difficulty of standardizing different types of materials within one document, i.e. the lower values of strain in the acceptance range are there to accommodate the polyether materials whilst the higher values accommodate the polysulphide materials. The significance of the value of strain in compression is that it gives an indication of the ease with which a set impression can be removed (less stiff material is easier) and an indication of the possibility that teeth may be fractured from models (greater stiffness gives a greater danger of fracture). For stiff materials it is important to use them in great enough thickness to allow sufficient deformation to occur under load.

The value of recovery from deformation (Table 19.6) gives an indication of the elastic characteristics of the material. It is determined by compressing a cylindrical sample by 30% of its height for one second at one minute after the end of its setting time (the time recommended by the manufacturer for removing the material from the mouth). The recovery is measured 40 seconds after removing the compressing load. All elastomeric impression mate-

Table 19.6 Requirements of ISO Standard for Elastomeric Impression Materials (ISO 4823).

Type*	Strain in compression (%)	Recovery from deformation (%)	24 h dimensional change (%)	Detail reproduction – width of line reproduced (mm)	
				in impression	in gypsum cast
0	0.8–20	96.5	0–1.5	0.075	0.075
1	0.8–20	96.5	0–1.5	0.050	0.050
2	2–20	96.5	0–1.5	0.020	0.020
3	2–20	96.5	0–1.5	0.020	0.020

* See Table 19.1.

rials are required to undergo at least 96.5% recovery in this test. In practice, most silicone and polyether materials give 99–100% elastic recovery and the lower limit of 96.5% recovery is set in order to accommodate the polysulphide materials. The latter products are markedly viscoelastic in nature and their recovery from deformation depends significantly on the time for which the deforming load is applied (i.e. the time the material is under stress).

The maximum dimensional change permitted by the ISO Standard is 1.5% for all materials. This is measured by recording the distance between two lines on a metal test block and comparing the measurement with an equivalent measurement in an impression of the test block which has been stored for 24 hours. The change in dimensions is negligible for polyether .and addition silicone products and more significant for the other materials – particularly for condensation curing silicones. The dimensional change of the latter materials can be correlated with a weight loss which occurs on standing. This is caused by loss of ethyl alcohol which is formed as a byproduct of the setting reaction. A small dimensional change (and weight loss) can be measured for polysulphides. This may be due to loss of water which is formed as a byproduct. The final major requirement of the ISO Standard is that the fine detail which is recorded in the impression can be retained in the gypsum cast.

Two approaches have been used to assess resistance to tearing. One involves measurement of tensile strength, the other involves measurement of elongation to break. Both approaches can be considered less than ideal and this probably explains why there is no test for tear resistance in the ISO Standard. Polysulphide materials invariably give the highest elongation at break (500% or more for regular-bodied material) but very little of this is 'usable' elongation as much of it will result in permanent deformation. On the other hand, the addition silicones give the highest values of tensile strength (2–5 MPa for regular-bodied materials). The strength of these products can be influenced by the presence of pre-existing notches in the material. Perhaps a more acceptable way to compare materials is, therefore, to use a specimen of the type shown in Fig. 18.4. On stretching the specimen, the force required to propagate a tear from the notch tip can be determined. This type of determination, which is commonly used in the rubber industry, reveals that there is little difference between the different material types.

Decontamination of elastomeric impression materials is sometimes required in order to prevent cross-infection. It is a requirement of the ISO Standard that the manufacturer provides details of a method which is suitable for any particular product. Typically, the method of decontamination involves rinsing followed by a short soak in a solution of hypochlorite or glutaraldehyde. Such treatment is unlikely to harm the silicone or polysulphide materials. However, the polyether materials are hydrophilic and great care must be taken when soaking impressions in aqueous solutions – lest the material absorbs water and swells.

Jaw Registration: Increasingly elastomeric materials (both polyether and addition cured silicone rubber)

Table 19.7 Comparison of the properties (qualitative) of elastometric impression materials.

Property	Polysulphides	Condensation silicones	Addition silicones	Polyethers
Viscosity	Available in three viscosities (no putty)	Available in four viscosities including putty	Available in four viscosities including putty	Available in a single viscosity (regular) + diluent + putty
Tear resistance	Adequate	Adequate	Adequate	Adequate
Elasticity	Viscoelastic material	Very good	Very good	Adequate
Accuracy	Good with special trays	Acceptable with stock trays	Good with stock trays	Good with special trays*
Dimensional stability	Adequate, but pouring of models should not be delayed[†]	Models should be poured as quickly as possible[†]	Very good[†]	Very good in low humidity conditions

* Can give good accuracy with stock trays, with care.
[†] Some manufacturers recommend a *short* delay in pouring models for these materials, either to allow elastic recovery to occur or to allow gaseous products to escape which would otherwise cause pitting of the model surface.

are being used to record the relationship between the upper and lower jaws. The materials are usually in a gun-mix format and of sufficient viscosity that they will not drip off the teeth when applied from the applicator. One clinical problem with their use is that the materials will record too much surface detail from the occlusal areas of the molar teeth which is not recorded and/or cannot be re-engaged by the registration when placed onto the working model. This results in folds of registration material being trapped against the surface of the casts making the whole process less accurate.

Table 19.7 gives a qualitative summary of the comparative properties of the materials.

19.7 Suggested further reading

Brown, D. (1973) Factors affecting the dimensional stability of elastic impression materials. *J. Dent.* **1**, 265.

Craig, R.G., Urquiola, N.J. & Liu, C.C. (1990) Comparison of commercial elastomeric impression materials. *Oper. Dent.* **15**, 94.

Wassell, R.W. & Abuasi, H.A. (1992) Laboratory assessment of impression accuracy by clinical simulation. *J. Dent.* **20**, 108.

ISO 4823 Dental Elastomeric Impression Materials.

Chapter 20

Requirements of Direct Filling Materials and Historical Perspectives

20.1 Introduction

Direct filling materials are used for chairside restoration of teeth. They differ from indirect restorations, such as crowns, bridges or inlays, because no laboratory stage is involved in the provision of the restoration.

Teeth may need restoring for a variety of reasons. Destruction of tooth substance caused by dental caries may result in the loss of considerable quantities of enamel and dentine. Trauma may cause fracture and loss of parts of teeth. In this case the anterior teeth are most vulnerable and those teeth affected may be otherwise sound and caries-free. A third factor causing loss of tooth substance is abrasion. This often arises due to overzealous brushing using an abrasive dentifrice but may also arise due to a peculiarity of the diet, working environment of habits of the patient.

The parts of teeth which require replacement by a restorative material vary in size, shape and location in the mouth. Thus, at one extreme, it may be necessary to restore a large cavity which extends over the mesial, occlusal and distal surfaces of a molar tooth. An entirely different situation is the restoration of the corner of an incisor which has been lost in an accident. The requirements of materials used in these and other applications vary and it is not surprising that no single restorative material is suitable for all cases. For some situations the strength and abrasion resistance of the material may be the prime consideration. In other situations appearance and adhesive properties may become more important.

The factor which is generally used to assess the success or failure of a restorative material for any application is *durability*. In this context the term refers to the life expectancy of the restoration and the life expectancy of the surrounding tooth sub-

stance and how it may be affected by the presence of the restoration. Durability depends on the physical and biological properties of the restorative material.

The acceptance of the material by the profession also depends on the ease with which it can be handled in the surgery.

20.2 Rheological properties and setting characteristics

Many restorative materials are supplied as two or more components which require mixing. Thorough mixing should be easy to accomplish in a reasonable time. After mixing, the ease of handling depends on factors such as *viscosity*, *tackiness* and setting characteristics such as *working time* and *setting time*. Different techniques must often be adopted to handle different materials. Whereas some materials readily flow into the prepared cavity under little pressure some products require 'packing' under considerable pressure. When materials remain tacky for some time after mixing they may be difficult to handle because they adhere to instruments. Working time should be sufficiently long to enable manipulation and placement of materials before the setting reaction reaches the stage at which continued manipulation is either difficult or would adversely affect the structure and properties of the final set material. Setting times should, ideally, be short for the comfort and convenience of both the patient and clinician.

20.3 Chemical properties

Filling materials are required to withstand the hostile environment of the oral cavity for many years without dissolving, degrading or eroding. Thus, the materials must withstand large variations in pH and a variety of solvents which may be taken into the mouth in drinks, foodstuffs and medicaments. In addition, metallic filling materials should not undergo excessive corrosion or be involved in the development of electrical currents which may cause *galvanic pain.*

20.4 Thermal properties

Filling materials should, ideally, be good thermal insulators, protecting the dental pulp from the harmful effects of hot and cold stimuli. The thermal insulating properties of filling materials are best characterized in terms of *thermal diffusivity* (p. 19) since this describes the behaviour of materials subjected to transient thermal stimuli. Hence, the value of thermal diffusivity should ideally be low. Materials having relatively high values of thermal diffusivity require the use of an insulating cavity base material.

The thermal expansion and contraction of a filling which occurs, for example, when a patient takes a hot or cold drink, should match that of the surrounding tooth substance. Thus, materials should have values of *coefficient of thermal expansion* (p. 21) similar to those of enamel and dentine. A large mismatch of values may result in leakage of fluids down the margin between the filling material and surrounding tooth.

20.5 Mechanical properties

The mechanical property requirements of filling materials vary considerably depending on the type of tooth and the particular surface being restored. For the restoration of large cavities, involving two or more surfaces of a posterior tooth, a *strong* material with adequate *abrasion resistance* is required to withstand the large stresses developed in that region of the mouth. When materials are subjected to direct masticatory loading they should also be able to resist plastic deformation or *creep*. For a small occlusal cavity in a posterior tooth the properties of the material may not be as critical since it is totally supported by enamel. For a small interproximal cavity in the anterior region the major factor for consideration may be abrasion resistance. That surface of the tooth is not involved in direct contact with other teeth but may be subjected to considerable toothbrush/dentifrice abuse.

It is recognized that the marginal seal between filling material and tooth substance may be destroyed if the material is able to undergo elastic deformation under loading. A high value of *modulus of elasticity* is therefore beneficial.

20.6 Adhesion

It is recognized that an adhesive bond between restorative material and tooth substance is desirable though not always attainable. Such a bond effectively seals the margin, preventing the ingress of fluids and bacteria. In addition, the adhesive bond potentially reduces the amount of cavity preparation required in order to achieve retention of the filling. The subject of adhesion and adhesive materials is dealt with in Chapter 24.

20.7 Biological properties

Filling materials, in common with all other dental materials, should be harmless, to both the operators and patients. The specific requirements of these products relate to their effect on the dental pulp. They should not, either directly or indirectly cause irritation to the pulp, nor should they contain substances which are able to leach out and cause irritation. It should be remembered that dentine contains many tubules which are capable of transporting chemicals from the base of fillings to the pulp. Biologically bland cavity bases or cavity linings are often used when filling materials are not sufficiently bland to be used directly.

20.8 Historical

Directly placed fillings offer the advantage of potential savings in time and cost coupled with greater convenience when compared with restorations which are constructed by an indirect process. Historically, the three earliest materials to gain acceptance as direct fillings were cohesive gold foil, dental amalgam and silicate cements. Of these, only amalgam is still widely used and its continued use is subject to considerable scrutiny as concerns over the use of heavy metals, and particularly mercury, increase. Cohesive gold is discussed in Section 7.2. Although it has some attributes its use is now very limited due to the cost of the material and the involved technique required.

Silicate cements were the first directly placed tooth coloured filling materials. They are now rarely, if ever, used but some important lessons can be learned from a consideration of their composition and properties. The materials were supplied as a powder (alumino silicate glass) and liquid (aqueous phosphoric acid) which were mixed together to bring about setting. Setting was through a complex series of acid–base reactions. One of the most crucial aspects of the manipulation of the cement was the need to protect from moisture during setting. Contamination could lead to a marked increase in solubility – a fact which also applies to some currently used cements which have similar setting reactions to that of the silicates. Dentists using silicates were aware of the highly acid nature of the cements and a lining was considered essential to protect the dentine and pulp from the phosphoric acid component. Pulpal problems were invariably attributed to the harmful effects of acid and this is of interest in respect of the modern trend to utilize acid treatments of dentine for conditioning prior to the placement of fillings. There has recently been a lot of work carried out to review the way in which the pulp reacts to chemical attack. It is now thought that many of the pulpal problems associated with silicates possibly had nothing to do with traumatization by acid but were more likely related to the fact that silicates offer no means of adhesion to the tooth and therefore cannot prevent microleakage from occurring.

Much of the evidence (some anecdotal) on the beneficial effects of fluoride release from fillings comes from experience of the use of silicates. The materials were able to release fluoride over a long time and the incidence of decay around silicate fillings was always low.

The mechanical properties of silicates were far from ideal. The materials were relatively weak and brittle compared with other materials and this limited their use to low-stress situations – particularly class III cavities. Experience with silicates clearly illustrated the importance of using the correct powder–liquid ratio for cements and pointed the way to the improvements which could be obtained with encapsulation. Silicate materials offered a very good example of the way in which material durability can depend on the oral hygiene and dietary habits of the patient. The solubility and erosion of the cements was very pH dependent. A well constructed restoration in a patient practising good oral hygiene and having a low acid content diet could survive 20 years or more. On the other hand, an acid environment arising from poor oral hygiene and/or a habitual acid drink intake caused rapid erosion of the filling. To some extent, the same is true of some modern day restorative cements. The use of silicates declined markedly with the advent of resin based products – particularly composites in the 1960s. Glass-ionomer cements, which have been used since the 1970s, bear some similarity to the silicates. They set by a similar acid–base reaction and have a glass component which is similar to that of the silicates.

Chapter 21
Dental Amalgam

*, Purified by distillation
, Mercury + silver - tin alloy

21.1 Introduction

An amalgam consists of a mixture of two or more metals, one of which is mercury. Dental amalgam consists, essentially, of mercury combined with a powdered silver–tin alloy. Mercury is a liquid at room temperature and is able to form a 'workable' mass when mixed with the alloy. This behaviour renders the material suitable for use in dentistry.

The reaction between mercury and alloy which follows mixing is termed an *amalgamation* reaction. It results in the formation of a hard restorative material of silvery-grey appearance. The colour generally limits its use to those cavities where appearance is not of primary concern.

Dental amalgam has been used for many years with a large measure of success, in fact, it is the most widely used of all the available filling materials.

21.2 Composition

Mercury used in dental amalgam is purified by distillation. This ensures the elimination of impurities which would adversely affect the setting characteristics and physical properties of the set amalgam.

The composition of the alloy powder is controlled by the ISO Standard for dental amalgam alloy (ISO 1559). The compositional limits allowed by the standard are given in Table 21.1. It can be seen that the major components of the alloy are silver, tin and copper. Small quantities of zinc, mercury and other metals such as indium or palladium may be present in some alloys. The compositional limit specified in the earlier version of the ISO Standard represented an attempt to control properties such as corrosion and setting expansion in the absence of any real understanding of the structure of amalgam. Materials having a composition which is in line with the pre-1986 standard are referred to as 'conventional' amalgam alloys. The change in the compositional limits specified in the current standard (post-

Table 21.1 Compositional limits of dental amalgam alloys specified in ISO 1559.

Metal	Weight (%)	
	Limits prior to 1986 ('conventional' alloys)	Current limits
Silver	65 (min)	40 (min)
Tin	29 (max)	32 (max)
Copper	6 (max)	30 (max)
Zinc	2 (max)	2 (max)
Mercury	3 (max)	3 (max)

1986) reflects a marked improvement in the understanding of structure–property relationships for the materials.

The quantities of silver and tin specified ensure a preponderance of the silver/tin intermetallic compound Ag_3Sn. This compound, known as the γ (gamma) phase of the silver–tin system, is formed over only a small composition range and is particularly advantageous since it readily undergoes an amalgamation reaction with mercury. Most conventional alloys contain around 5% copper, which has a significant strengthening effect on the set amalgam.

The role of zinc is as a *scavenger* during the production of the alloy. The alloy is formed by melting all the constituent metals together. At the elevated temperatures required for this purpose there is a tendency for oxidation to occur. Oxidation of tin, copper or silver would seriously affect the properties of the alloy and amalgam. Zinc reacts rapidly and preferentially with the available oxygen, forming a slag of zinc oxide which is easily removed. Many alloys contain no zinc. They are described as *zinc-free alloys* and oxidation during melting is prevented by carrying out the procedure in an inert atmosphere.

The majority of alloy powders contain no mercury.

*Zinc scavenger + 2=0
So no rust or oxidation*

157

Those products containing up to 3% mercury are called *pre-amalgamated alloys*. They are said to react more rapidly when mixed with mercury.

The shape and size of the alloy powder particles vary from one product to another. Two methods are commonly used to produce the particles. Firstly, filings of alloy may be cut from a prehomogenized ingot of alloy. These *lathe-cut* alloy powders are irregular in shape (Fig. 21.1a) and are graded according to size, being described as fine-grain or coarse-grain. Secondly, particles may be produced by *atomization*. Here, molten alloy is sprayed into a column filled with inert gas. The droplets of alloy solidify as they fall down the column. Particles produced in this way are either *spherical* or *spheroidal* in nature (Fig. 21.1b).

(a)

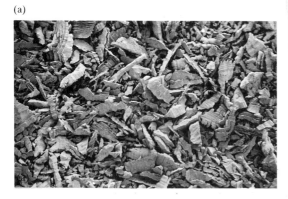

(b)

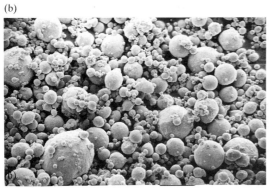

Fig. 21.1 Dental amalgam alloys. (a) Lathe-cut alloy particles ($\times$ 100). (b) Spherical alloy particles ($\times$ 500).

Lathe-cut alloys are normally subjected to two heat treating procedures. The first of these is a homogenization heat treatment (see Section 6.5) normally carried out on the alloy ingot before lathe-cutting and designed to produce homogeneous grains in which the Ag_3Sn intermetallic compound predominates. During the formation of the ingot of

alloy there is a tendency for phase separation to occur and for a cored grain structure to be formed. The heat treatment involves heating to about 420°C for several hours. The resulting alloy contains relatively large grains of γ phase material. The second heat treatment is carried out after lathe-cutting. This is a lower temperature treatment typically involving heating the alloy powder to approximately 100°C for about 1 hour. This treatment is referred to as alloy ageing; it is thought to remove residual stresses introduced during cutting and ensures that the alloy remains stable during future storage.

For spherical alloys the method of manufacture dictates that each small sphere is like an individual ingot. Thus homogenization is normally carried out for the reasons outlined above.

Many alloy powders are formulated by mixing particles of varying size or even shape in order to increase the packing efficiency of the alloy and reduce the amount of mercury required to produce a workable mix.

After the discovery in the 1960s that some of the properties of 'conventional' amalgam materials could be improved by the inclusion of great quantities of copper (in place of silver) a new class of materials was developed and became available for use by the dentist. The ISO Standard finally recognized this change in composition when the 1986 version of ISO 1559 was published. As shown in Table 21.1, these newer alloy powders have the same basic ingredients as the conventional products but they contain much greater concentrations of copper, typically 10–30% compared to less than 6% in the conventional materials. These newer alloys are referred to as *copper-enriched alloys*. In addition to the increased copper levels some alloys also contain small quantities of other metals such as palladium. Higher copper levels in alloy powders may be produced by the manufacturer in one of several ways. Lathe-cut, spherical or spheroidal powders can be produced in which the manufacturer alters the ratio of metals at the melting stage. Hence the resulting alloy particles are similar in shape and size to conventional alloys but simply contain a higher copper content. These are *single-composition, copper-enriched alloys*. An alternative approach is to blend particles of conventional alloy with those of, for example, a silver–copper alloy in order to achieve a higher overall copper content. Such blends are called *dispersion-modified, copper-enriched alloys* and one widely used product contains two parts by weight of a lathe-cut alloy of conventional composition (less than 6% copper) and one part by weight of spherical silver–copper eutectic particles (Fig. 21.2). The latter

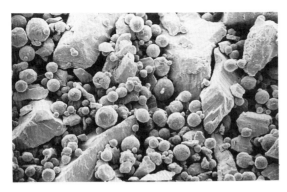

Fig. 21.2 Dispersion-modified alloy powder. Lathe-cut particles of conventional alloy and spherical particles of silver-copper eutectic alloy ($\times$ 500).

particles contain 72 parts silver and 28 parts copper and the overall copper content in the blended alloy is 12%.

21.3 Setting reactions

The reaction which takes place when alloy powder and mercury are mixed is complex. Mercury diffuses into the alloy particles; very small particles may become totally dissolved in mercury. The alloy structure of the surface layers is broken down and the constituent metals undergo amalgamation with mercury. The reaction products crystallize to give new phases in the set amalgam. A considerable quantity of the initial alloy remains unreacted at the completion of setting. The structure of the set material is such that the unreacted cores of alloy particles remain embedded in a matrix of reaction products.

In simplified terms, the reaction for conventional amalgam alloys may be given by the following unbalanced equation:

$$Ag_3Sn + Hg \rightarrow Ag_2Hg_3 + Sn_xHg + Ag_3Sn$$
$$\text{or} \quad \gamma + Hg \rightarrow \gamma_1 + \gamma_2 + \gamma$$

The primary reaction products are a silver–mercury phase (the γ_1 phase) and a tin–mercury phase (the γ_2 phase). The γ_2 phase has a rather imprecise structure and the value of x in the formula Sn_xHg may vary from seven to eight. The equation emphasizes the fact that considerable quantities of unreacted alloy (γ phase) remain unconsumed.

For copper-enriched alloys the reaction may be represented by:

$$Ag_3Sn + Cu + Hg \rightarrow Ag_2Hg_3 + Cu_6Sn_5 + Ag_3Sn$$
$$\text{or } \gamma + Cu + Hg \rightarrow \gamma_1 + Cu_6Sn_5 + \gamma$$

The essential difference between this and the reaction for conventional alloys is the replacement of the tin–mercury, γ_2 phase in the reaction product with a copper–tin phase. The copper–tin phase may exist in the form of Cu_6Sn_5 (η phase) or Cu_3Sn (ε phase) depending on the precise formulation of the alloy. In either case, the elimination of the γ_2 phase has a profound effect on the properties of the set material.

In the case of the dispersion-modified, copper-enriched materials, it is believed that the particles of conventional lathe-cut alloy initially react to form γ_1 and γ_2 phases. The γ_2 phase then reacts with copper from the silver–copper eutectic spheres to form the copper-tin phase. Thus, in these materials, the γ_2 phase exists as an intermediate reaction product for a short time during setting. The reaction rate is quite slow and sometimes takes several days or even weeks to reach completion. This is reflected in the rate of development of mechanical properties.

21.4 Properties

Some of the important physical and mechanical properties of amalgam are specified as tests and requirements in the ISO specification for dental amalgam alloy (ISO 1559). The requirements are given in Table 21.2.

Table 21.2 Physical and mechanical properties of dental amalgam specified in ISO 1559.

Property	Required value
Dimensional change (%)	–0.1 to +0.2
Compressive strength (MPa)	
at 1 hour	50 (minimum)
at 24 hours	300 (minimum)
Creep (%)	3.0 (maximum)

Dimensional changes: The setting reaction for amalgam involves a dimensional change. If cylindrical specimens of material are prepared and allowed to set in unrestrained conditions, plots of dimensional change versus time are akin to those shown in Fig. 21.3. Curves (a) and (b) are typical of results obtained for commonly used materials. A small contraction takes place during the first half hour or so. This corresponds to the stage during which mercury is still diffusing into the alloy particles. The upturn in the curve begins when crystallization of new phases becomes the predominant feature of the setting reaction. The outward thrust of growing crystals

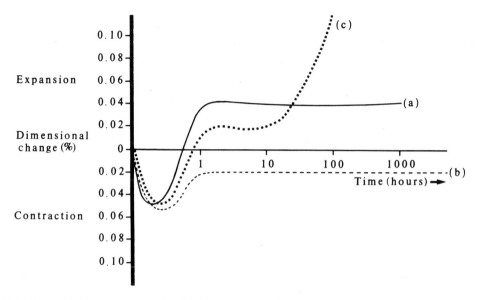

Fig. 21.3 Dimensional change versus time for dental amalgam. Measurements started soon after mixing. (a) and (b) Examples of normal behaviour. (c) Example of moisture-contaminated material.

causes the expansion. The overall effect may cause a slight final expansion as shown in curve (a) or a slight final contraction as in curve (b). Factors which affect the amount of expansion of contraction include the type of alloy used, the particle size and shape and, most significantly, manipulative variables such as the pressure used to condense the amalgam into the cavity. It is important that the final set filling should not have dimensions which are very different from that of the cavity. A large contraction would result in a marginal-gap down which fluids could penetrate. A large expansion would result in the protrusion of the filling from the cavity. Hence, standard specification tests for dental amalgam permit only a small expansion (typically 0.1% maximum) or a small contraction (typically 0.1% maximum).

A far greater expansion than the maximum value given above may result if a zinc-containing amalgam is contaminated with moisture during condensation. Zinc reacts readily with water producing hydrogen:

$$Zn + H_2O \rightarrow ZnO + H_2$$

The liberation of hydrogen causes a considerable *delayed* expansion as illustrated by curve (c) in Fig. 21.3. This confirms the need for adequate moisture control when using these materials.

In order to facilitate a good marginal seal between amalgam fillings and the cavity wall it is suggested that a cavity varnish is used. Such varnishes consists of solutions of natural or synthetic resins in a volatile solvent such as ether. The varnish is applied to the cavity walls and after evaporation of the solvent a thin layer of resin covers the dentine. The amalgam is condensed against the varnish which helps to seal the cavity walls and to take up some of the strain if the amalgam expands. In order to effectively seal the cavity the varnish should be water resistant, a property which is not achieved in some of the natural resin varnishes.

Strength: The strength of dental amalgam is developed slowly. It may take up to 24 hours to reach a reasonably high value and continues to increase slightly for some time after that. At the time when the patient is dismissed from the surgery, typically some 15–20 minutes after placing the filling, the amalgam is relatively weak. It is necessary, therefore, to instruct patients not to apply undue stress to their freshly placed amalgam fillings. The requirements of the ISO Standard (Table 21.2) reflect the slow development of the strength which can occur with dental amalgam. The requirement for strength at 24 hours is six times the requirement at 1 hour.

Spherical particle alloys and copper-enriched alloys develop strength more rapidly than conventional lathe-cut materials. Fine-grain, lathe-cut products develop strength more rapidly than coarse-grain products (Fig. 21.4). There is little difference in the ultimate compressive strength values of the materials – all being adequate in this respect.

The tensile strength and transverse strength values of amalgam are very much lower than the compres-

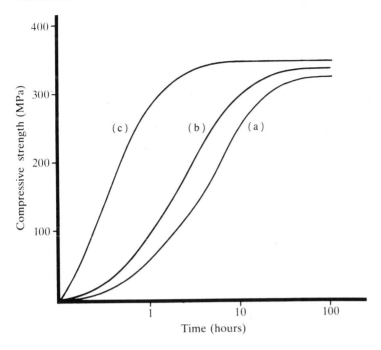

Fig. 21.4 Graph showing increase in compressive strength as a function of time. (a) Coarse-grain, lathe-cut material. (b) Fine-grain, lathe-cut material. (c) Spherical particle material.

sive strength. The material is weak in thin sections and unsupported edges of amalgam are readily fractured under occlusal loads. Due regard must be paid to the mechanical properties of amalgam when considering cavity preparation. The material should be considered essentially brittle in nature, requiring adequate support from surrounding structures and occasionally requiring reinforcement with metal pins embedded in dentine. Technique may play an important part in determining the final strength of amalgam. There is good correlation between strength and mercury content. Optimum properties are produced for amalgams containing 44–48% mercury. Since most materials are initially proportioned at more than 50% mercury it is necessary to reduce this level during manipulation.

Table 21.3 gives mechanical properties of a typical lathe-cut amalgam along with those of enamel and dentine for comparison. It can be seen that in many respects the material is a relatively good replacement for the natural tooth substance. Values of modulus of elasticity, tensile strength and hardness lie between those of the materials being replaced. The hardness of amalgam is somewhat lower than that of enamel, a factor that may be responsible for amalgam restorations developing surface facets when they make contact with cusps of opposing teeth. Despite having a surface hardness which is over three times lower than that of enamel, amalgam appears to have adequate resistance to intra-oral abrasion and rarely fails by this mechanism.

Plastic deformation (creep): Amalgam undergoes a certain amount of plastic deformation or creep when subjected to dynamic intra-oral stresses. The tendency for a material to creep is, however, normally

Table 21.3 Mechanical properties of a lathe-cut amalgam compared with tooth substance.

Property	Enamel	Dentine	Amalgam
Modulus of elasticity (GPa)	50	12	30
Compressive strength at 7 days (MPa)	250*	280	350
Tensile strength at 7 days	35[†]	40–260[‡]	60[†]
Vickers hardness	350	60	100

* Value for enamel cusp.
[†] Diammetral test.
[‡] Higher values calculated from flexural test.

Tarnish due to sulfide layer.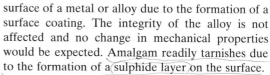

measured in the laboratory using a *static creep* test. (See p. 14.) Creep is determined by applying an axial compressive stress of 36 MPa to a cylinder of amalgam 6 mm long and 4 mm in diameter. The specimen is stored at 37°C for 7 days before testing. After loading, the change in length of the specimen is monitored for 4 hours and the creep is calculated as the change in length between 1 hour and 4 hours as a percentage of the original length.

The significance of creep can be explained by reference to Fig. 21.5. Creep causes the amalgam to flow, such that unsupported amalgam protrudes from the margin of the cavity (Fig. 21.5b). These unsupported edges are weak and may be further weakened by corrosion. Fracture causes the formation of a 'ditch' around the margins of the amalgam restoration. The phenomenon is often referred to as the *ditching* of amalgam. The γ_2 phase of amalgam is primarily responsible for the relatively high values of creep exhibited by some materials. The copper-enriched amalgams, which contain little or no γ_2 in the set material, have significantly lower creep values and clinical trials show they are less prone to ditching. Amalgams produced from copper-enriched alloys containing small quantities of metals such as palladium or indium have lower values still. This suggests that although the γ_2 phase may be implicated as being responsible for high creep it is not the only factor involved. Typical values of static creep for three types of amalgam are given in Table 21.4. These values can be compared with the maximum value accepted in standards (Table 21.2).

Corrosion: The term corrosion should be distinguished from the often misused term tarnish. Tarnishing simply involves the loss of lustre from the surface of a metal or alloy due to the formation of a surface coating. The integrity of the alloy is not affected and no change in mechanical properties would be expected. Amalgam readily tarnishes due to the formation of a sulphide layer on the surface.

Corrosion is a more serious matter which may significantly affect the structure and mechanical properties.

The heterogeneous, multiphase structure of dental amalgam makes it prone to corrosion. Electrolytic cells are readily set up in which different phases form the anode and cathode and saliva provides the electrolytes (p. 26).

The γ_2 phase of a conventional amalgam is the most electrochemically reactive and readily forms the anode in an electrolytic cell. The γ_2 phase breaks down to give tin-containing corrosion products and mercury which may be able to combine with unreacted alloy (γ phase). Not all the mercury formed during corrosion is able to combine rapidly with unreacted alloy and small quantities inevitably become ingested. This source of ingested mercury is a worry to those concerned about the cumulative toxic effects of mercury in the body. The proposed mechanism for the release of mercury during corrosion would suggest that this problem should be less acute for the copper-enriched, γ_2 free materials. For these products the most reactive phase, and the one most likely to form the anode in a corrosive couple, is the Cu–Sn phase. The rate of corrosion is accelerated if the amalgam filling contacts a gold restoration. The large difference in potential results in a significant corrosion current being established.

Corrosion produces a restoration with poor appearance and may significantly affect mechanical properties. The chances of ditching are increased, particularly if creep has also occurred. The level of corrosion can be minimized by polishing the surfaces of restorations. Smooth surfaces are less prone to concentration cell corrosion.

The corrosion products are thought to produce one beneficial result. They are thought to gather at the restoration-tooth interface and to eventually form a seal which prevents microleakage. This proposed mechanism is supported by the fact that, in laboratory tests, microleakage is observed to

Table 21.4 Values of static creep for amalgam.

Material type	Creep (%)*
Conventional lathe-cut	2.5
Dispersion-modified, copper-enriched	0.2
Copper-enriched, containing 0.5% palladium	0.06

* Creep after 7 days, stress of 37 MPa applied for 4 hours.

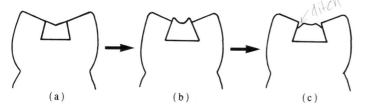

(a)   (b)   (c)

Fig. 21.5 Diagram showing how creep of amalgam causes the formation of unsupported edges which can fracture. (a) Initial restoration. (b) Following creep. (c) Following marginal fracture.

decrease with time if amalgam restored teeth are stored in a corrosive environment.

Copper-enriched amalgams contain little or no γ_2 phase. The copper–tin phase, which replaces γ_2 in these materials, is still the most corrosion-prone phase in the amalgam. The corrosion currents produced, however, are lower than those for conventional amalgams.

It is now generally accepted that copper-enriched amalgams perform better than conventional materials in terms of corrosion and that this may be a factor involved in the lower incidence of ditching reported for these materials. There are no reports of increased marginal leakage for the copper-enriched materials, indicating that sufficient quantities of corrosion product are produced to seal the margins.

Thermal properties: Amalgam has a relatively high value of *thermal diffusivity*, as would be expected for a metallic restorative material. Thus, in constructing an amalgam restoration, an insulating material, dentine, is replaced by a good thermal conductor (Table 21.5). In large cavities it is necessary to line the base of the cavity with an insulating, cavity lining material prior to condensing the amalgam. This reduces the harmful effects of thermal stimuli on the pulp.

Table 21.5 Thermal properties of amalgam and dentine.

	Thermal diffusivity $\times\ 10^{-3}\ cm^2\ s^{-1}$	Coefficient of thermal expansion $\times\ 10^{-6}\ °C^{-1}$
Amalgam	78	25
Dentine	2	8

The *coefficient of thermal expansion* value for amalgam is about three times greater than that for dentine (Table 21.5). This, coupled with the greater diffusivity of amalgam, results in considerably more expansion and contraction in the restoration than in the surrounding tooth when a patient takes hot or cold food or drink. Such a mismatch of thermal expansion behaviour may cause microleakage around the filling since there is no adhesion between amalgam and tooth substance. The occurrence of decay in the dentine which surrounds an amalgam filling is the major cause for replacement of such restorations. It is likely that microleakage plays an important part in initiating such lesions.

Biological properties: Certain mercury compounds are known to have a harmful effect on the central nervous system. The patient is briefly subjected to relatively high doses of mercury during placement, contouring and removal of amalgam fillings. A lower, but continuing, dose results from ingestion of corrosion products. Some studies have shown a higher concentration of mercury in the blood and urine of patients with amalgam fillings than those without. Levels of mercury were generally within acceptable limits however, and some studies have been unable to demonstrate a difference between patients with amalgam fillings and those without. Despite this there have been reports linking mercury from dental amalgams with a variety of ailments, ranging from fairly mild behavioural problems to major psychiatric disturbances and multiple sclerosis. Many of the claims are unsubstantiated and are often based on unscientific evidence. There are some documented cases, however, in which symptoms appear to subside after a patient's amalgam fillings are removed. This is a surprising observation that goes a long way towards proving that the original symptoms had little or nothing to do with mercury since the removal of amalgam fillings would ensure a marked increase in the body burden of mercury. This is caused by release of mercury vapour during the grinding of amalgam.

Another concern has been associated with reports that mercury can be concentrated in the placenta and then be passed from mother to fetus, potentially causing spontaneous abortion or abnormalities in the new-born child. Scientific evidence suggests that there are no grounds for such concerns. Despite the wealth of scientific evidence some authorities have advocated avoidance of the exposure of pregnant women to dental amalgam. Concerns over mercury release from amalgam fillings should have become less of an issue since the introduction and widespread use of non-γ_2 alloys. These alloys have significantly better corrosion resistance and the corrosion process involves the liberation of far less mercury than the γ_2-containing products.

Another potential problem concerns allergic reactions to mercury in dental amalgam. Such allergic reactions, usually manifested as a contact dermatitis, are well documented and can normally be explained by previous sensitization of the patient with mercury-containing medicaments. Despite the vast numbers of amalgam fillings placed every year the number of reported allergic reactions is very small and will presumably decrease further if the use of mercury-containing sensitizing agents (e.g. certain eye ointments) declines.

Whilst it is generally agreed that amalgam fillings cause little damage to patients, concern has been expressed over the possible effects of long-term exposure of dentists and assistants to mercury vapour. Mercury vapour may be released into the atmosphere during trituration, condensation or during the removal of old amalgam restorations. In addition, spillages of mercury in the surgery can cause long-term contamination of the atmosphere. It should be remembered that the vapour pressure of mercury increases markedly with temperature. The levels of atmospheric mercury will increase if an attempt is made to sterilize instruments contaminated with mercury or dental amalgam. Mercury-containing material should always be stored well away from any heat source. Spillages of mercury which occur near any source of heat, such as radiator or oven, will cause a marked increase in the concentration of mercury in the atmosphere.

Serious problems can be avoided by ensuring that the surgery is well ventilated and that flooring of a suitable type is chosen such that accidental spillages can be readily dealt with. Excess, waste or scrap amalgam should be stored, under water or chemical fixative solution, in a sealed container in order to prevent another possible source of contamination. Mercury or freshly mixed amalgam should never be touched by hand. Mercury is readily absorbed by the skin, a fact which was obviously not appreciated in the days when it was normal practice to 'mull' the material in the hand before condensation. In addition to being hazardous this practice leads to contamination of the amalgam.

Despite the increased exposure of dental personnel to mercury vapour, examinations of the health, mortality and morbidity rates for dentists have shown that they are not significantly different from those of the general population, a fact which should go a long way towards reassuring those who harbour fears over mercury toxicity.

21.5 Clinical handling notes for dental amalgam

Cavity design: Many designs of cavity have been used for amalgam restorations, starting with modification of Black's design for cavities for gold restorations. Over the years the cavity design has been refined to minimize destruction of sound tooth tissue and to give an appropriate form to the restoration to ensure that the physical properties of the material are optimized in the end product.

Amalgam has no intrinsic ability to bond to enamel and dentine, hence cavities have to be used which are undercut, i.e., the cavity is wider within the structure of the tooth than at its surface, in order that the material should be mechanically retained. *At all times the cavity should be no wider than is compatible with removal of caries from the dentine, removal of any unsupported enamel and adequate access to pack the amalgam into the cavity.* All internal line angles should be rounded to minimize internal stresses within the restoration and to facilitate adaptation of the material to the cavity walls. The floor of the cavity, both that overlying the pulp and at the gingival extent of any box, should be flat to permit condensation of amalgam.

The cavo-surface margin is of particular importance for amalgam restorations. Amalgam is weak in thin section and hence a cavo-surface angle of approaching 90° is desirable. This can be difficult to achieve, particularly on a cusp slope, whilst retaining a reasonable quantity of tooth tissue. Local modifications to the cavity margin, in enamel, may help to surmount this problem.

It is always necessary to remove unsupported enamel once any carious dentine has been removed. This is relatively easy to achieve on the clearly visible cavity surface, but it should be remembered that the enamel prism orientation close to the gingival margins is apical. Hence this area of the tooth needs to be finished using a gingival margin trimmer. Failure to remove unsupported enamel will result in an intrinsic weakness at the margins of the restoration. The unsupported tissue could fail either during function or under the pressure applied by a steel matrix band whilst the restoration is being packed (Fig. 21.6). Such failure would result in very rapid marginal ditch formation and probable early failure of the restoration through recurrent decay.

Small cavities rely upon the undercut between opposing walls of the tooth for retention. If one or more cusps has fractured off a tooth it may be necessary to use an alternative form of retention for the amalgam. One method is to prepare pits and grooves in the remaining dentine into which the amalgam can be condensed. These act as retentive features if positioned correctly in relation to the remaining tooth tissues. Alternatively dentine pins can be used. A pin hole is prepared in the dentine and a pin is cemented, pressed or threaded into place. Nowadays, the most common form of pin is the self-threading pin in which a thread on the pin acts as its own *tap* to cut a thread into the dentine. In practice the quality of the thread cut into the dentine is poor and such pins are retained by tightly packed dentine chips. Pins which have a shoulder which engages the tooth tissue before the threaded shaft of the pin contacts the base of the pin hole cause less

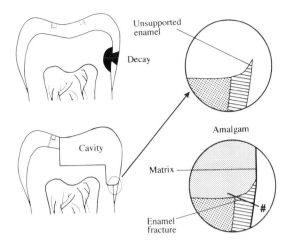

Fig. 21.6 Preparation of cavity margins with round-tipped cutting instruments can lead to the production of a marginal lip of unsupported enamel. If this lip is not removed prior to adaptation of the matrix the band will apply considerable pressure to the enamel which will tend to fracture. The fractured portion will be held in place by the matrix, but will be lost relatively rapidly after matrix removal, resulting in a marginal defect at the base of the box.

damage to the tooth. Pins need to be placed with care to avoid the pulp and the periodontium. At the same time adequate space needs to be available between the pin and the location of the surface of the restoration to permit the condensation of an appropriate bulk of amalgam. Finally pins should not be placed too close together. All dentine pins weaken the restoration in which they are placed so they should be used sparingly. The most recent innovation for retention of amalgam is the use of chemically-active adhesive resins as an adhesive between tooth structure and the restoration. These materials are covered in Sections 23.9 and 27.2.

Matrices: If an external wall of a tooth is breached by a cavity a steel matrix band needs to be applied to the tooth to provide a surface against which the amalgam can be condensed. In addition to forming the external wall of the cavity the matrix should adapt very closely to the gingival margin of the cavity to prevent the production of ledges of amalgam outside the cavity during packing.

Matrices either come with some form of holder or can be made from stainless steel tape held in place using impression compound.

It is important when rebuilding the proximal surfaces of any tooth to restore its contact relationship with any adjacent tooth. Obviously the use of a matrix may compromise this objective as the thickness of the matrix is interposed between the filling material and the tooth. This problem is surmounted when using amalgam in two ways. First, having adapted the matrix to the tooth it is burnished outward to try to achieve a contact with the adjacent tooth. Second, a wooden or metal wedge should be inserted between the teeth if possible. This has a dual benefit in that it helps to maintain adaptation of the band to the tooth surface cervically and it separates the teeth slightly. Once the wedge is in place the matrix can be loosened slightly to facilitate burnishing against the adjacent tooth.

21.6 Manipulative variables

The manipulation of amalgam involves the following sequence of events.

(1) Proportioning and dispensing;
(2) Trituration;
(3) Condensation;
(4) Carving;
(5) Polishing.

The way in which each of these operations is carried out has an effect on the properties of the final restoration.

Proportioning and dispensing: Alloy/mercury ratios vary between 5:8 and 10:8. Those mixes containing greater quantities of mercury are 'wetter' and are generally used with hand mixing. Those mixes containing smaller quantities of mercury are 'drier' and are generally used with mechanical mixing. For any given alloy/mercury ratio, the nature of the mix may vary depending upon the size and shape of the alloy particles. Spherical particle alloys, for example, require less mercury to produce a workable mix.

For optimum properties the final set amalgam should contain less than 50% mercury. Those materials used at alloy/mercury ratios at or approaching 5:8 require the removal of excess mercury following trituration and during condensation.

The optimal final mercury content ranges from an average of 45% for lathe-cut materials to an average of 40% for spherical materials. Hence, the amount of mercury required to produce a workable plastic mass of material is generally greater than that required to produce optimal properties in the set material. If too much mercury is present in the final set amalgam it is likely that too much of the relatively hard γ phase will be converted into relatively weak and soft γ_2 phase and that a considerable amount of mercury will remain unreacted. If, on the other hand, an attempt is made to use too little mercury there may not be enough to wet the surface of the alloy particles and produce sufficient matrix phase material to bind the unreacted γ cores together. This would result in porosity being present in the set material.

Various methods of dispensation are available. The most accurate method is to weigh the mercury and alloy components using a balance. This method is rarely used however, and both are commonly proportioned using volume dispensers.

The simplest type of volume dispenser consists of a glass bottle with a plastic, screw-top cap. The cap has a spring-loaded plunger which releases a known volume of either mercury or alloy when depressed. This method of dispensation is relatively accurate and reproducible for mercury but less so for the powdered alloys since the amount of alloy released depends on the way in which the particles are packed together in the container.

An alternative method of dispensation for the alloy is preproportioned as a powder in a small sachet or envelope or as a tablet in which the powder particles are compressed together. Mixing involves the use of either the contents of one envelope or one tablet with a given volume of mercury.

Perhaps the most commonly used method of dispensation involves the use of semi-automatic dispensers which also carry out the mixing or trituration. These devices typically have two hoppers. One is filled with alloy, the other with mercury. The alloy/mercury ratio can be set by the operator and the required amount of each component is released into a mixing chamber on the throw of a switch or the press of a button.

Another convenient method of dispensation involves the use of encapsulated materials. Each capsule contains both alloy and mercury in proportions which have been determined by the manufacturer. The two components are initially separated by an impermeable membrane which is readily shattered using a purpose-built capsule press or on starting to vibrate the capsule in a mechanical mixer. Capsules which do not require the use of a press are called self-activating capsules.

Trituration: The mixing or trituration of amalgam may be carried out by hand, using a mortar and pestle, or in an electrically powered machine which vibrates a capsule containing the mercury and alloy.

For hand trituration, a glass mortar and pestle with roughened surfaces are normally used. A low alloy/mercury ratio (around 5:8) is often required to produce a workable mix and care must be taken not to use excessive pressure during trituration in order

to prevent splintering of alloy particles which may change the character of the mix.

The trituration time may have an effect on the properties of the final set amalgam. Some products require at least 40 seconds trituration in order to achieve full 'wetting' of alloy particles by mercury and optimal properties in the amalgam. Following trituration it is necessary to reduce the mercury content of the mix before condensing. This is normally done by placing the amalgam into a strip of gauze or chamois leather and squeezing to express excess mercury which appears as droplets on the outside.

Trituration by hand is not extensively practised in developed countries nowadays. Mechanical mixing is far more widely used. There are three levels of sophistication which may be employed. Following proportioning, the mercury and alloy may be placed in a capsule which is vibrated on a purpose-built machine, often referred to as an amalgamator. Alternatively, mechanical mixing in a semi-automatic machine, which also proportions mercury and alloy, is possible. The use of encapsulated, preproportioned materials is probably the most convenient, although also the most expensive option. For all three options, trituration times of 5–20 seconds are normal. The trituration time will vary according to the nature of the alloy and the alloy: mercury ratio. For uncapsulated products the mercury and alloy are separated by a diaphragm which commonly has to be broken mechanically before the material can be triturated. Manufacturer's instructions should be followed at all times for length of trituration.

The advantages of mechanical trituration are as follows.

(1) A uniform and reproducible mix is produced.
(2) A shorter trituration time can be used.
(3) A greater alloy/mercury ration can be used.

This negates the requirement to express excess mercury before condensing. Encapsulated materials have the extra advantage that they are proportioned by the manufacturer.

Another potential advantage of using encapsulated materials is that they may help to reduce the risk of atmospheric mercury contamination. In order for this potential advantage to be realized it is essential that the capsules do not release mercury during trituration. If the capsule is not properly sealed, considerable amounts of mercury may escape as the temperature within the capsule increases during mechanical mixing. A further precaution is recommended when trituration is complete and the capsule is opened. The contents remain warm at this stage and the capsule should be opened away from the face in well-ventilated conditions.

Condensation: Following trituration, the material is packed or condensed into the prepared cavity. A variety of methods have been suggested to condense amalgam including ultrasonic vibration and mechanical condensing tools. The mechanical tools apply quite high loads with a reasonably large amplitude of movement of the condensing tool. As a consequence they may be associated with damage to teeth, notably cuspal fracture during condensation.

Ultrasonic condensers tend to produce local heating of the amalgam with detrimental effects both in terms of mercury vapour release and modification in the setting reaction of the material.

The most widely used method of condensation is with a hand instrument called an amalgam condenser. These are flat-ended and come in a variety of styles. The shape and size of the condenser should be chosen with the size of the cavity in mind. The condenser must be able to fit within the cavity outline and should be able to get reasonably close to the peripheral margin of the restoration. This can be a problem with boxes on the surface of a tooth as a large round condenser will not pack the amalgam well into the box walls close to the matrix. It is often better to use a smaller diameter round condenser or an ovoid instrument to facilitate this first stage of packing. The amalgam is packed in increments, each increment being equivalent to the volume of material which can be carried in an amalgam 'gun'. This is the device used to transfer the material from the mixing vessel to the prepared cavity. During condensation, a fluid, mercury-rich layer is formed on the surface of each incremental layer. The cavity is overfilled and the mercury-rich layer carved away from the surface. This effectively reduces the mercury content of the filling thus improving its mechanical properties.

The technique chosen for condensation must ensure the following.

(1) Adequate adaptation of the material to all parts of the cavity base and walls.
(2) Good bonding between the incremental layers of amalgam.
(3) Optimal mechanical properties in the set amalgam by minimizing porosity and achieving a final mercury content of 44–48%.

There should be a minimal time delay between trituration and condensation. If condensation is commenced too late, the amalgam will have achieved a certain degree of set and adaptation, bonding of increments and final mechanical properties are all adversely affected.

There is good correlation between the quality of an amalgam restoration and the energy expended by the operator who condenses it. For lathe-cut amalgam alloys best results are achieved by using a high condensing force at a rapid condensing frequency and continuing to condense until the amalgam feels hard and a mercury-rich layer has been formed at the surface. Amalgams made from spherical alloy particles have very different condensation characteristics to their lathe-cut counter parts. They require lower condensation pressures to achieve the same degree of homogeneity and physical strength. Indeed, there is a risk when condensing spherical alloys of using too great a condensation pressure. If this occurs the alloy particles roll over each other and are displaced by the condenser rather than being condensed into an homogenous mass. Recently some manufacturers have started to sand blast the spherical alloy particles. This has the effect of giving the material a similar handling characteristic to lathe-cut alloys but still retaining their ease of condensing with low pressure.

Carving: The objectives of carving an amalgam restoration are to remove the mercury-rich layer on the amalgam surface and to rebuild the anatomy of the tooth, re-establishing contact with the opposing dentition. Obviously a knowledge of normal tooth anatomy is necessary for this purpose.

Soon after condensing the amalgam, the surface layer, which is rich in mercury, is carved away with a sharp instrument. Carving should be carried out when the material has reached a certain degree of set. If attempts are made to carve too soon there is a danger of 'dragging out' significant amounts of material from the surface. If carving is delayed too long the material may become too hard to carve and there is a danger of chipping at the margins. It is useful to try to retain a mental picture of the extent of the cavity when carving. The amalgam needs to be cut back to the cavity margins. If this is not done, long fine-tapered extensions of amalgam will lie on top of the enamel surface. These will be poorly supported and will fracture rapidly if under occlusal load producing a positive margin (the amalgam stands proud of the tooth structure).

It will be necessary to check the pattern of occlusal contacts whilst carving a restoration. When the amalgam is still soft, rubbing the surface with cotton wool produces a matt finish, if the subject then gently taps their teeth together or moves them from side to side in contact, any areas of contact will show up as bright burnished spots and can be removed/reduced as required. If carving is not complete by the time that the amalgam has become hard, occlusal contacts need to be marked using thin articulating tape. High areas can be removed using steel instruments or ultimately a bur, usually a steel bur in a slow hand piece.

Spherical amalgams are easier to carve than lathe-cut materials and fine-grain products easier than coarse-grain.

Removal of the matrix: If a matrix has been used to help form a large amalgam restoration this should be removed during the carving process. The amalgam must be sufficiently set that removal of the band will not result in bulk failure of the restoration. Equally, the materials should be sufficiently soft that any marginal excesses can be removed easily once the band has been removed. It is important to check that excess amalgam has not been forced beyond the matrix band gingivaly during condensation. This would otherwise result in a marginal ledge formation which could lead to periodontal disease as a consequence of inadequate cleansibility.

Polishing: Polishing is carried out in order to achieve a lustrous surface having a more acceptable appearance and better corrosion resistance. The fillings should not be polished until the material has achieved a certain level of mechanical strength, otherwise there is a danger of fracture, particularly at the margins. The strength which should be attained before polishing is commenced is not certain but many products require a delay of 24 hours between placing and polishing. It is claimed that some faster setting materials can be polished soon after placing.

Gross irregularities in the surface are reduced using multi-bladed steel burs in a slow hand piece. This stage should result in a smooth surface contour. Fine polishing to produce a lustre is then undertaken using graded abrasives, either flours of pumice followed by zinc or ceric oxides with water as a carrier or by using abrasive impregnated rubber points and wheels. Pastes need to be applied using a rubber cup or brush, but are less frequently used now that impregnated points are available. One beneficial effect of using a rubber carrier for the abrasive (either a cup or a point) is to burnish the surface of the restoration, improving its marginal adaptation.

21.7 Suggested further reading

Eley, B.M. (1997) The future of dental amalgam: A review of the literature. *Br. Dent. J.* **182**, 6 parts.

Greener, E.H. (1979) Amalgam – yesterday, today and tomorrow. *Oper. Dent.* **4**, 24.

ISO 1559 Alloys for dental amalgam.

Jones, D.W. (1993) The enigma of amalgam in dentistry. *J. Can. Dent. Assoc.* **59**, 155.

Chapter 22
Resin-based Filling Materials

22.1 Introduction

The development of filling materials based on synthetic polymers has been initiated by two major driving forces, in addition to the obvious commercial ones. Firstly, there was a requirement to produce a material which could overcome the major deficiencies of the silicate materials, namely, erosion, brittleness, acidity and a moisture sensitivity which demanded very careful manipulation. Secondly, developments in polymer technology produced resins which could be readily cured at mouth temperature and, with the aid of pigments and fillers, could be made to resemble the natural tooth in appearance.

The first materials to be widely used were the *acrylic resins.*. These are, essentially, similar to resins used in denture construction (Chapter 13). The unfilled acrylic resins have now been superseded by a myriad of *composite materials* consisting of a heterogeneous blend of organic resin and inorganic filler.

22.2 Acrylic resins

These are supplied as a powder and liquid which are mixed together. The composition is similar to that given in Table 13.1 for denture base materials. Briefly, the materials consist of a powder and liquid. The powder contains beads of polymethylmethacrylate (< 50 µm), chemical initiator (often a peroxide) and pigment, whilst the liquid consists of methylmethacrylate monomer and a chemical activator (often a tertiary amine). The pigments used are, generally, white, yellow or brown, in order to match natural tooth shades, as opposed to the pink pigments used in denture base polymers. The setting reaction involves a free radical addition polymerization as described in Chapter 12.

The amine which is often used as a chemical activator in acrylic resins remains largely unconsumed at the end of the setting reaction. One such amine which has been widely used is N, N' dimethyl-p-toluidine. This has very poor colour stability, particularly in ultraviolet light, and gradually changes from clear to brown, causing a consequent change of colour in the material itself; hence some acrylic filling materials have been reported as having very poor colour stability. Attempts to overcome this problem have involved the use of UV absorbers and more stable amines as well as other types of activators and initiators. Peroxide/alkylborane systems have been used as an alternative to peroxide/amine. This system was claimed to produce a material with adhesive properties although this has never been extensively evaluated.

Other materials utilized a peroxide/mercaptan initiation system whilst peroxide/sulphinic acid was used in other products. The latter system is complicated because the sulphinic acid (normally p-toluene sulphinic acid) is unstable and can inadvertently cause premature polymerization of the monomer if incorporated in the liquid. This problem is overcome by incorporation of a salt of the sulphinic acid in the powder with the peroxide. A small quantity of methacrylic acid is incorporated in the liquid. This rapidly converts and sulphinic acid salt to the free acid when powder and liquid are mixed together. The sulphinic acid then reacts with the peroxide to activate the polymerization process.

Advantages: The acrylic resin materials are *less prone to erosion* than silicates. They have low solubility over a wide range of pH values. They are *less acidic* than silicates though cannot be considered biologically bland due to the presence of residual methylmethacrylate monomer. They are *less brittle* than silicates although their mechanical properties are far from ideal.

The materials are good thermal insulators having a *low value of thermal diffusivity*, 1.0×10^{-3} cm^{2}s^{-1} as opposed to 2.0×10^{-3} cm^{2}s^{-1} for dentine. The ability to match the appearance of tooth substance is, initially, very good, although some products have a tendency to discolour gradually with time. Discoloration at the margins is also observed with many restorations.

Disadvantages: Although the acrylic materials do not contain any strong acids, some products contain methacrylic acid, used to modify setting characteristics, and all contain a certain level of residual methylmethacrylate monomer which is *irritant.* This, coupled with a significant *temperature rise* during setting caused by a highly exothermic polymerization reaction, necessitates the use of a protective cavity base material. The material of choice is a setting calcium hydroxide type. Products containing eugenol should be avoided since they retard the setting of the resin and cause discoloration.

The materials undergo a considerable *setting contraction* (6% by volume). If uncontrolled, this could produce a significant marginal gap down which fluids could penetrate. The problem may be partially alleviated by filling the cavity with small increments and allowing the contraction to occur towards the walls of the cavity before the next increment is added (Fig. 22.1). Another approach is to overfill the cavity and place the setting material under strong finger pressure with a matrix strip during setting.

The *coefficient of thermal expansion* value for acrylic resin is some ten times greater than that for tooth substance. The potential for *percolation* of fluids down the restoration–tooth interface when the patient takes hot or cold food and drink is, therefore, significant.

The mechanical properties of acrylic resin compare unfavourably with those of the natural tooth material which it replaces (Table 22.1). The low value of *modulus of elasticity* indicates that acrylic resin is a far more flexible material than either enamel or dentine. Flexing of restorations under load can lead to marginal breakdown. The lower

Table 22.1 Some mechanical properties of acrylic resin, enamel and dentine.

	Acrylic resin	Enamel	Dentine
Modulus of elasticity (GPa)	2	50	15
Compressive strength (MPa)	70	250	280
Hardness (Vickers)	20	350	60

compressive strength and *hardness* values of acrylic resin are reflected in a *poor durability*, particularly when restorations are subjected to abrasive forces. Material loss by *wear* is a phenomenon associated with these relatively soft materials.

Current status: Acrylic resins are now rarely used as permanent filling materials. They overcome the major problems associated with silicates but have many other disadvantages which preclude regular use. The materials are still in use for temporary crown and bridge construction.

22.3 Composite materials – introduction

A composite material is a product which consists of at least two distinct phases normally formed by blending together components having different structures and properties. The purpose of this is to produce a material having properties which could not be achieved from any of the individual components alone. The two main components of composite filling materials are the resin phase and the reinforcing filler. The beneficial properties contributed by the resin are the ability to be moulded at ambient temperatures coupled with setting by polymerization achieved in a conveniently short time. The disadvantages of using resin alone have been given in the previous section. The beneficial properties con-

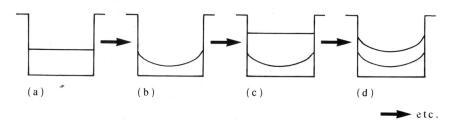

(a)   (b)   (c)   (d)

→ etc.

Fig. 22.1 Diagrammatic representation of incremental layers of acrylic resin filling material, used to partially overcome polymerization contraction. (a) First increment placed. (b) Shrinkage occurs towards base and walls of cavity. (c) Second increment added. (d) Further shrinkage.

tributed by the filler are rigidity, hardness, strength and a lower value for the coefficient of thermal expansion. In addition, if the filler occupies a significant proportion of the volume of a composite material it markedly lowers setting contraction. The effect of filler depends on the type, shape, size and amount of filler incorporated and, often, the existence of efficient coupling between the filler and resin.

When particulate glass fillers are incorporated in acrylic resins, three properties, namely, coefficient of thermal expansion, setting contraction and surface hardness, depend almost linearly on the filler content, as shown in Fig. 22.2.

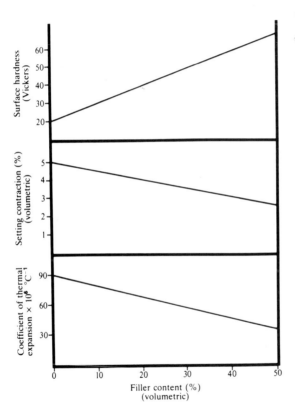

Fig. 22.2 Variation of surface hardness, setting contraction and coefficient of thermal expansion with inorganic filler content for acrylic resins.

Other thermal and mechanical properties may vary in a similar way. Strength and modulus of elasticity generally increase with addition of filler, as does abrasion resistance, probably as a result of increased surface hardness. If the added filler is translucent, the optical properties of the resin are improved and a more lifelike appearance produced.

The resins used in composite materials are invariably based in methacrylate monomers. Simple methylmethacrylate was used in some early products but most materials now utilize dimethacrylates. These monomers undergo a small contraction on setting and form a highly cross-linked three dimensional network with properties which are generally better than those of polymethylmelthacrylate.

22.4 Classification and composition of composites

All dental composites consist of a blend of resin and inorganic filler. Methods used to characterize materials are based upon the method used to activate polymerization of the resin and on the particle size distribution of filler. Figure 22.3 shows the polished surface of a composite in which the filler particles embedded in a matrix of resin are clearly visible.

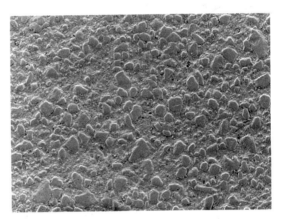

Fig. 22.3 Polished surface of a dental composite showing filler particles embedded in a matrix of resin ($\times$ 1445).

Resins: The nature of the resin may alter slightly from one product to another, although, essentially, they all contain a modified methacrylate or acrylate. Figure 22.4 gives the molecular structures of two of the most commonly used monomers, Bis GMA and urethane dimethacrylate, together with that of triethylene glycol dimethacrylate (TEGMA) which is a comonomer often used to control the viscosity of the unmixed materials. It can be seen from Fig. 22.4 that the monomer and comonomer molecules are difunctional methacrylates. Each carbon–carbon double bond is able to take part in a free radical addition polymerization, to give a highly cross-linked resin after setting.

Bis GMA is a difunctional methacrylate which is

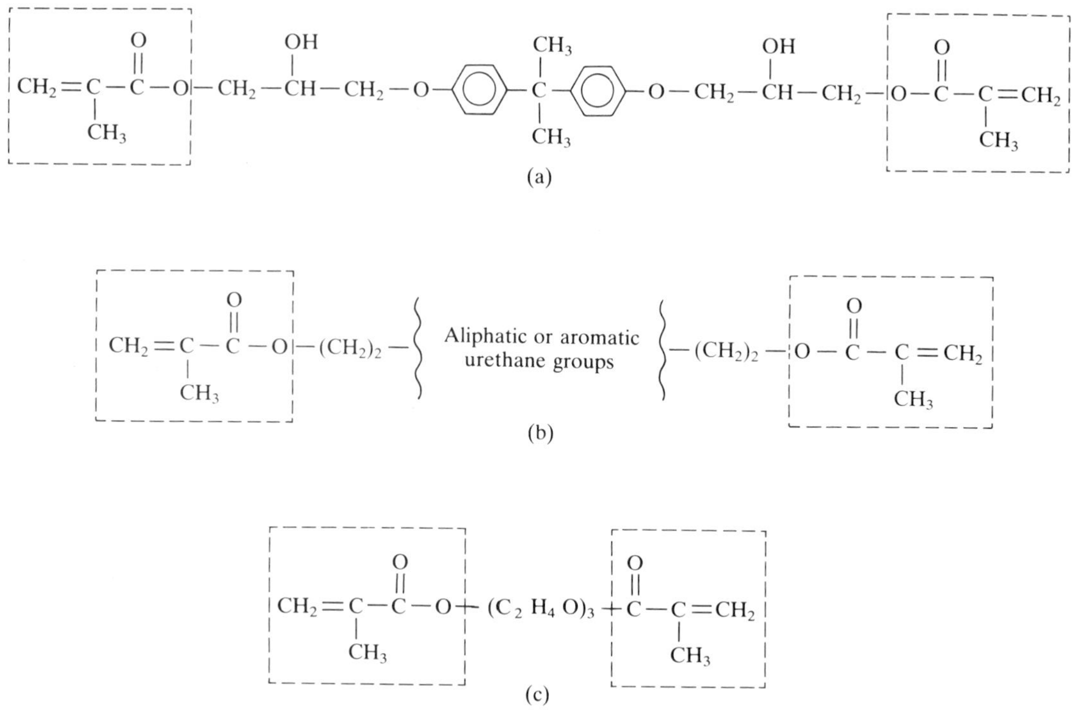

Fig. 22.4 Molecular structures of three modified methacrylate or acrylate resin monomers used in composite materials. (a) Bis GMA (addition product of BisPhenol A and glycidylmethacrylate). (b) Urethane dimethacrylate. (c) Triethylene glycol dimethacrylate.

normally formed by a reaction between bisphenol A and glycidylmethacrylate. It has two phenyl groups which lend a degree of rigidity to the molecule and the hydroxyl groups are thought to give some intermolecular hydrogen bonding. These features give Bis GMA a consistency which is similar to that of thick treacle at room temperature. Blending of filler particles with a material of this consistency is difficult and the manufacturers normally have to use a fluid diluent monomer such as TEGMA to reduce the viscosity. A mixture of three parts Bis GMA and one part TEGMA is typically blended with filler. Bis MA monomer is used in some products. This is very similar to Bis GMA but contains no hydroxyl groups.

The urethanedimethacrylate monomers may be aliphatic or aromatic in nature. The central group in Fig. 22.4 is typically:

$$-O-CO-NH-CH_2-CH(CH_3)-CH_2-C(CH_3)_2$$
$$-CH_2-CH_2-NH-CO-O-$$

in a commonly used aliphatic dimethacrylate monomer. Monomers of this type have relatively low viscosity and do not require the use of a diluent monomer although some manufacturers do blend various monomers together. Urethanedimethacry-

late monomers containing aromatic groups have a slightly more complicated structure and are often more viscous, normally requiring the presence of a diluent monomer.

The size of the monomer and comonomer molecules, coupled with a rapid increase in viscosity during setting, causes a relatively high concentration of acrylate or methacrylate groups to remain unreacted after setting. This results from the fact that reactive methacrylate groups find it increasingly difficult to migrate to the reaction sites as viscosity increases. When the glass transition temperature of the polymerizing mass approaches the ambient temperature the rate of diffusion diminishes markedly and little further reaction is possible. Further reaction could be encouraged by heating the material to a temperature well above the ambient temperature in order to regenerate mobility of reactive groups. Heat treatment of this type is not feasible for direct composite filling materials but may be used to enhance the properties of composite inlay materials.

Methods of activation: Polymerization may be activated *chemically*, by mixing two components, one of which typically contains an initiator and the other an activator, or by an external *ultraviolet* or *visible light* source.

For chemical activation, many different methods of dispensation are available. The most popular is the 'two paste' system. Each paste contains a blend of resin and filler. One paste contains about 1% of a peroxide initiator, such as benzoyl peroxide, whilst the other paste contains about 0.5% of a tertiary amine activator, such as N, N' dimethyl-*p*-toluidine or *p*-tolyl diethanolamine. The ensuing reaction is a free radical addition polymerization as described in Chapter 12.

Other systems which rely on chemical activation are as follows:

(1) Powder/liquid systems, in which the powder contains filler particles and peroxide initiator whilst the liquid contains monomer, comonomer and chemical activator.

(2) Paste/liquid materials in which the paste contains monomers, comonomers, filler and peroxide whilst the liquid contains monomers and chemical activator.

(3) Encapsulated materials in which the filler, mixed with peroxide, is initially separated within a capsule from the monomers and comonomers containing the chemical activator. On breaking the seal between the two parts of the capsule the reactive components come into contact and are mixed mechanically.

Light-activated materials are generally supplied as a single paste which contains monomers, comonomers, filler and an initiator which is unstable in the presence of either ultraviolet (uv) or high-intensity visible light. For uv-activated materials, the most commonly used initiator is benzoin methyl ether. At certain selected wavelengths within the uv range, this molecule is able to absorb radiation and undergo heterolytic decomposition to form free radicals. The radicals initiate polymerization which then continues in much the same way as that described for vinyl monomers (p. 88).

The use of uv-activated materials has diminished greatly since the possible dangers of longterm exposure to ultraviolet radiation were highlighted.

For visible light-activated materials the initiator system comprises a mixture of a diketone and an amine. Camphorquinone is a commonly used diketone which rapidly forms free radicals in the presence of an amine and radiation of the correct wavelength and intensity.

Light-activated materials require the use of a specialist light source, capable of delivering radiation with the appropriate characteristics to the surface of the freshly placed material *in situ*.

Care must be taken in the storage of unused pastes since exposure to sunlight, or particularly to the surgery operating light, may be sufficient to activate a slow initiation process which causes the paste to thicken and become unworkable. For materials which are supplied in pots it is essential to replace the lid quickly after removing the required amount of paste.

Many materials are supplied in syringes which will enable the operator or his assistant to expel sufficient material for one restoration. The material remaining in the syringe is not exposed. Another method of dispensation is in the form of 'compules'. Each compule contains sufficient paste for at least one restoration and is extruded into the cavity by placing the compule into a press.

Fillers: The type, concentration, particle size and particle size distribution of the filler used in a composite material are major factors controlling properties.

Fillers commonly used include quartz, fused silica and many types of glass including aluminosilicates and borosilicates, some containing barium oxide.

The first generation of composite materials typically contain 60–80%, by weight, of quartz or glass in the particle size range of 1–50 µm. The particle size distribution may vary, within this range, from one product to another, some containing relatively greater amounts of larger particles, approaching 50 µm, others containing larger quantities of smaller particles. Materials containing filler particles of this type are normally referred to as *conventional* composites. The filler particles are subjected to a special pretreatment prior to blending with the resin. This involves laying down a surface coating of a *coupling agent* on the particles to enhance bonding between the filler and resin matrix. The coupling agent most commonly used is γ-methacryloxypropyltrimethoxysilane:

$$CH_2 = CCH_3CO_2(CH_2)_3Si(OCH_3)_3$$

This is a difunctional molecule which at one end has the characteristics of a methacrylate monomer whilst at the other it has a silane group capable of interacting and bonding with glass or quartz surfaces. Hence, it is able to set up a bond between the resin and filler components in a composite system.

Since the composite filling materials were introduced in the mid-1960s, there has been a trend towards the use of fillers with smaller particle size. Many of the currently available products with glass or quartz fillers contain particles in the more limited range of 1–5 µm.

Another development has been the introduction of a number of products containing submicron particles of silica. These materials are referred to as *microfilled composites* and contain silica particles in the range 0.01–0.1 µm with a typical mean diameter of 0.04 µm. The very small particle size produces a massive increase in available surface area for a given volume of filler (typically 10^3–10^4 times more surface area). Consequently, it is not possible to incorporate very high filler loadings of this small particle size and products which are available contain only 30–60% filler by weight. Even at these lower levels, calculations show that many filler particles must be present as agglomerates and not as individual particles surrounded by resin.

The method of incorporating the smaller particles varies, direct blending with resin being difficult. The most widely used method is to prepare pre-polymerized blocks of resin containing a high filler loading of silica. The block is splintered and ground to give particles of resin up to 100 µm in diameter, each containing silica. These particles are blended with monomer, comonomers, initiators or activators to form pastes.

A third series of composite materials contain a blend of both conventional glass or quartz particles together with some submicron, particulate silica. These products are referred to as *hybrid* composites. Using filler loadings of about 75% conventional size (1–50 µm) and 8% submicron size (0.04 µm average), a total filler content of 83% or greater can be achieved. Some hybrid products contain a blend of at least three different particles sizes of filler. These allow efficient packing of filler into the smallest possible volume and enable filler loadings of up to 90% by weight to be achieved.

Figure 22.5 shows diagrammatically the microstructure of the three main groups of materials.

Conventional, microfilled and hybrid composites are all available as either chemically activated or light-activated products.

The ISO Standard for resin-based restorative materials (ISO 4049) classifies materials as being of two types depending upon the intended application. Type 1 is claimed by the manufacturer to be suitable for the restoration of cavities involving occlusal surfaces. Type 2 includes all other polymer-based filling and restorative materials. The standard further sub-divides materials into three classes as follows:

- Class 1 comprises self-curing materials whose setting is activated by mixing an initiator and an activator.
- Class 2 materials are those whose setting is effected by application of energy from an external source such as blue light or heat. These materials are further sub-divided as follows:
    Class 2 group 1 – materials whose use requires the energy to be applied intra-orally.
    Class 2 group 2 – materials whose method of use requires the energy to be applied extra-orally.
  The latter materials are specifically designed for the production of composite inlays and onlays.
- Class 3 materials are dual-cure materials which have a self-curing chemical mechanism but are also cured by the application of external energy.

22.5 Properties of composites

Some of the properties of resin-based restoratives are included within the tests and requirements of the ISO Standard (ISO 4049). This standard sets minimum standards of quality in relation to the following:

(1) The working time and setting time of class 1 materials.
(2) The sensitivity to ambient light and depth of cure of class 2 materials.

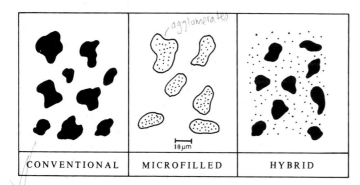

Fig. 22.5 Diagrammatic representation of the size of filler particles used in the three main groups of composite resins.

(3) The flexural strength of type 1 and 2 materials; water absorption, solubility, shade, colour stability and radiopacity of all materials.

Setting characteristics: For chemically activated materials, setting commences immediately after mixing the two components (paste and paste or paste and liquid etc.). The rate of set is uniform throughout the bulk of the material causing a gradual increase in viscosity at room temperature. Hence, the materials have a limited working time and must be inserted into the prepared cavity before they become unmanageable. In ISO 4049 the working time is determined using a thermocouple located at the base of a small cavity (6 mm deep by 4 mm diameter). The working time is taken as the time when the exothermic heat of reaction for the mixed material causes a noticeable rise in temperature. The standard requires that the working time (timed from start of mixing) should be at least 90 seconds.

After insertion, the materials are held under pressure with a plastic matrix strip and setting is normally completed within two or three minutes. Since setting occurs uniformly throughout the material it is safe to assume that a hard surface indicates that the material has set right through to the base of the cavity. Any material which is not covered by the matrix during setting is likely to have a tacky surface layer due to inhibition of the polymerization reaction by oxygen. In ISO 4049 the setting time is determined using the same apparatus as that described for measuring working time. For setting time determinations the equipment is maintained at mouth temperature (37°C). The setting time is defined as the time to reach the peak temperature in the exothermic setting reaction. The setting time measured by this method must be no more than 5 minutes.

For light-activated materials, only a minimal increase in viscosity takes place before the material is exposed to the activating light source. With these products the operator has, therefore, a longer working time. It should be remembered, however, that visible light-activated materials do begin to set slowly after exposure to light, particularly light of high intensity such as the surgery operating light. Therefore, insertion of the material into the cavity should not be delayed longer than necessary. In ISO 4049 light-activated materials are required to be tested for sensitivity to ambient light. When subjected to lighting equivalent to a dental operating light they should show no detectable change in consistency after 60 seconds exposure. After being covered with a matrix strip and exposed to the light

source, polymerization is often very rapid. Exposure times of between 10 seconds and one minute are, typically, required to cause setting. This ability to set rapidly after exposure to a light source is termed *command setting.*

The pattern of setting for light-activated materials is dictated by the fact that activation is first achieved in the surface layers of material where the light intensity is greatest. The potential for activation declines exponentially as a function of the distance from the surface of the filling. The intensity of light I_x at a distance x from the surface is given by the function

$$I_x = I_0\, e^{-\mu x}$$

where I_0 is the light intensity at the surface and μ is the absorption coefficient of the material. Since a certain level of intensity is required to cause activation it follows that light-activated materials have a *limited depth of cure.* The high viscosity of the pastes retards the diffusion of active free radicals from the surface layers to the lower unactivated layers, hence, material which is not activated initially may take a considerable time to set or may remain unset indefinitely. In ISO 4049 depth of cure is evaluated simply using a *scrape* test. Material is packed into a cylindrical mould and cured from one end for the time specified by the manufacturer. Immediately after curing, the mould is opened and any soft uncured material is removed using a plastic spatula. The height of the remaining hard, cured material is used to indicate depth of cure. In recognition of the fact that the method is quite crude and that material near the centre of the mass of material cures to a greater depth than the edges, the measured value is divided by 2 to give the final calculated depth of cure. This should be no less than 2 mm for most materials. A lower value of 1 mm is allowed for opaqueing materials.

Manufacturers of light-activated composites can control depth of cure by formulating the products in such a way that they more readily allow light penetration. In addition, they can supply or recommend a light source of adequate intensity and stipulate the exposure time required to give a certain depth of cure. Darker and more opaque shades of materials cannot be cured to the same depth as light and translucent shades. As an example, the light paste of one material can be cured to a depth of 2.5 mm using a 30 second exposure to light. The brown, opaque paste of the same material can only be cured to a depth of 1 mm using the same exposure time. Increasing the exposure time has very little effect on the depth of cure. If a material cures to a depth of

2.5 mm following a 30 second exposure it will not be cured to a significantly greater depth by increasing the exposure time to 1 or 2 minutes. On the other hand, the depth of cure can be significantly reduced by using a light exposure time of less than that recommended by the manufacturer.

The compatibility of light sources and composite materials has been the subject of several studies and debates. Most currently available light-activated composite materials utilize a similar catalyst system and most light-activation units are designed to deliver radiation which has a high intensity at the relevant wavelength. There are marked differences in performance between the units however, with a variation in intensity of light at 470 nm of up to ten times (130–1300 lux at 470 nm). Since depth of cure values which are supplied by manufacturers have normally been measured with a specific light source, it cannot be guaranteed that the same depth of cure could be achieved with a different light source.

Other factors can be controlled by the operator. The distance of the light source from the surface of the material is important. Depth of cure decreases significantly as this distance increases. The operator should never attempt to cure a greater depth of material than that recommended by the manufacturer, nor should he attempt to use a shorter exposure time. When large cavities are being restored the composite material should be cured in increments to ensure proper curing.

The polymerization reaction which causes setting of composite materials is exothermic in nature. The heat liberated can cause a significant temperature rise within the material. If the temperature rise is excessive and the pulp is not effectively insulated, irritation, sensitivity or more serious irreversible damage may be caused. The heat of reaction for chemically activated and light-activated materials is of similar magnitude but the resulting temperature rise varies considerably. In the case of a typical chemically activated material the temperature rise is expected to be in the range 1–5°C for an average size of restoration. For light-activated materials the temperature rise is typically 5–15°C depending upon the monomer system used and the filler content. The temperature rise is much higher for light-activated materials because the heat of polymerization is liberated over a much shorter time-scale. In addition, the heating effect of the light-activation unit further increases the temperature of the composite material when it is illuminated. In order to minimize the latter effect, manufacturers incorporate filters into their light-activation units. These filters are designed to remove the 'hotter' parts of the white light which

occur at the red end of the visible spectrum. Hence, the radiation used in most units appears blue.

Light activation units: The purpose of the light activation unit is to deliver high intensity radiation of the correct wavelength to the surface of the material in order to activate polymerization. The critical wavelength used by the vast majority of units and materials is 470 nm which corresponds to the blue region of the visible spectrum. Two approaches have been used to deliver this blue light to the mouth. The first is to use a 'light-gun' system in which the lamp producing the light is housed inside the hand-held 'gun' which has a short light guide to transmit the light to the tooth surface. Between the lamp and the light guide is housed the filter which removes the unwanted red and ultra-violet light. The alternative system involves the housing of both the lamp and filter inside a box of electronics and the light is transmitted along a cable which is packed with glass fibre strands. The latter light units have the advantage that the hand-held unit from which the light eventually emerges is about the same size as other dental instruments and is therefore less obtrusive. One drawback is that if the fibre-optic cable is not treated with respect, fibres can fracture and cause deterioration in the performance of the unit. Both systems generally include some means of cooling the lamp and a device for timing the curing exposure time.

An ISO Standard for dental curing light units has been in preparation for several years. Difficulties in preparing an acceptable standard arise from the fact that it is difficult to divorce the performance of the lamp from that of the material. Nevertheless, manufacturers have produced a number of devices which can be used to monitor the quality of light-curing units. Many consist of light-sensitive diodes which are used as light-intensity meters. When the reading falls below a critical value it suggests that the unit needs attention – perhaps a bulb needs replacing. Another approach to quality control is to carry out a depth of cure test using the chosen light unit/composite combination. Such testing performed on a regular basis is probably the best way to monitor the performance of both curing unit and material. At least one manufacturer supplies an easily assembled three-part mould to enable this determination to be made.

Setting contraction: The setting contraction of composite resins is considerably smaller than that observed for unfilled acrylic resins. Two factors contribute to this reduction. Firstly, the use of larger monomer and comonomer molecules effectively reduces the concentration of reactive groups in a given volume of material. Secondly, additions of fillers which take no part in the setting reaction further reduce the concentration of reactive methacrylate groups.

The setting contraction depends on the number of addition reactions which take place during polymerisation and is therefore much smaller for composite materials. Values of around 1.5–3.0 volumetric contraction are typical as opposed to 6% for acrylics. The setting contraction varies from one type of composite to another. Products with higher filler loadings undergo less shrinkage since there are fewer reactive groups participating in the setting reaction. Heavily filled hybrid materials exhibit the lowest shrinkage values. Microfilled materials generally have lower shrinkage values than would be expected from their low filler contents. It should be remembered however that these materials contain prepolymerized resin filler in addition to the inorganic filler material. The total volumetric proportion of combined inorganic and resin filler is often equal to, or greater than, that present in conventional or hybrid products and gives a value of shrinkage which can compare favourably with that for other materials. The type of resin used may influence shrinkage. Bis GMA has a relatively low setting contraction but this is increased proportionately according to the amount of diluent monomer (e.g. TEGMA) used. High molecular weight urethanedimethacrylate monomers which are often fluid enough to be used without diluents may give a lower value of contraction.

Shrinkage can compromise marginal seal and rupture adhesive bonds created at the tooth-restorative interface. The total amount of volumetric contraction which occurs depends upon the bulk of material used and hence on cavity size and clinical technique. Some materials are expected to perform quite well in small cavities where the contraction may be small enough to ensure that marginal adaptation is maintained. The same product may undergo sufficient contraction to cause breakdown of marginal seal in larger cavities. Layering techniques, particularly applicable to use with light-activated materials, can be used to limit the damaging effects of shrinkage. In addition, it has been claimed that the slight expansion, due to absorption of water, which gradually occurs in some materials over a period of several weeks following placement can help to partially off-set the effects of shrinkage.

Another potentially serious effect of shrinkage is thought to be the stress placed on tooth substance, particularly on the residual cusps of posterior teeth when composite materials are used in relatively large class II cavities. Such stresses, caused by the composite material 'pulling-in' cusps to which it may adhere, is thought to be responsible for some cases of post-operative pain experienced after placement of so-called posterior composites. In extreme cases the stress on the tooth may be great enough to cause cuspal fracture.

The direct measurement of the volumetric shrinkage of composites during setting has proved difficult – a fact which probably explains the lack of a test for this property in the ISO Standard. Simple dilatometric methods are difficult for various reasons including the high initial viscosity of the composite pastes and the setting characteristics which allow inadequate working time to set up a dilotometer (for chemically-activated products) or require access for a light-activation unit (for light-activated products). The method which has emerged as being most practical has been to sandwich the composite paste between two glass plates and to measure the reduction in the plate separation distance as the material sets. Since the vector of shrinkage is normal to the interface between composite paste and glass plates, virtually all the shrinkage is constrained in one direction and the linear shrinkage across the plates reflects the volumetric shrinkage of the composite.

Measurements of shrinkage made using this or similar methods have led to other important observations. First, if the material is allowed to set between two plates which are constrained the contraction stress can be calculated. This gives an indication of the stress which would be set up at a cavity margin or wall and may be a significant factor in determining whether an adhesive bond is disrupted or whether cusp deflection occurs, etc. Measurements of shrinkage stress indicate that the initial shrinkage which takes place whilst the material is still fluid may be of little clinical significance as it can be compensated by the flow of the material. It is the 'post-gelation' rigid contraction which is significant and when we measure shrinkage it is important to identify this component of the overall shrinkage.

Second, the ability of a resin-based filling material to compensate for shrinkage by flow depends on the cavity configuration. When there is a small ratio of contact surface area to free surface area flow occurs readily over the free area in order to minimize the stress at the interface. When there is little free surface area of material, little flow can occur and a larger stress at the interface results. The ratio of bonded free area can therefore be used to predict interfacial stress caused by shrinkage. The ratio has become known as the C-factor or configuration factor. Further insight into the C-factor can be obtained by reference to Fig. 22.6. If a cube of composite

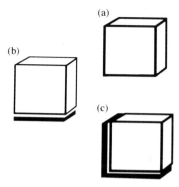

Fig. 22.6 Diagrammatic illustration of the configuration (C) factor. A cube of resin having six faces, is completely free in (a), bound at one face (b) or bound at two of its faces (c). The C factors for these situations are 0, 0.2 and 0.5, respectively.

material is completely unconstrained (as in A) it can flow readily in all directions in order to minimize the shrinkage stress. The C-factor for this situation is zero. In example B the material is bound to a surface across one of the six faces of the cube. There are five free faces over which flow can readily occur (a C-factor of 0.2) and the stress at the interface with the bonded surface will be relatively small. In example C the cube of material is constrained at two of the six faces giving a C-factor of 0.5. This will result in a greater stress at the interface as flow can only occur over 67% of the area of the cube. When the material is constrained over five of the six surfaces of the cube (giving a C-factor of 5) flow can only occur at the one free surface and the stress at the five remaining surfaces is much greater. Hence, the C-factor gives an indication of the potential for stress to develop. It is possible to make approximate calculations of the C-factor values which would apply for different cavity configurations, i.e. a class IV cavity approximates to Fig. 22.6C and therefore has a C-factor of 0.5 whereas a class I cavity approximates to a cube constrained on five out of six sides and thus has a C-factor of about 5. The greatest C-factor values will apply when materials are used in thin, constrained layers, such as occurs when the material is used as a luting agent. In this situation C-factor values of greater than 10 may apply.

Thermal properties: The thermal properties of composite materials depend primarily on the inorganic filler content. Table 22.2 gives values of thermal diffusivity and coefficient of thermal expansion for a conventional composite, microfilled composite, unfilled acrylic resin and dentine for comparison. It can be seen that as the filler content increases the coefficient of thermal expansion decreases, although even for convention composites, with 78% filler, there is still a considerable mismatch in values compared to dentine. This mismatch may cause percolation of fluids down the margins when patients take hot or cold foods. The amount of mismatch which can be tolerated without causing clinically significant problems is not precisely known. It is significant, however, that the microfilled composites have values some six or seven times greater than tooth substance.

The thermal diffusivity also depends on filler content although the values for all the materials are close to that measured for dentine and they can all be considered adequate thermal insulators.

Mechanical properties: The mechanical properties of composite materials depend upon the filler content, the type of filler, the efficiency of the filler–resin coupling process and the degree of porosity in the set material.

Light-activated composites, supplied as single pastes, contain very little porosity whereas chemically-activated composites requiring the mixing of two components contain, typically, 2–5% porosity. The porosity is introduced during mixing. A correctly cured, light-activated, conventional composite may, typically, have a compressive strength value of 260 MPa, whereas an equivalent chemically activated material, containing 3% porosity, is likely to have a compressive strength of 210 MPa. Porosity

Table 22.2 Thermal properties of typical composite resins.

	Filler content (% by weight)	Thermal diffusivity $\times 10^{-3}$ cm^2 s^{-1}	Coefficient of thermal expansion $\times 10^{-6}$ °C^{-1}
Conventional composite	78	5.0	32
Microfilled composite	50	2.5	60
Unfilled acrylic	0	1.0	90
Dentine	—	2.0	9

also has a significant effect on the fatigue limits of composite materials. Non-porous products have a higher fatigue limit and longer fatigue life than porous ones. This may have some bearing on the durability of materials in certain applications.

The lack of an adequate coupling agent pretreatment of the filler may have a dramatic effect on properties. Both the compressive strength and fatigue limit are reduced by about 30% when the coupling agent is not used.

Heavily filled, conventional composites undergo brittle fracture. As the filler content is reduced a transition to a more ductile failure is observed. Microfilled composites, which generally have a filler content of 50% by weight or less, normally exhibit a yield point at a stress considerably lower than that for fracture. Values of compressive strength for microfilled materials are often similar to or even higher than those for conventional composites, but the lower yield stress value is probably more significant for these products since it represents the point of irretrievable breakdown of the material.

The hybrid composites have mechanical properties very similar to those of conventional materials. Strength and modulus values are often slightly higher but not significantly so. Table 22.3 gives values of certain mechanical properties for typical products from each of the three groups of composite materials. The values of compressive strength are for a porosity-free material.

Table 22.3 Mechanical properties of composite resins.

	Typical conventional composite	Typical microfilled composite	Typical hybrid composite
Compressive strength (MPa)	260	260	300
Yield stress (MPa)	260	160	300
Tensile strength (MPa)	45	40	50
Flexural strength (MPa)	110	80	150
Modulus of elasticity (GPa)	12	6	14
Hardness (VHN)	60	30	90

In the past a lot of emphasis has been placed on the compressive strengths of dental restorative materials. Nowadays more emphasis is placed on tensile and flexural strength as it is recognized that these modes of fracture may be more clinically relevant. Table 22.3 shows that the flexural strength and tensile strength of hybrid composites tend to be greater than for the microfilled products. Table 22.4 gives the values of flexural strength required by the ISO Standard (ISO 4049) for different types of material. Type 1 materials (for use on occlusal surfaces) are required to be stronger than type 2 materials (more limited use). Type 1 class 2 (group 2) products which are subjected to extra-oral curing are required to have even higher strength. These products are used to produce composite inlays and onlays. Most commercially available materials have values of strength well above the minimum values allowed by the standard.

Table 22.4 Flexural strength of resin-based restorations as required by ISO 4049.

Type	Class	Minimum value of flexural strength (MPa)
1	1	80
1	2 (group 1)	80
1	2 (group 2)	100
1	3	80
2	1	50
2	2 (group 1)	50
2	3	50

The significantly lower value of modulus of elasticity for the microfilled materials may have clinical significance. These products may potentially deform under stress, leading to a breakdown of the marginal seal. This is recognized as a problem with unfilled acrylics, where a modulus value of 2 GPa is normal. Whether or not the increase from 2 GPa to 6 GPa is sufficient to prevent breakdown is not known.

Fracture toughness testing is being used increasingly to give an indication of mechanical strength (see Section 2.2). Tests are carried out on notched specimens and the results indicate the *critical stress intensity factor*. This factor gives an indication of elastic stress distribution near a crack tip when a force is applied of sufficient magnitude to cause fracture. It provides a means of comparing the ability of different materials to resist crack propagation. The value of fracture toughness for a typical conventional composite material is around $1.2 \text{ MNm}^{-1.5}$, whilst that for an unfilled acrylic resin is around 1.0 $\text{MNm}^{-1.5}$. Some heavily filled hybrid composites have values approaching $2.0 \text{ MNm}^{-1.5}$. These can all be considered to be relatively low values when compared with that for mild steel of $100 \text{ MNm}^{-1.5}$.

Surface characteristics: Surface hardness, roughness and abrasion resistance are properties which are mainly controlled by the filler content and particle size.

The resin and filler have characteristic hardness values which remain independent of filler content. The bulk hardness value of the composite, however, increases as the filler content increases. The Vickers hardness number for unfilled resin is about 18 whereas that for a heavily filled hybrid composite approaches 100. The microfilled materials have values around 30–40.

The surface of a composite material is initially very smooth and glossy due to contact with a matrix strip during setting. The surface layer is initially richer in resin than the bulk of the material and few, if any, filler particles are exposed at the surface. Any process of abrasion, however, has a tendency to cause surface roughening as the relatively soft resin matrix is worn preferentially leaving the filler particles protruding from the surface. This is a particular problem with the conventional and hybrid materials which contain relatively large particles (Fig. 22.7). One advantage of the microfill materials is that they retain a relatively smooth surface following abrasion, due to the fact that the hard inorganic particles are very small. Another factor which contributes towards surface roughness is the exposure of porosity voids at the surface by abrasion. This is observed for all types of chemically activated composites, and is illustrated in Fig. 22.8 for a microfilled material.

Surface roughness may be caused by abrasive forces exerted on materials during service, for example, from foodstuffs, dentifrices etc. Alternatively, roughening may occur during contouring

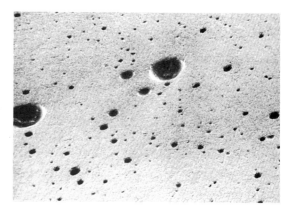

Fig. 22.8 Scanning electron microscope photograph of the abraded surface of a microfilled composite material showing exposed porosity ($\times$ 325).

and polishing. The surface cured against the matrix strip should be left intact if possible, but removal of excess material followed by polishing is often necessary. Table 22.5 gives roughness average values of materials, following polishing by one of three commonly used methods. Values for the smooth, matrix surface are given for comparison.

It can be seen that all of the polishing procedures produce a significant increase in roughness compared to the matrix surface. This is accompanied by a loss of gloss. The increase is greatest for the conventional and hybrid materials and the polishing method which appears most damaging is the use of silicone rubber points which are impregnated with abrasive.

A smooth surface can be restored to a roughened composite by using a *glazing agent.* These consist of resins which are identical to composites except that they do not contain filler particles. The glaze is applied to the surface of the composite and sets to form a smooth surface layer of about 100 μm thickness. The material is very soft, however, and is soon abraded, revealing the composite surface again.

If the rate of material loss due to abrasion becomes excessive it may cause a change in the anatomical form of the restoration. Abrasion of this magnitude may, conceivably, be caused by one of a variety of mechanisms and is of particular importance when considering the use of composites in posterior cavities. Here, the forces exerted on materials are relatively high and abrasive wear may take place at a rapid pace due to either two-body contacts, normally involving the restorative material and an opposing tooth cusp, or three-body contacts in which an abrasive foodstuff maybe involved as the

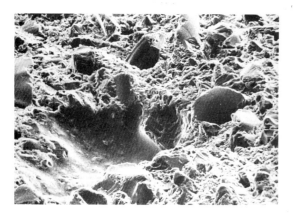

Fig. 22.7 Scanning electron microscope photograph of the roughened surface of a conventional composite material showing protruding filler particles ($\times$ 750).

Table 22.5 Roughness average (Ra μm) values of composite materials following polishing.

Surface treatment	Conventional composite	Microfilled composite	Hybrid composite
None (matrix surface)	0.04	0.02	0.03
Aluminium oxide-impregnated finishing disc	0.15	0.10	0.20
White stone	0.30	0.20	0.30
Silicone rubber point	1.10	0.45	1.00

third body between the material and opposing tooth cusp. Cyclic masticatory loadings also offer a potential for fatigue wear in which surface failure occurs following the development of small surface or subsurface cracks over a period of time. The process of wear, whether occurring by a fatigue or abrasive mechanism, may be accelerated by chemical factors. Certain solvents occurring naturally in some drinks and foodstuffs may soften the resin component of the composite. Other chemical agents, particularly acids, may cause degradation of the filler component and this process is probably accompanied by, or preceded by, the breakdown of the filler–matrix bond. Indeed, following storage of some composite materials in erosive media it is often possible to detect metallic ions from the composite filler in the storage liquid. These chemical processes may significantly affect the perceived rate of wear.

Wear resistance of composites designed for use in posterior cavities has improved markedly over the past few years. Most modern products wear at a rate of 10–30 μm per annum. Some products undergo a generalized loss of material including that at the cavity margins (Fig. 22.9). This type of wear is rela-

tively easy to detect and monitor using a sharp probe either directly in the mouth or on a cast. Wear which takes place primarily in the occlusal contact areas is more difficult to evaluate and is likely to be more rapid.

Appearance: Composite materials, when freshly placed, offer an excellent match with surrounding tooth substance. The availability of a variety of shades, combined with a degree of translucency imparted by the filler, enables the dentist to achieve a very pleasing result. Polishing reduces the gloss, however, and abrasion may further increase surface roughness. The surface may eventually become stained due to deposition of coloured foodstuffs or tobacco tars. The microfilled products are capable of maintaining a smoother surface than either the conventional or hybrid materials. Providing the resin of the material is inherently colour stable or contains effective stabilizers these products should be more resistant to surface staining.

Cavity linings: Although monomers employed in composite materials may be considered potentially harmful to the pulp, they are generally strongly bound in a highly cross-linked network following setting. Despite this, it is normal practice to line cavities prior to placement of a composite restoration. The material of choice is normally a calcium hydroxide product. Manufacturers of composite materials deter operators from using eugenol-containing liners because of the possible, though not definitely proven, adverse effects that eugenol may have on the setting and colour stability of the resin.

Recent developments in the bonding of resin-based materials to dentine have re-opened the debate over the need for linings beneath composite restorations. Some authorities now doubt the need for a lining, provided the restoration is able to fully seal the cavity such that marginal leakage is prevented.

Adhesion: Composites do not inherently form a durable bond with tooth substance. Retention of the

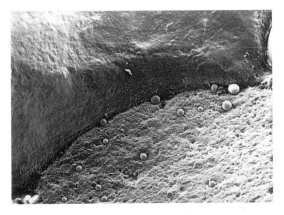

Fig. 22.9 Scanning electron microscope photograph of the margin of a composite restoration showing loss of material due to wear (× 83).

material is generally achieved by using undercut cavities. This often involves removing significant quantities of sound tooth substance.

Methods of establishing a bond between composites and enamel or dentine are discussed in Chapter 23. Such techniques greatly increase the number of potential applications of the materials and also offer a means of preventing microleakage.

22.6 Clinical handling notes for composites

One of the greater failings amongst dentists is their failure to adopt new techniques which are appropriate to new materials. New products are often used in the same way as existing materials without due thought being given to modifying technique and applications to maximize the physical performance of the materials concerned. Whenever dentists are faced with a new material they should ask 'What are the properties of this product?'. 'How can I or should I change what I usually do to maximize the performance of any restoration I produce with this material when compared to the one I have used previously?' These are questions that have been answered historically only after a material has been unsuccessful when used in a 'classical' manner. This can result in a material gaining a bad reputation undeservedly and in a delay in its acceptance by the profession to the detriment of patient care. A case in point are the dental composites. These materials are very different in physical characteristics to their predecessors (either dental silicate cements or amalgam) and yet were used initially in *amalgam cavities* where their performance was less good than it is now that attempts have been made to adopt cavity design and placement techniques better suited to their physical characteristics and handling properties.

Cavity design and bonding to enamel

The ability of composites to form a durable seal to both enamel and dentine has allowed modifications to cavity design to both minimize the destruction of otherwise sound enamel and dentine and to maximize the performance of these restorations. Access through enamel should be sufficient to permit removal of underlying decayed dentine.

Composite resins exhibit good flow characteristics in their prepolymerized form. Cavities should be designed to use this property with rounded internal line angles and smooth flowing contours. Smaller cavities produced as a result of caries removal alone will help to reduce the potential for wear of the composite, as a consequence of the remaining tooth structure providing some protection from functional contact. Traditional cavity design has included the removal of deep tortuous fissures adjacent to areas of decay as these were regarded as being at high risk from carious attack. This is not required when using a composite as these areas can be prepared and then sealed using a compatible fissure sealant system to achieve *extension for prevention.*

Cavities designed for tooth-coloured restorations rely heavily on their bonding to enamel and/or dentine to achieve retention and resistance to displacement. If a restoration is to be placed under high functional load it may be sensible to augment this chemical attachment by the preparation of macro-mechanical undercuts where possible. It is just as important, however, to remove unsupported enamel from cavity margins with composites as it is with amalgam, although for different reasons. The margins of a cavity for a composite restoration are treated to achieve a chemical and/or mechanical link between resin and tooth. Once this link is established then the forces that are generated by polymerization shrinkage of the composite are transmitted to the tooth through the enamel margins. If the enamel at these margins is unsupported then there is an increased risk that the enamel prism structure will be disrupted by the shrinkage of the resin, resulting in a failure of marginal seal.

Once any unsupported enamel has been removed, the cavity margins need to be designed to maximize the bond strength that can be achieved with either enamel or dentine. Attachment of composites to enamel is achieved primarily by etching the enamel surface with acid as described in the next chapter. This etching process results in preferential dissolution of either the enamel prism cores or the prism boundaries, producing a microporous enamel surface with high surface energy. The pattern and quality of etching depend on the acid used and also on the orientation of the enamel prisms in relation to the cavity margin. Classically, enamel is etched with between 30 and 37% phosphoric acid, although more recently a wider variety of acids have been used including 10% phosphoric, nitric and maleic. The etching time is specific to a given acid and hence manufacturer recommendations should be followed with care. Enamel prisms can be etched in any orientation. However, the quality of the etch pattern is better when they are etched perpendicular to their long axes as opposed to parallel to the prism orientation. Unfortunately the production of a 90° cavo surface angle giving well supported enamel margins will result in prisms being exposed for etching parallel to their long axes. Production of a cavo surface angle of the order of 120° will help to overcome this problem by exposing a combination etch pattern, although it is not as easy to finish a tooth-coloured restoration accurately to an oblique margin.

This approach (the 120° cavo surface angle) is acceptable for cavities where a tightly adapted matrix band is not required during the initial stage of restoring the cavity. This is not the case for class II cavities (those involving two surfaces of molar or premolar teeth) where a matrix in a band holder is used to help form the shape of the tooth surface. In this situation the unfilled resin that is used to initiate the bond between composite and tooth tends to pool in the V-shaped defect formed between the matrix and an obtusely finished cavity margin (Fig. 22.10). This produces a marginal finish formed from unfilled resin which is both weak and prone to wear/degradation in function in an area where both problems are to be avoided if possible. In this circumstance a 90° cavo surface angle is preferable.

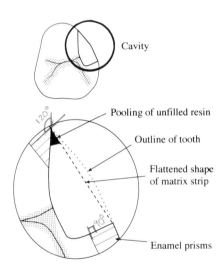

Fig. 22.10   If a class II cavity is prepared with an oblique finishing margin there is a risk of unfilled resin pooling in the narrow cleft at the edge of the box. This is a particular problem when clear matrix strips are used as these tend to flatten across the proximal box, making the cleft even narrower.

Etching the enamel surface produces a clean higher energy surface that is highly receptive to wetting. Attachment to the etched surface is established best using either an unfilled resin (the resin which forms the basis of the composite) or a *dentine bonding agent* (DBA). Although DBAs are designed to attach composite to dentine, they also bond well to enamel. Indeed, the bond strength of composite to etched enamel using a DBA as the intermediary layer is often greater than that when using a simple unfilled resin. It is essential to use an unfilled resin as the intermediary between etched enamel and the composite. Modern composites contain sufficiently small quantities of resin that they cannot wet the enamel surface adequately without the intermediary resin layer.

Etching a prepared enamel surface is relatively straightforward. If part of the enamel to be etched has not been prepared then it is necessary to extend the etching time. Enamel that has been exposed in the mouth has an amorphous mineralized layer on its surface as a result of intra-oral maturation. (This occurs as a consequence of the regular cycle of surface de- and re-mineralization associated with acids in diet and those produced as a consequence of intake of fermentable sugars. As a consequence the surface layers of enamel have high levels of trace minerals and fluoride, making them more resistant to etching, and are without a regular prismatic structure.) The same caveat applies to enamel on teeth that have recently erupted into the mouth where there is also an amorphous layer on the surface. Such amorphous layers need to be removed before the etching process can produce an appropriately microporous surface to achieve micromechanical retention at the enamel interface.

The high energy enamel surface produced by etching will also actively attract saliva and its contained protein. If an etched surface becomes contaminated with saliva then its surface energy is dramatically reduced and effective bonding with a resin system is prevented. The precipitated protein can be removed by further acid treatment of the enamel surface. The etching time required to remove such protein contamination is less than that required for initial enamel preparation (typically 15 seconds compared with 30 for treatment with 37% phosphoric acid).

The bonding of composites to dentine

The reader is encouraged to refer to Chapter 23 of this book *before* undertaking any consideration of the clinical handling of bonding systems. Dentine has a very different structure to enamel. It has much higher levels of organic component with reduced mineral. In addition the structure and composition vary considerably as the dentine surface under consideration gets closer to the pulp. There are two reasons for the alteration in mineralization and structure. Dentine maturation is greater as the dentine gets close to the root surface or the amelo-dentinal junction. This results in increased mineralization of intertubular dentine and extensive deposition of intratubular deposit. This latter has the effect both of increasing local mineral content and reducing the relative areas of mineralized dentine and patent dentine tubules. As the dentine gets closer to the pulp the mineralization of intertubular dentine decreases, as do the deposits of intratubular mineral. Furthermore, all tubules originate at the pulp and then radiate outwards towards the periphery of the tooth/root. Consequently, the tubule density per unit surface area of a cut dentine surface increases markedly the closer that surface gets to the pulp (Fig. 22.11).

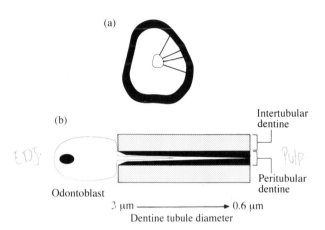

Fig. 22.11   The area of a cross-section of dentine occupied by dentine tubules is reduced as the dentine approaches the amelo-dentinal junction for two reasons: (1) The dentine tubules radiate outwards from the pulp towards the enamel, reducing the number per unit area. (2) The diameter of the dentine tubule reduces dramatically as it progresses towards the pulp as the peritubular dentine increases in thickness.

The bulk of the water that is contained in dentine is located in the dentine tubules, hence the water content of the dentine increases the closer to the pulp. All vital dentine contains some moisture and hence a hydrophilic resin (e.g. DBA) is required to achieve adequate attachment. The DBA can be designed to bond to either the organic or the inorganic elements of dentine, although the latter is more common. Current concepts of dentine bonding also include the creation of an interpenetrating resin structure with collagen fibres originating within the dentine becoming invested in resin to form the *hybrid layer*. Theories of bonding are covered in greater detail in Chapter 23.

In order to achieve bonding the surface of the dentine needs to be demineralized using an acid. This results in removal of the smear layer (a layer of loosely attached cutting debris from surface preparation) and then demineralization of the dentine, exposing collagen. Simultaneously the plugs of cutting debris that occlude dentine tubule openings are removed and the tubule orifice widened.

Care is required in handling this prepared surface to achieve reliable bonding. If the surface of the dentine is desiccated during drying the cavity the collagen network collapses, producing a dense mat of collagen fibres lying on the surface of the dentine. This collagen thatch is very difficult to penetrate with a resin to achieve bonding. Equally, if the dentine surface is too wet, even the hydrophilic resins used in DBAs cannot cope with the water volume and the DBA tends to form an emulsion with the water rather than displacing it. This emulsion cannot polymerize adequately and hence bond strengths are reduced. There is an optimum dampness of dentine which maintains an expanded collagen structure but at which level homogeneity of the DBA is maintained. The methods of achieving this optimum *in vivo* are two-fold:

(1)   If the cavity is confined to dentine alone then the wet dentine surface should be blotted dry with cotton wool rather than air dried.
(2)   If there are both enamel and dentine surfaces involved there is a need to dry the enamel to check the quality of enamel preparation (well etched enamel has a *frosty* surface appearance). The drying is likely to result in a formation of a collagen thatch. The dentine surface is then rehydrated with water before blot drying with cotton wool to achieve the required dampness.

Prevention of salivary contamination of prepared dentine surfaces is again important to ensure adequate bonding. For both enamel and dentine bonding the best way of achieving this quality of isolation is the use of a rubber dam. Rubber dam can be difficult to place for cavities with deep subgingival margins. In this circumstance it may be possible to use a combination of cotton rolls and gingival retraction cord to control moisture. If it is not possible to control moisture contamination, particularly at the gingival extent of a cavity, then the operator should question seriously whether composite is the appropriate material to use for a given cavity. A lack of bonding of composite to enamel and/or dentine will result in a significant marginal gap forming and an associated risk of sensitivity and recurrent decay.

Material placement

There are two considerations to be taken into account when placing composites in a cavity: maximizing quality of cure and minimizing the adverse effects of polymerization shrinkage on the tooth. All currently available composites shrink on setting by between 1.5 and 3% by volume (depending on filler type and loading). The pattern of shrinkage and quality of cure depends upon the method of initiation of polymerization (see above). In summary, chemically activated resins shrink towards their centre and will cure in bulk. Visible light cured (VLC) resins shrink towards the curing light and can only be cured in thin section. These latter properties can be exploited when placing VLC resins to help to maximize the chance of obtaining a marginal seal and minimize the effects of polymerization shrinkage on tooth tissue by directing cure towards tooth/resin interfaces and placing the material in small increments. This is particularly appropriate and important for class II cavities, where material bulk is greater and tooth deformation associated with wall-to-wall polymerization contraction has been implicated in causation of post-operative sensitivity.

Maximizing quality of cure

It is necessary to place VLC resins in increments of not more than 2 mm in depth to ensure adequate cure using currently available curing units. The 2 mm cure depth is dependent upon the colour and translucency of the resin, the distance the light tip is away from the surface of the composite and whether or not the curing is being performed through another tissue (e.g. enamel or dentine). Incremental depths should be reduced for dark shades, where the light tip has to be some distance from the resin or when cure is being attempted through tooth tissue. One particular problem is achieving adequate cure at the base of the gingival floor of a class II cavity. Some light-curing units have interchangeable fibre-optic light guides with small tip diameters to allow the tip of the curing light to get as close as possible to the resin surface. Alternatively light-transmitting wedges can be used in conjunction with a transparent matrix band to direct light towards the gingival floor of the cavity and material present in that area.

Minimizing the adverse effects of polymerization shrinkage

The adverse effects of polymerization shrinkage include distortion of the tooth and failure to establish a marginal seal, both of which can result in post-operative sensitivity.

Incremental placement techniques: The dimensional changes associated with polymerization affect composite resins in two ways. Whilst the material remains plastic it will flow in association with contraction, whereas once a certain level of rigidity is achieved the material undergoes a formal shrinkage process. Plastic flow occurs towards *bound surfaces* (usually those where the resin is in contact with another material, e.g. enamel or dentine) and away from surfaces exposed to air. If a given volume of material is cured in increments then there are multiple opportunities for this plastic flow to occur hence, although the overall proportional shrinkage of the resin filling a cavity will be the same for bulk or incremental placement, more of that shrinkage will be taken up by plastic flow with an incremental approach. An explanation of this is given by consideration of the section on setting contraction.

There have been two techniques for incremental curing described, the herringbone and lateral filling methods (Fig. 22.12). Both techniques minimize the wall to wall effects of shrinkage.

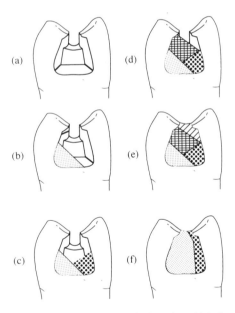

Fig. 22.12 Composites should be introduced into large cavities in increments to maximize quality of cure and help to reduce polymerization stress. On completion of the cavity (a) composite is placed in the cavity in diagonal increments, producing a herringbone effect (b–e) to restore the defect. An alternative approach is a lateral incremental filling technique (f).

Directional curing techniques: VLC materials start to cure at the surface closest to the curing light and then shrink towards that light. This can be used to help establish and maintain a marginal seal. At the base of a box, curing can be initiated by using a light-transmitting wedge to cure the increment closest to the cervical margins first. Curing of the remainder of the increment will then be undertaken from the occlusal aspect. When the herringbone approach is used the initial curing application of the curing light should be through the tooth from the lateral aspect if possible. This will establish the link between the composite and tooth before once again curing the bulk of the increment from the occlusal.

Increasing the effective filler loading: One of the principal methods of reducing polymerization shrinkage in composites is to increase the relative proportion of filler to resin. Unfortunately there are practical limits in increasing the filler loading after which the material becomes so viscous that it cannot be handled clinically. It is, however, possible to increase the effective filler loading by incorporating either a pre-polymerized piece of composite into the restoration or by using commercially available quartz inserts to achieve the same effect. The logical extension of this approach is to make a composite or porcelain inlay and lute the inlay using a composite luting agent. Unfortunately there comes a stage where the geometry of the restoration negates the beneficial result of reducing the volume of resin undergoing a polymerization reaction. This effect is associated with the configuration or C-factor, as discussed in Section 22.5.

Matrix techniques and the establishment of proximal contacts

A surface matrix has three benefits: it helps to guide the formation of a peripheral profile of the restoration, it isolates the resin from the atmosphere which helps to minimize the effect of air inhibition of cure of the resin at the surface and the layer of material immediately adjacent to the matrix is resin-rich, producing a high gloss surface giving optimal appearance on placement.

Two materials are used to produce clear, flexible matrix structures for use with composites, cellulose acetate and polyester film (Mylar® or Melinex®). Cellulose acetate is thicker and more fragile than the polyester products. In addition there have been some suggestions that the plasticizer in cellulose acetate strips may cause some softening of the resin surface,

making it more susceptible to early loss of resin and hence the high gloss matrix finish.

Matrixes for proximal cavities on anterior teeth should be placed between teeth after the enamel has been prepared for bonding but before the DBA or unfilled resin is applied to the prepared tooth tissues. If the matrix is not applied before the DBA/resin there is a risk that the unfilled resins will flow between adjacent teeth, linking them together and making subsequent matrix placement difficult if not impossible. This approach applies even when an incremental build-up technique is being used, even though the matrix does not come into use until the increments begin to restore the peripheral contour of the tooth.

Transparent matrixes for cervical restorations are more difficult to use. Those that are commercially available are pre-formed to produce the buccal convexity of the root surface. They can exhibit some flexibility to allow them to adapt to different root contours; however, there remains a tendency for the matrix to 'fit where it touches' with an associated risk of producing marginal overhangs that need to be removed after the restoration has been cured.

Matrix techniques for proximal cavities on molar teeth involve placing a band around the tooth with some form of tightening mechanism. If a tooth only has one proximal box and the opposite surface is intact, forming a good contact with an adjacent tooth, it can be difficult to pass a transparent band through such a contact as the matrix material is relatively fragile. Pressing a wedge home between pairs of teeth in this position can help to separate the contact and facilitate band placement. Obviously, a transparent band is essential if the concepts of directional polymerization described earlier are to be used. As a last resort a metallic matrix can be used, but it must be recognized that the ability to achieve a satisfactory marginal seal may be compromised as a consequence.

Obviously, when restoring a proximal surface it is desirable to establish an appropriate contact relationship between any adjacent tooth and the restoration. This can be a difficult task when using a composite as compensation has to be achieved both for the thickness of the matrix band itself and also for the shrinkage of the resin on setting. The use of a proximal wedge to help to hold the cervical extent of the band against the root face will help with this process as the wedge will tend to separate adjacent teeth and also extrude the teeth from their socket slightly. On removing the wedge the teeth will rebound into their original position, coming closer together in the process. Once the wedge is in place, it is essential to ensure that the matrix band is in contact with the adjacent tooth in their separated state, to optimize the chance of a contact being achieved. One further possibility is to make a small pellet of pre-cured composite which can be wedged into the proximal box between the axial wall of the box and the adjacent tooth. Obviously this will not shrink on further polymerization and hence will facilitate the formation of a contact.

Finishing and polishing

Once material is placed, there will usually be a requirement for finishing and polishing in some form, either as a consequence of marginal excess or to define and refine the position and pattern of tooth to tooth contact. Composites can be finished immediately after placement using rotary cutting tools. Bulk changes in profile are best achieved using small particle size diamond burs, either in an airotor or a speed accelerating hand piece on a conventional motor (the latter accelerates the rotational speed by between 3 and 5 to 1, giving a burr speed of up to 120–200 000 rpm from a 40 000 rpm air or electromotor). These burs are delicate and should be used with care and with copious water cooling to prevent damage to the diamond abrasives. Such small particle diamond burs are produced in a variety of shapes and grit sizes of diamond. The basic principle of surface finishing – commencing with the large particle size abrasives and progressing downward in grit size – should be observed. Multi-fluted tungsten carbide burs are an alternative to diamond abrasives. These have between 20 and 40 cutting blades as opposed to 6 or 8 for conventional cavity preparation instruments.

The ease of identification of cavity margins, particularly on the occlusal surface of molar teeth, during finishing will depend on the design of the enamel finishing line. Enamel margins that are finished at or close to a 90° angle are easier to identify than those that are prepared with a very marked marginal bevel. In addition such margins are less likely to develop marginal strain with time. (This is probably a reflection of the relative fragility of thin films of composite and their very different thermal properties compared to enamel on dentine.) The desirability for ease of identification of a margin and structural integrity of the periphery of the completed restoration given by marginal bulk must be weighed against the desire to achieve optimal bonding by etching enamel prisms perpendicular to their long axes. A finishing angle of about 120° gives a reasonable compromise between these two ideals.

Once bulk contour has been achieved using burs then finishing can continue with either disc-mounted abrasives or abrasive-impregnated rubber wheels, cones or points. There are a large number of commercially available systems for fine polishing of composite, some of which are material-specific and some more generic in nature. Once again, each system comes in a variety of abrasive particle sizes and the larger abrasive size should be used first. Polishing is achieved by gradually reducing the particle size of the abrasive. Some composite manufactures recommend an abrasive paste in a slurry for final polishing.

The objective of polishing is to produce as smooth a surface as possible whilst maintaining the required morphology of the restoration. The quality of surface finish that can be achieved depends upon both the skill of the operator and the nature of the composite, as described in Section 22.5. Microfilled composites are inherently more polishable than those with larger/harder filler particles. One secondary benefit of the polishing process is an increased toughness of the surface layer of the composite. This is brought about due to local heating when using rubber or disc-based abrasives without water cooling. The local rise in temperature often exceeds the glass transition temperature of the resin, producing some smearing of the resin surface with altered physical characteristics.

22.7 Applications of composites

Composite resins may be used as alternatives to silicate filling materials for the restoration of class III cavities. Other applications, such as the restoration of fractured incisal edges, depend upon the use of special techniques in which adhesion between restorative material and tooth substance is achieved. These are discussed in Chapter 23.

There is a growing tendency to consider composite resins for use as alternatives to amalgam in posterior cavities. Materials are available which appear to match amalgam in terms of physical properties, however, the technique of placement for composites in posterior teeth, without incorporating voids, is difficult. In addition, the durability of composites appears to be inferior to that of amalgam, particularly in class II cavities where considerable loss of anatomical form can take place due to wear. For class I cavities, where the material is fully surrounded by enamel, the wear is less noticeable. Improvements in the quality of materials have to some extent overcome the problems related to wear resistance in that other factors such as chipping, ditching, fracture and leakage have become more noticeable.

There is some question over which group of composite materials offers the best chance of success in posterior teeth. Some clinical trials report encouraging results for microfilled composites after a year or two. However, many of the products offered commercially as alternatives to amalgam are hybrid materials, particularly the light-activated variety. Materials containing barium glass fillers or other fillers containing heavy metal atoms are most promising since they are radiopaque. They offer the practitioner the chance to confirm that the cavity has been correctly filled and also to check for the presence of caries in the surrounding dentine at subsequent examinations.

Good marginal seal is considered to be a major requirement of a restorative material in order to reduce or eliminate the chances of microleakage. The attainment of a good seal depends upon the formation of adhesive bonds between the restorative resin and tooth substance and upon minimal shrinkage of the resin during curing. In larger cavities the total amount of shrinkage is greater and the chance of maintaining a good marginal seal reduced. Class I and II cavities in molars and premolars may be large enough in some cases to cause significant stress to be placed on the tooth-restoration interface with a subsequent breakdown of adhesion, particularly at restorative-dentine margins. Inadequate marginal seal in large cavities is still considered a potential disadvantage of posterior composite materials, particularly when a seal to dentine is required. Adhesive materials and specialized techniques, including the so-called sandwich technique are discussed in Chapters 23 and 24.

Composite inlays: Another approach to overcoming the effects of shrinkage and the resulting microleakage that may occur is the use of *composite inlays.* The principle behind these materials is that shrinkage occurs before the material is finally seated into the prepared cavity using a luting resin. Two approaches are possible, using either a chairside technique or an indirect, laboratory-based technique. For the chairside technique, an inlay cavity is cut by the dentist and the walls of the cavity coated with a release agent. The cavity is then filled with a composite resin – a light-activated material would normally be used. After initial curing the inlay is removed from the cavity; a process which is facilitated by proper cavity preparation and the use of the release agent. At this stage an opportunity may be taken to enhance the properties of the composite material by subjecting it to treatment with intense light and heat or pressure and heat to increase the degree of polymerization. The principle of this post-curing or annealing treatment is to heat the material to above the glass transition temperature of the resin in order to cause sufficient molecular mobility to allow further polymerization and cross-linking to occur. This treatment has been shown to cause only a moderate improvement in hardness and flexural strength. Care must be taken not to induce an excessive amount of cross-linking as this causes the material to become more brittle. Hence, post-curing must be carried out under controlled conditions. The indirect approach is similar except that the inlay is formed on a model constructed from an impression. The composite inlay is seated back into the prepared cavity using a composite resin luting cement. Most cements used for this purpose are of the dual-cure variety, they have relatively low filler content giving the fluidity required to enable seating of the inlay. They set rapidly at the exposed margins when illuminated by a polmerization activation light but also undergo slow chemically activated polymerization within the unexposed bulk. The completed inlay therefore consists of a bulk of well-polymerized composite material for which the margins are sealed by a thin layer of the luting product. Only the shrinkage of the luting material can contribute towards marginal leakage gaps and the thin section of this material ensures that such gaps should be minimal. Although only a thin layer of luting resin cement is used, its shrinkage can result in a relatively large stress at the surface with both the tooth and the inlay due to the large C-factor which applies to this type of situation. The magnitude of the stress can be great enough to disrupt adhesive forces which may not have matured sufficiently to withstand the effects of shrinkage.

Another potential problem with composite inlays is related to the differential wear rates of the relatively hard inlay material compared to the relatively soft luting material. This is caused by a combination of the lower filler content and lower degree of polymerization of the latter. It can cause the formation of a ditch around the inlay as the softer material is preferentially worn.

22.8 Suggested further reading

Burke, F.J.T., Watts, D.C., Wilson, N.H.F. & Wilson, M.A. (1991) Current status and rationale for composite inlays and onlays. *Br. Dent. J.* **170**, 269.

ISO 4049 Polymer-based filling and restorative materials.

Jones, D.W. (1990) Composite restorative materials. *J. Can. Dent. Assoc.* **56**, 851.

Leinfelder, K.F. (1995) Posterior composite resins. *J. Am. Dent. Assoc.* **126**, 663.

Lutz, F. & Phillips, R.W. (1983) A classification and evaluation of composite resin systems. *J. Prosthet. Dent.* **50**, 480.

Chapter 23
Adhesive Restorative Materials: Bonding of Resin-based Materials

23.1 Introduction

The development and regular use of adhesive materials has begun to revolutionize many aspects of restorative and preventive dentistry. Attitudes towards cavity preparation are altering since, with adhesive materials, it is no longer necessary to produce large undercuts in order to retain the filling. These techniques are, therefore, responsible for the conservation of large quantities of sound tooth substance which would otherwise be victim to the dental bur. Microleakage, a major dental problem which is probably responsible for many cases of secondary caries, may be reduced or eliminated. New forms of treatment, such as the sealing of pits and fissures on posterior teeth, the coverage of badly stained or deformed teeth in order to improve appearance and the direct bonding of brackets in orthodontics have all grown from the development of adhesive systems.

Section 2.5 deals briefly with the general mechanistic aspects of adhesion. Three major approaches can be identified. First, bonding through micromechanical attachment; in dentistry this is best illustrated through the bonding of resins to enamel using the *acid-etch technique*. Second, bonding through *chemical adhesion* to either enamel or dentine can be identified in many systems based on the use of coupling agents or cements containing polyacids. Third, bonding through a complex mechanism involving wetting, penetration and the formation of a layer of bound material at the interface between the restorative and the substrate. The latter describes the mode of action of many modern dentine bonding agents.

23.2 Acid-etch systems for bonding to enamel

The surface of enamel is smooth and has little potential for bonding by micromechanical attach-ment. On treatment with certain acids, however, the structure of the enamel surface may be modified considerably. Figure 23.1 shows the surface of human enamel following one minute of etching with a 37% solution of phosphoric acid, which is the acid of choice for most applications of the acid-etch technique. Solutions of phosphoric acid are difficult to control when applied to enamel, some acid inevitably contacts areas which are not required to be etched. One improvement in acid-etching procedures has been the development of acidified gels. These contain phosphoric acid in aqueous gel which is viscous enough to allow controlled placement in the required area. In addition, the gel is normally pigmented, a feature which further aids control.

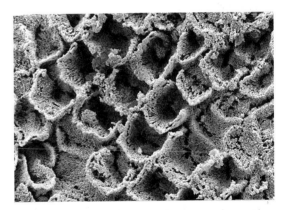

Fig. 23.1 Scanning electron microscope photograph of an enamel surface following one minute of etching with 37% aqueous phosphoric acid solution (original margin fixation × 750) (× 1786 magnification).

The pattern of etching enamel can vary. The most common (type 1) involves preferential removal of the enamel prism cores, the prism peripheries remaining intact. The type 2 etching pattern is the opposite of the type 1, involving preferential removal of the peripheries with the cores being left intact. The type 3 etching pattern contains areas which resemble both type 1 and type 2 along with some less distinct areas where the pattern of etching appears to be unrelated to the enamel prism morphology.

The individual features evident in Fig. 23.1 correspond to the ends of enamel prisms, each being about 5 μm in diameter. This surface is now suitable for micromechanical attachment since it contains a myriad of small undercuts into which resins can gain ingress, set and form a *mechanical lock*. The three major factors which affect the success or failure of acid-etch bonding systems are as follows:

(1) The etching time. This should be sufficient to cause effective etching as evidenced by a white, chalky appearance on the treated section of enamel after washing and drying. Etching should not continue long enough for dissolved apatites to reprecipitate as phosphates onto the etched surface. The etching time normally used is between 10 and 60 seconds.

(2) The washing stage. Following etching the enamel surface should be washed with copious amounts of water to remove debris. The washing time usually used is 60 seconds.

(3) The drying stage. The surface of the etched enamel should be very thoroughly dried using oil-free compressed air and maintained in a dry, uncontaminated state prior to application of the resin.

The type of resin applied to the etched enamel surface depends upon the specific application being used. For composite resins the mixed material may be applied directly to the etched enamel surface. Resin from the composite flows into the etched enamel and sets, forming rigid tags, typically 25 μm long, which retain the filling. Many manufacturers supply a fluid *bonding resin* which may enhance the adhesive bond strength. It consists of a resin similar to that used in the composite material but contains no filler particles. It is very fluid and readily flows into the etched enamel surface. The bonding resin may be a single component which is activated by light or may consist of two fluid resins, one containing initiator and the other activator, which require mixing before being applied to the etched enamel. The composite filling material is applied directly to the surface of the bonding resin. The need for the use of the intermediary layer of unfilled bonding resin varies depending upon the type of composite material used. For conventional compo-

sites it is likely that the materials contain sufficient excess resin to satisfy the requirements for attachment to etched enamel without the presence of the intermediate resin. For the more heavily filled and viscous products (mainly hybrid-type composites) it is necessary to use the unfilled resin layer in order to achieve adequate penetration of the etched enamel surface.

Bonding readily occurs at the unfilled resin to composite interface. This is aided by the fact that surface layers of resins polymerized by a free radical mechanism remain soft and unpolymerized due to the inhibiting effect which oxygen has on the polymerization mechanism. On applying a composite material to the surface of a 'cured' unfilled resin, mixing of the two resin systems occurs at the interface followed by a degree of copolymerization and entangling which effectively bonds the filled and unfilled resins together. The resulting shear bond strength achieved between etched enamel and restorative resins is 16–20 MPa.

The way in which the enamel etch pattern affects bonding has never been conclusively proven. The nature of some enamel bonding systems has changed over recent years as some manufacturers have produced materials which can be used for both enamel and dentine bonding. Hence, some enamel bonding resins now contain primers and solvents which enable bonding to moist enamel to be achieved. This is contrary to the previous situation in which thorough drying of enamel was essential for effective bonding. This theme is developed further in Section 23.8.

23.3 Applications of the acid-etch technique

The acid-etch technique has many applications in dentistry. It is now widely used for most composite fillings as a means of aiding retention and reducing or preventing microleakage. For *class IV cavities* the acid-etch technique has replaced the gold inlay as the treatment of choice for restoring the tooth contours and function. In this example the use of an adhesive system allows the conservation of considerable quantities of tooth substance which would otherwise be lost in cavity preparation. Bonding of resins using the acid-etch technique has also been used as a means of strengthening or *splinting* teeth which have been weakened by cavity preparation. It can readily be shown that a tooth having a prepared cavity is weakened relative to an unprepared tooth. Under stress, fracture of the tooth is likely with cusp fracture being the most likely occurrence. Restoring the cavity with a non-adhesive restoration has little beneficial effect on the strength of the tooth whereas the use of an adhesive material will strengthen the tooth and help to prevent cusp fractures.

Fissure sealants are now widely used for preventing pit and fissure caries. The majority of products are based on dimethacrylate resin systems such as Bis GMA or urethane dimethacrylate. The simplest products consist of two liquid components, each containing the dimethacrylate monomer or a mixture of the monomer and a diluent monomer such as triethylene glycol dimethacrylate (see Fig. 22.4). In addition, one component contains a peroxide initiator whilst the other contains an amine activator. The normal procedure is to mix together one drop of each liquid component in order to activate the polymerization of the methacrylate groups. Chemically, these products are almost identical to the intermediary resin bonding agents referred to in the previous section. The mixed material is applied to the etched enamel of the occlusal surface of the selected tooth where it typically takes a few minutes to harden. The surface layer remains tacky due to air inhibition of the polymerization and is generally wiped away to expose the fully cured material underneath.

Some products contain additives such as titanium dioxide in order to make the sealant more readily visible *in situ*. With the unpigmented material the sealant can be difficult to detect on inspection due to the translucent nature of the resin. There has also been a trend towards adding glass filler to improve durability and those products containing filler may be considered as lightly filled composites. The filler content remains somewhat lower than that found in composite filling materials so that the viscosity is low enough to enable the materials to flow into the fissure pattern of the occlusal surface of the tooth.

Not surprisingly, the development of light-activated fissure sealant materials has followed the development of light-activated composites. One of the most popular materials in use until a few years ago was activated using ultraviolet radiation. This is no longer used and has been replaced by products which are activated by light within the visible range. The visible light activation units which are used for curing composites can also be used to activate curing of fissure sealants so it is convenient for dentists who have such a unit to use it for several applications. The problems of limited depth of cure do not apply to these materials which are used in thin sections. The efficacy of fissure sealants is measured in one of two ways. One way is to monitor the survival of the sealant as a function of time. Apparent sealant loss

may be due to detachment or wear. The other way is to monitor the caries reduction on sealed teeth compared with a group of unsealed control teeth. Surprisingly the two approaches do not produce the same result. Sealants, being unfilled or lightly filled resins, are relatively soft and readily undergo abrasive wear, although this is minimized in practice due to the fact that the material is in a protected environment in which it is unlikely to come under direct occlusal loads. In any event, wear of the sealant does not impair its efficacy since the surface enamel remains impregnated with resin. Likewise, if a sealant becomes detached it may still have some beneficial effect if it leaves behind an enamel surface which is resin impregnated.

The success of fissure sealants is mainly dependent on initial placement conditions and techniques. In order to get good resin tag formation the enamel must be properly etched and washed and thoroughly dried before the sealant is applied. It is the variability in levels of moisture content which causes the wide variation in success rates recorded for fissure sealants. Attempts have been made to produce fluoride containing sealants so that the benefits of surface sealing can be combined with those of a sustained fluoride release. Release of fluoride from resin-based materials is difficult to achieve and the rate of release is generally much lower than is observed for glass ionomers. Fluoride releasing resin-modified glass ionomers (see Chapter 25) offer a potential for achieving the ideal of effective bonding durability and sustained fluoride release.

Most recently, chemically active luting resins have become available which will bond to oxide layers on the surface of non-precious metals and to copper oxide on heat treated gold casting alloys (see Section 23.9)

Resin systems are now widely used for attaching *orthodontic brackets*. These resins are normally supplied as two components carrying relatively high loadings of initiator and activator respectively. One component is applied to the etched enamel surface and the other to the bracket. When the two are pressed together rapid setting takes place. Alternatively, conventional composite resin materials can be used for this application.

Composites are gaining in popularity for the attachment of *bridges*. This involves a more conservative technique than the traditional methods, which involve considerable destruction of the abutment teeth in order to achieve retention. The principle of the resin-bonded systems is that the composite bonds mechanically to the etched enamel of the tooth and also to the surface of the cast alloy framework of the bridge. There are various means of achieving mechanical attachment between the resin and the alloy. One system employs the use of perforated 'wings' on the cast alloy bridge framework. The composite used for bonding flows through the perforations giving a mechanical lock onto the framework. Attachment to the abutment tooth is through resin penetration of acid-etched enamel. This type of bridge is known as a Rochette bridge. Another approach is to etch the wings of the bridge to produce a roughened surface with a myriad of small undercuts similar in appearance to the surface of etched enamel (Fig. 23.2). This surface is suitable for achieving mechanical attachment with a composite. Etching may be carried out electrolytically or with a strong acid. This second type of bridge is normally referred to as a Maryland bridge. Recently, chemically active resins capable of attaching to both metals and tooth have been used to bond sandblasted metal retainers to the supporting tooth.

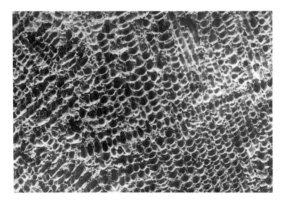

Fig. 23.2   A scanning electron micrograph of an electrolytically acid-etched metal surface showing the irregular etch pattern that can give micromechanical retention for attachment (× 124).

Another application of the acid-etch technique is the attachment of acrylic or porcelain labial veneers in order to improve the appearance of stained, discoloured or misshapen teeth. Acrylic veneers may be produced in a range of standard shapes and sizes which can be customized by heat adaptation to a cast of the patient's teeth. A composite of the correct shade is used to attach the veneer to the etched enamel surface. The fitting surface of the veneer is softened with a solvent primer to aid bonding between the veneer and composite. The acrylic laminate veneers have limited lifetime due to the fact that the acrylic resin is soft and readily abrades to expose regions of the underlying composite resin.

Also the bond between the composite resin and veneer has a tendency to fail, probably due to stresses set up at the interface as a result of the differing values of the coefficient of thermal expansion and water sorption for the two materials. The use of porcelain veneers is covered in Section 11.8. Essentially the veneers are custom made and bonding to the composite is achieved by etching the fitting surface of the veneer with hydrofluoric acid and using a silane coupling agent to chemically link silica groups in the porcelain to methacrylate groups in the resin. Porcelain veneers are much harder and more resistant to abrasion than acrylic veneers. Providing that etching and silane treatment is carried out carefully the bond to composite appears adequate. The brittle nature of the porcelain must be taken into account when considering the design of veneers if chipping at the incisal edge is to be avoided.

23.4 Bonding to dentine – background

The mechanism of bonding to enamel involves the penetration of resin into the relatively porous surface layer of the etched enamel to create a mechanical interlocking. It was recognized many years ago that a similar mechanism could be used with dentine. This would involve etching of the surface of exposed dentine with acid to expose the patent dentinal tubules which could be penetrated by resin to form tags. Until quite recently this mechanism of bonding to dentine was rejected by most authorities as being both ineffective and unacceptable for the following reasons.

(1) Concerns over the potentially damaging effect of acids on vital dentine: these concerns were related to what was considered a well established fact that acid-containing restoratives placed in contact with vital dentine cause irritation and/or irreversible pathological change to the pulp. Much of the evidence for these concerns involved experience with silicate restorative materials which contain phosphoric acid. Current philosophy on this important point is that most cases of pulpal irritation were not related to direct chemical traumatization with phosphoric acid but were as a result of ineffective sealing of cavity margins due to lack of adhesion. Hence, most authorities now accept that the dentine and pulp are able to withstand a greater chemical insult with acids than was once thought to be acceptable.

(2) Etching dentine opens dentinal tubules and encourages dentinal fluid flow. In view of the fact that most restorative resins are relatively hydrophobic, any increase in the moisture content of the

surface of dentine is likely to make bonding more difficult to achieve. Ever since attempts to bond resins to dentine were first attempted the inability of resins to 'wet' moist dentine and adapt closely enough to achieve bonding has been recognized as a major problem which has hindered development. Experience of bonding to enamel suggested that 'dryness' of the substrate was essential in order to achieve an effective bond, so it is easy to appreciate why the etching of dentine was considered unlikely to help in the production of an effective bond to this substrate. Most early attempts to achieve bonding emphasize the drying of dentine as an important step in the bonding procedure. Current thinking appreciates the damage which can be caused by desiccation of dentine and tries to overcome the moisture problem by the use of primers and solvents.

(3) The dentinal tubule openings occupy only about 5% of the cut dentine surface in superficial dentine (near the amelodentinal junction). This rises to near 20% in deep dentine. Hence, it was suggested that in inserting resin tags into dentinal tubules the effectiveness of the bond to dentine would be limited by the relatively small proportion of the area being utilized. It is currently accepted that whereas tags in dentinal tubules can contribute to bonding, other mechanisms involving all the exposed dentine surface are at least equally as important.

In the 1970s and 1980s, when dentine bonding was considered desirable but when etching of dentine was considered unacceptable, emphasis was placed on trying to achieve bonding to dentine through the formation of chemical links between restoratives and chemical moieties in the dentine surface.

23.5 Attempts at chemical bonding

When attempting to form chemical links with the tooth surface it is obviously necessary to pay some attention to the chemical nature of the substrate tooth material. Dentine contains approximately 50% hydroxyapatite and 30% polypeptides (e.g. collagen), the balance being aqueous solutions which occupy the dentinal tubules. Enamel, on the other hand, contains only about 1% protein and 97% hydroxyapatite. Forming chemical links with enamel therefore inevitably involves forming a union with hydroxyapatite. Adhesive systems which attach to hydroxyapatite will form links with both enamel and dentine, although the bond to enamel for such materials is generally significantly stronger than the bond to dentine. Dentine offers the possibility of utilizing reactive groups, such as –NH which are

present in dentine proteins, for achieving chemical union with adhesives. For adhesives of this type a significant bond strength may be demonstrated with dentine but no appreciable adhesion is observed with enamel.

In order to bridge the gap between the tooth surface and the resin-based restorative a series of difunctional chemical coupling agents were developed. Resin-based restorative materials may be bonded to either dentine or enamel using coupling agents. The principle of the coupling agent is that it consists of a difunctional molecule, one part of which enters into chemical union with the tooth surface whilst the other attaches to the resin, as illustrated in Fig. 23.3. The method of use is to apply the coupling agent to the clean, dry tooth surface followed by the resin filling material, normally a composite. The coupling agents all have a general formula of the type shown in Fig. 23.4 where M represents a methacrylate group which

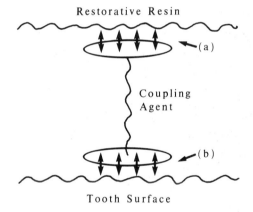

Fig. 23.3 Diagram illustrating the principle of bonding with a coupling agent. (a) Part of molecule which enters into bonding with restorative resin. (b) Part of molecule which enters into bonding with tooth surface.

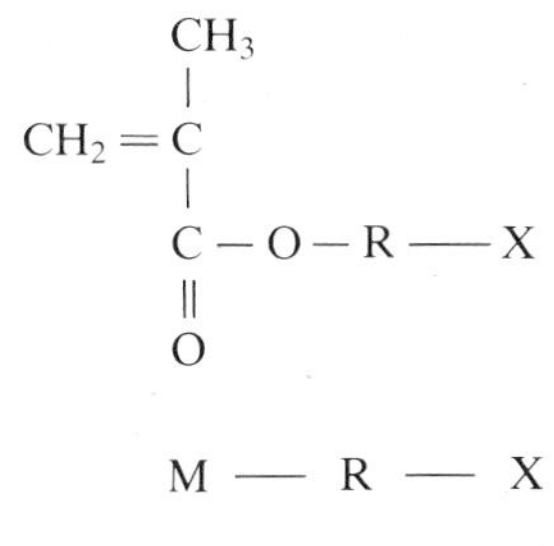

$$CH_2 = \overset{\overset{\displaystyle CH_3}{|}}{\underset{\underset{\displaystyle O}{\parallel}}{\overset{\displaystyle |}{C}} - O - R - X}$$

$$M - R - X$$

Fig. 23.4 General structural formula of a resin–tooth coupling agent. X represents a chemical group which interacts with enamel or dentine. R represents a linking group which joins X to the methacrylate (M).

eventually becomes bound to the resin by co-polymerization, X represents a reactive group which interacts with the tooth surface and R is a linking and spacing group.

Bonding to the inorganic component of dentine

One of the earliest molecules to be used for this purpose was *N*-phenylglycine-glycidylmethacrylate, NPG-GMA (Fig. 23.5). A chelate bond between the *N*-phenylglycine group and the calcium of the tooth (Fig. 23.6) is postulated whilst the methacrylate group becomes incorporated into the resin during polymerization. By relating the structure of NPG-GMA to the general formula given in Fig. 23.4 it can be seen that the X group in this case is *N*-phenylglycine. Since bond formation is primarily with the calcium of tooth substance, coupling agents of this type form stronger bonds to enamel than to dentine.

Another coupling system which can potentially work by chelating with calcium is 4-methacryloxyethyltrimelliticanhydride (4-META) (Fig 23.7). The bond strengths of NPG-GMA and 4-META to dentine can be increased by pretreatment with certain *mordant* ions such as ferric and aluminium ions, normally in the form of aqueous solutions of their chloride or oxalate salts. A strongly bound surface layer concentrated in ions capable of reacting with the chelating species is formed.

Other coupling agents which may bond to the inorganic component of dentine contain reactive phosphate groups. One such product has the structure shown in Fig. 23.8. The interfacial bond may be established through attractions between the negative charges of the oxygens on the phosphate and the positively charged calcium at the dentine surface, as indicated by the arrows. It is not certain how durable the bond is likely to be in a moist environment. The R–O–P bond is thought to become hydrolysed leading to a gradual reduction in bond strength.

Most of the coupling agents referred to above are polymerizable monomers containing groups capable of interacting with the tooth surface. In the presence of the required initiators and activators the monomers are readily polymerized to form resins. Hence some of the products are supplied as two compo-

nents, one containing a chemical activator (e.g. a tertiary amine), the other containing a polymerization initiator (e.g. a peroxide). Over the years there has been a trend for chemically activated resin systems to be replaced by light-activated materials. As a result, some products are supplied as one component containing the adhesive and a light-sensitive polymerization activator.

The adhesive systems described above work primarily through affinity for calcium in the organic component of dentine. Consequently, whereas each material was primarily designed as a dentine adhesive they all form a more tenacious bond to enamel. Some direct bonding between reactive groups in dentinal collagen and reactive groups in the adhesives is thought possible.

Some adhesive systems have been developed specifically with the aim of grafting to the organic collagenous component of dentine. Collagen has several reactive groups which make this a feasible proposition. The groups which have received most attention are the hydroxyl and amine groups. One commercial product relied on the addition reaction which occurs between isocyanate groups and both hydroxyl and amine groups. Another commercial product relied on the reaction which readily occurs between aldehyde groups and amine groups.

Attempts at bonding restorative resins to dentine by direct chemical coupling led to limited clinical success in the absence of any form of dentine pretreatment or conditioning. Table 23.1 shows values of shear bond strength to acid-etched enamel and unconditioned dentine. The significantly lower bond strengths to dentine explain the lack of clinical efficacy. Microleakage studies also showed that a less than perfect marginal seal to dentine was achieved, indicating that close adaptation between the

Table 23.1 Shear bond strength of various bonding systems to etched enamel or unconditioned dentine.

Bonding system	Bond strength (MPa)
Acid-etched enamel + resin	16–20
Dentine + phosphate modified resin	3–5
Dentine + NPG-GMA + resin	2–5
Dentine + 4-META	2–5

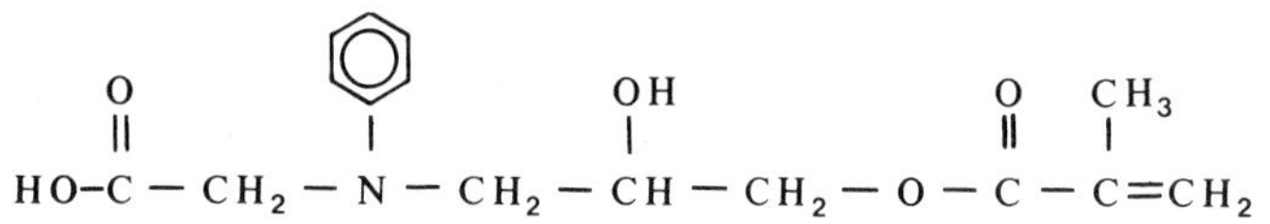

Fig. 23.5 Structural formula of *N*-phenylglycine-glycidylmethacrylate (NPG-GMA). Used as a coupling agent to link composite resin restorative materials with tooth substance.

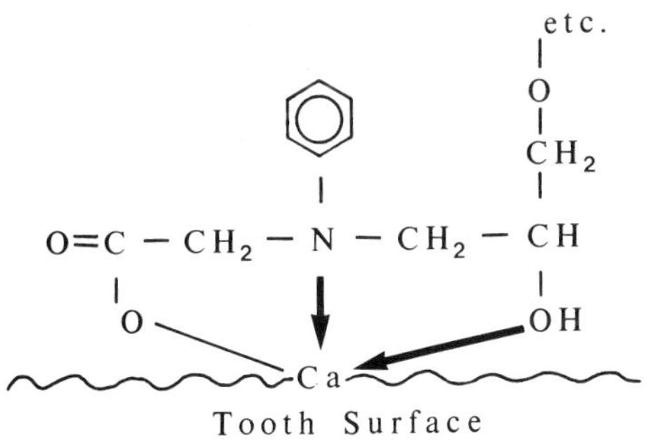

Fig. 23.6 Diagram illustrating the probable mechanism of adhesion between NPG-GMA and the tooth surface.

restorative and dentine had not been developed over a significant proportion of the dentine surface.

Improvements in the ability to bond to dentine and to form an effective seal at the tooth restoration interface were not possible until a greater understanding of the nature of the dentine surface and the changes which could be produced by *conditioning* was achieved. For those materials discussed in this section, drying of the dentine surface was considered a prerequisite for effective bonding. The higher values of shear bond strength to dentine (Table 23.1) were achieved only after effective drying. Work on dentine conditioning and the use of *primers* was to cause a complete re-think of how bonding to dentine is best achieved.

23.6 Dentine conditioning – the smear layer

There are several possible reasons why the bond strength to dentine was so much lower than that which could be achieved with enamel (Table 23.1). The proposed mechanism was different and relied upon the very close adaptation of bonding agent to substrate in order to allow chemical bonding to occur. The inherent problem involved in bonding a hydrophobic resin to a hydrophilic substrate was thought to be a major factor in this regard. It became clear, however, that one of the most significant factors which limits bonding, in the absence of any form of dentine pre-treatment, is the presence of the dentine smear layer. This layer, which is 3–15 µm thick, prevents interaction of the adhesive with the bulk dentine and this prevents the formation of any effective or durable bond. Any bond which is formed is to the surface of the smear layer itself and since this may not be strongly bound to the underlying dentine the bond strength and sealing ability are compromised. The smear layer (Fig. 23.9) is formed by the process of cavity preparation and extends over the whole prepared surface of the dentine and into the dentinal tubules (smear plug). It is a loosely bound layer of cutting debris including dentine chips, micro-organisms, salivary protein and collagen from the dentine. A smear layer is present on the surface of freshly cut dentine irrespective of the method of mechanical tooth preparation.

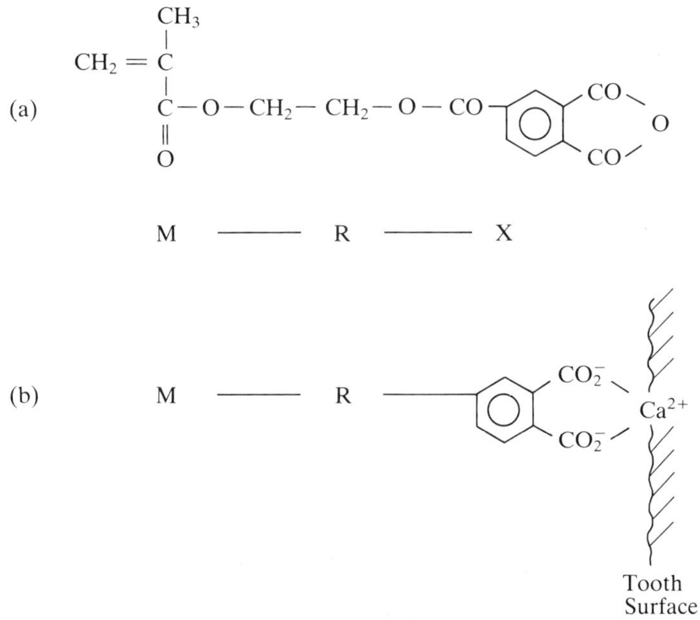

Fig. 23.7 Structure of 4-META (4-methacryloxyethyltrimelliticanhydride) and its mode of bonding to tooth substance. (a) Structure of 4-META. (b) 4-META bound to calcium in tooth substance.

(a)

$$CH_2 = \underset{\underset{O}{\underset{\|}{\overset{\underset{|}{C-O-CH_2-CH_2-O-P=O}}{C}}}}{\overset{\overset{CH_3}{|}}{C}}$$

M — R — X

(b)

M — R — O, O⁻ ... P⁺ ... Ca²⁺ ... O O⁻

Tooth
Surface

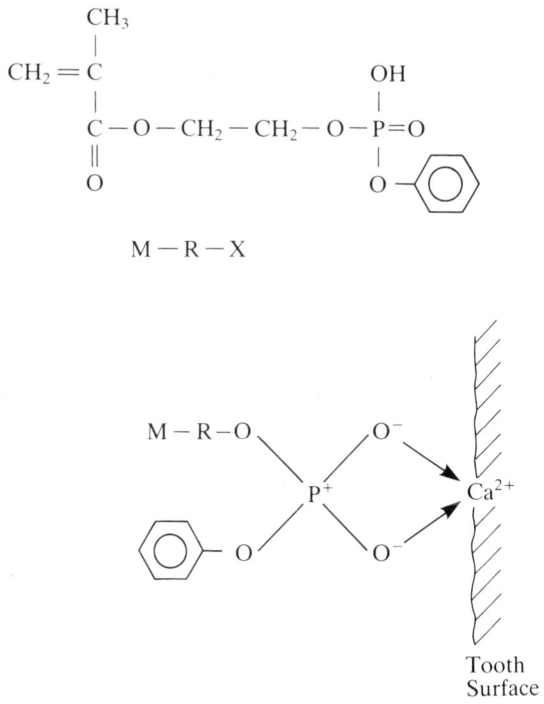

Fig. 23.8 Structure of a phosphate ester suggested as a dental adhesive. (a) Structure of the ester which is essentially a product of an aromatic phosphate and hydroxyethylmethacrylate (HEMA). (b) Proposed method of bonding to tooth substance.

Table 23.2 Commonly used dentine conditioners.

35–37% Phosphoric acid
10% Phosphoric acid
10% Maleic acid
17% EDTA
10% Citric acid + 3% ferric chloride

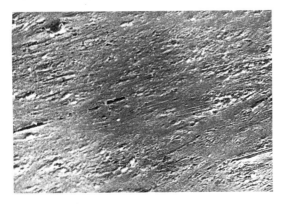

Fig. 23.9 Surface of the dentine smear layer formed after cavity preparation.

It is now recognized that in order to form an effective bond and seal between a restorative resin and dentine the smear layer must be removed, disturbed or modified in some way which allows access to the underlying bulk dentine. The liquids used for dentine pre-treatments prior to bonding are called *conditioners*. They are generally acid solutions which are capable of dissolving or at least *solubilizing* the smear layer, exposing the underlying dentine to the bonding agent. Many acidic solutions have been employed as conditioners. Some of the more common agents are listed in Table 23.2

It is advantageous if the acid used for dentine conditioning can also be used for acid-etching enamel and there is a growing trend now for manufacturers to supply a single agent for both purposes. Since 37% phosphoric acid has a proven track record as an enamel etchant its popularity as a dentine conditioner is increasing. In many ways, dental research has come full circle in accepting acidic dentine conditioning using strong etchants as part of a normal treatment regime. There is mounting evidence that etching can be tolerated, without adverse effects, even in the deepest dentine and the use of cavity liners under resin-based restorative materials is declining. A prerequisite to the tolerance of acidic dentine conditioning is the ability to form a strong bond with an adequate seal at the end of the treatment.

The option for removing or just disturbing the smear layer depends on whether the manufacturer recommends rinsing after the conditioning stage. A rinse at this stage is likely to remove the smear layer completely, leaving a relatively smooth dentine surface with patent dentinal tubules (Fig. 23.10). When there is no rinsing stage after conditioning the smear layer becomes re-deposited on the dentine surface. The latter approach is used when manufacturers attempt to reduce the number of steps required to form a bond. The conditioning stage can be viewed as the first of three stages – the other two being priming and bonding. Many manufacturers now try to combine at least two of the three stages.

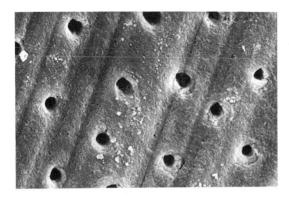

Fig. 23.10 Surface of dentine after conditioning with 37% phosphoric acid followed by rinsing. The smear layer is removed, the dentinal tubules opened and the intertubular dentine partially decalcified (× 1690).

23.7 Priming and bonding

Having conditioned the dentine in order to remove or modify the smear layer, the next stage is the priming stage. This stage is a key stage in the procedure as it is designed to change the chemical nature of the dentine surface and to overcome the normal repulsion between the hydrophilic dentine and the hydrophobic resin. The priming agents are similar in nature to the di-functional chemical coupling agents described in Section 23.5. Their nature is described in general terms in Fig. 23.4. They are difunctional materials with a methacrylate group (having affinity for the resin) and another reactive group having affinity for the dentine. This other reactive group may be an amino group, a phosphate group or a 4-META group as described in Section 23.5. However, the most commonly used primer is hydroxyethylmethacrylate (HEMA) in which the R–X group in Fig. 23.4 is simply a C_2H_4OH group. It is the hydrophilic nature of the hydroxyl group which makes HEMA such an effective priming agent. Much more emphasis is now placed on the affinity

between the reactive groups and the dentine and less emphasis is placed on the ability to form a chemical bond with components of dentine, although this is still recognized as being a possibility with some materials. After priming, the nature of the dentine surface is significantly changed – it being more hydrophobic and ready to accept the resin-based bonding agent.

The bonding agent is normally a fluid resin similar in composition to the products described for enamel bonding (Section 23.2). The fluid resin is able to flow over and *wet* the primed surface to complete the formation of an effective bond. Curing of the bonding agent is activated by light for single component materials or chemically for two component materials.

Manufacturers have responded to the needs of clinicians by trying to simplify the application procedures for conditioners, primers and bonding agents and by combining these procedures into one in some cases. Hence, the primer is sometimes incorporated with the conditioner and following the combined conditioning/priming the smear layer is incorporated within the primer which now has direct contact with the bulk dentine surface. Alternatively, the primer may be incorporated with the bonding resin and the combined liquid applied to the conditioned and rinsed dentine surface. A previously unmentioned component of the priming agent is the solvent carrier. The role of this solvent becomes evident when the overall concept of bonding is considered.

23.8 Current concepts in dentine bonding – the hybrid layer

In Sections 23.6 and 23.7 the importance of dentine conditioning and priming has been stressed. Modern dentine bonding systems are able to produce bond strength values equivalent to or greater than the value obtained in bonding resins to acid-etched enamel. An indication of the tenacious nature of the bond which can be achieved is obtained from the mode of failure during bond testing. This is often cohesive in nature – either within the adhesive or within the dentine. Table 23.3 gives an indication of the bond strength values which can be achieved with some systems. Values of this magnitude suggest that the mechanism of bonding must involve something other than weak interfacial bonding caused by good wetting and close adaptation.

Painstaking work in Japan and the USA has gone some way towards explaining the mechanism of bonding of most modern materials and the reason why high bond strength values are achieved. It is now

Table 23.3 Shear bond strength of various bonding systems to conditioned and primed dentine.

Bonding system	Bond strength (MPa)
Maleic acid/HEMA/polyacid	17–24
Phosphoric acid/NTG GMA[1] BPDM[2]	20–30
Citric acid + ferric chloride/4-META/MMA	15–25
Phosphoric acid/PENTA[3] – moist	20–30
Phosphoric acid/PENTA – dry	10–20

(1) *N*-tolylglycine-glycidylmethacrylate.
(2) Biphenyldimethacrylate.
(3) Phosphonated penta-acrylate ester.

believed that efficient dentine conditioning not only involves removal of the smear layer and smear plug but also causes a significant decalcification of inter-tubular dentine to a depth of a few microns. The decalcification process leaves a three-dimensional collagenous network which can be infiltrated by primer and resin to form a *resin infiltrated/reinforced layer* or *hybrid layer* at the interface between the bulk dentine and the resin. This hybrid layer is illustrated in Fig. 23.11 and can be considered to have a composite structure of two continuous phases, the resin phase and the fibrous collagenous phase, which when the resin is polymerized, strongly binds the resin and dentine together. In Fig. 23.11 it can be seen that the resin also penetrates the dentinal tubules and this is likely to contribute to the overall efficacy of the bond.

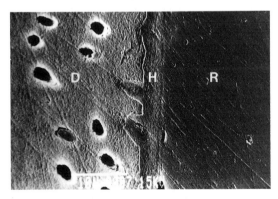

Fig. 23.11 Interface of conditioned, primed dentine and resin bonding agent illustrating the presence of the resin reinforced or hybrid layer. (Kindly supplied by Professor N. Nakabayashi. Originally published in *Oper. Dent.* Suppl. 5, 197 (1992), reproduced with permission from the editor.) In this case bonding was achieved using a 4-META system (× 1472).

The ability of primers and resins (or mixtures of the two) to penetrate the demineralized dentine surface is the key to the formation of the hybrid layer. Following demineralization the collagenous network is supported only by moisture and any attempt to rigorously dry the dentine at this stage will lead to the collapse of collagen fibres and impair the formation of a hybrid layer. Most manufacturers now recommend that dentine is maintained in a moist state immediately prior to application of the primer in order to prevent collapse of the demineralized collagenous network. This represents a strange turn of events for dentists who had previously believed dryness to be critical when bonding to both enamel and dentine. Published results for many products confirm that the bond strength to moist dentine is often greater than that to dry dentine. This is confirmed for at least one product by reference to Table 23.3. The ability of primer solutions to wet and penetrate moist dentine is a function of the hydrophilic group in the primer molecule and the presence of a solvent such as acetone. This type of solvent is able to 'chase' away the water in the porous dentine surface, allowing the spaces to be filled by primer and resin. Before curing of the resin the solvent is lost by evaporation. Another approach to wetting and penetration is to use aqueous primer solutions in which infiltration of primer is achieved by diffusion.

The mechanism of bonding which involves the formation of the hybrid layer produces some impressive values of bond strength, as shown in Table 23.3. Most bond failures above 20 MPa occur through fracture within dentine (cohesive failure). Comparison of the values in Table 23.3 with those in Table 23.1 illustrates the marked improvement in bond strength which has followed the improvement in the understanding of the structure of the resin–dentine interface. The thickness of the hybrid layer is not considered an important factor which controls bonding. In most cases the layer is thought to be 2–10 μm thick and the important feature as far as bonding is concerned is that the demineralised dentine is completely infiltrated to give close adaptation of the resin to the irregular surface of the bulk dentine.

It is not known what value of bond strength is required in order to prevent debonding during the setting of a composite restorative. The stress set up caused by shrinkage during setting is a function of cavity shape and size as well as the nature of the material, as described in Section 22.3. One method adopted by some manufacturers to prevent the disruption of bonding resins by polymerization shrinkage of composites is to incorporate elastomeric resins into the bonding material. These may allow the bonded layer to deform elastically without destroying the bond. Another approach is to advise the application of multiple layers of bonding resin in order to create a more flexible buffer layer between the tooth and the composite. Since dentists demand the availability of bonding systems which can be used simultaneously with both dentine and enamel the products described in this section have become widely used as enamel bonding agents. The mechanism of bonding to enamel is essentially similar to that for conventional enamel bonding systems (Section 23.2). Application of the conditioning (or etching) agent results in the familiar change in the surface of the enamel (Fig. 23.1). This is then impregnated by the primer and bonding resin. The developments in dentine primers, which are now also used for enamel bonding, have led to the emphasis on enamel dryness becoming less of an issue with these modern systems. Also, there is evidence that an enamel–resin hybrid layer analogous to the dentine hybrid layer can form during enamel bonding. Figure 23.12 shows the interface of a resin–enamel bond after partial removal of enamel with hydrochloric acid. The area at the interface where resin had impregnated the porous enamel surface is clearly visible.

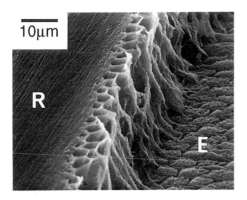

Fig. 23.12 The interface of a resin–enamel bond (mediated by a 4-META primer) after partial removal of enamel with hydrochloric acid. (Kindly supplied by Professor N. Nakabayashi. First published in *Dent. Mat.* **8**, 175 (1992), reproduced with permission from the editor (× 1000).

23.9 Bonding to alloys, amalgam and ceramics

In the previous sections, emphasis has been placed on the use of enamel and dentine bonding agents

used to improve bonding to tooth substance during the placement of direct composite restorations. In Section 23.3 reference was made to the fact that composite type materials are used for bonding of orthodontic brackets and resin-retained bridges. In these situations the bond between the composite and metal may rely upon mechanical retention, either by building in retention into the design of the metal structure (e.g. the base of the orthodontic bracket) or by creating a retentive surface through electrolytic etching or abrasion. For these and other applications where a strong durable bond is required in the absence of any natural retentive forces a resin-based luting agent may be preferred to a conventional cement. The ability of the resin to achieve a chemical union with the alloy may improve retention whilst at the same time reducing the amount of preparative work required to be performed on the alloy.

Virtually all the bonding agents described in the previous section can be used to achieve bonding with a variety of alloys – normally in conjunction with a low viscosity composite luting cement. Some specialist resin-based adhesive luting cements have become widely used over recent years. One such system, originally supplied as a powder and liquid, was essentially a self-curing composite in which the powder was primarily a quartz filler along with some initiator and the liquid consisted of a mixture of dimethacrylate monomers and a methacrylate–phosphate coupling agent along with a small amount of a chemical activator. The mixed material combined adhesive characteristics with an ideal consistency for luting purposes. A material of similar composition is now available in two-paste form. One feature of this particular type of resin-based cement was a marked sensitivity of the polymerization reaction to the presence of oxygen. In order to enable the material to set properly oxygen must be excluded from the exposed surface of the cement. This is achieved by the application of a gel-type barrier which can be washed away after setting.

Another powder–liquid type luting cement in common use is based upon the 4-META system referred to in the previous section. The powder contains polymethylmethacrylate (PMMA) whilst the liquid contains a mixture of methylmethacrylate monomer (MMA), 4-META and tri-butylborane (TBB). The TBB liberates free radicals on contact with moisture (e.g. on the tooth surface) and causes polymerization of the MMA.

The nature of the metal surface required for bonding has received some attention – particularly with regard to crown and bridge alloys. Bonding of most materials to base metal alloys appears to be quite straightforward with bond strengths in excess of 20 MPA being normal. The naturally formed oxide layer on the alloy surface is thought to be involved in the bonding process and the only preparation required is a moderate roughening using sand blasting followed by steam cleaning. Bonding to precious alloys can be more difficult. Tin plating is recommended for some products in order to generate an oxide layer. It is not clear whether this treatment aids bonding by producing a surface suitable for chemical bonding or through the formation of a roughened surface coated with tin oxide crystals. For other alloy/adhesive systems heating of the alloy to 400°C in air for 10 minutes generates a copper oxide layer on the metal surface, whilst other products claim to bond adequately to a sand blasted alloy surface.

Bonding of base metal alloys opened up the possibility of achieving union between dental amalgam and tooth substance. One specialist product based on 4-META and several of the materials referred to in Section 23.6 are now advocated by the manufacturers for this purpose. This has led to the *bonded amalgam* restoration. The potential advantages are that the cavity does not need to be so retentive and that the adhesive provides a means of reducing leakage. Other applications of these systems are in amalgam repairs (bonding amalgam to amalgam) and in amalgam core build-up (bonding amalgam to dentine).

Systems which bond to ceramics can be used to bond ceramic inlays, onlays, veneers and ceramic orthodontic brackets. The surface to be bonded may be initially prepared using a diamond bur, sand blasting or etching with hydrofluoric acid. The latter is an extremely caustic substance so the etching procedure is often performed in the laboratory rather than in the clinic. The priming agent comprises a solution of a silane–methacrylate coupling agent such as γ-methacryloxypropyltrimethoxysilane (as described in Section 22.3) in a volatile solvent such as acetone. The solution is applied to the surface of the ceramic material and air drying rapidly removes the solvent to leave a layer of bound silane coupling agent. Very high values of bond strength (>20 MPa) to ceramic can be achieved using composite luting cements. In orthodontics concern has been expressed that ceramic brackets are bonded to enamel so strongly that debonding can result in fracture through the ceramic or, more seriously, fracture through the tooth. There is a suggestion that silane coupling becomes less effective with time as the silane may be subjected to hydrolysis.

23.10 Bond strength and leakage measurements

It is recognized that the most meaningful test of a new adhesive system involves long-term clinical use as part of a formal clinical trial or as part of a prospective or retrospective audit procedure. *In vitro* testing of adhesives can be used as a means of ensuring that only relatively promising materials are subjected to clinical testing. The two methods most widely used for assessing adhesives in the laboratory are bond strength and leakage. Bond strength testing involves the measurement of tensile or shear bond strength (the latter has been quoted in Tables 23.1 and 23.3). These tests produce results which are notoriously variable, particularly for natural substrates such as enamel and dentine. Variations in the value of bond strength may result partly from imperfections in the testing equipment (e.g. imperfect alignment in a tensile bond test rig) or from variations in the substrate material. For example, bond strength to dentine varies with the type of tooth, age of patient, depth of dentine, time of storage after extraction, nature of the storage medium, etc. These variations can be dealt with in one of two ways – either by controlling the distribution of variables between test groups or by using teeth at random but using sufficiently large numbers of test specimens which will make biased distributions unlikely. The International Standards Organization has recognized these problems in its technical report on testing adhesion to tooth substance (ISO TR 11405). This report makes recommendations as to the nature of the teeth to be used in testing and to the method of storage, the method of forming and testing the bond. Even when the guidelines are followed a coefficient of variation of 50% is not unusual and this can cast some doubt over the reliability of some of the systems. The results of these tests suggest that there is always a reasonable probability of getting an unusually low value of bond strength and these examples when translated into clinical practice may account for some of the observed failures with otherwise 'good' materials.

In addition to the value of bond strength the mode of bond failure is normally quoted and this is often considered a more important parameter. The mode of failure may be adhesive, i.e. occurring at the adhesive/substrate interface, cohesive, i.e. occurring entirely within the substrate or adhesive or mixed, i.e. occurring partly at the interface and partly cohesively. A value of bond strength without any indication of the mode of failure is almost meaningless. Recently techniques have been developed to simulate dentine tubular fluid flow perfusion during bond strength testing. The surface of dentine that has been etched will be wet as a result of tubular fluid flow and it is important to simulate this if possible.

Leakage studies are designed to give an indication of the ability of a material to form an effective seal against fluids and bacteria at the tooth/adhesive interface. Tests are normally performed by placing restorations in restored teeth and then subjecting them to storage, normally with an element of thermal cycling, in a solution of dye-stuff or other marker (e.g. radioisotope). At the end of the prescribed period of testing the restoration and tooth are sectioned and the effectiveness of the seal is judged by how far the dye (or other marker) has penetrated down the margin towards the cavity floor. Guidelines for leakage testing are also included in ISO TR 11405.

23.11 Suggested further reading

Swift, E.J., Perdigao, J. & Heymann, H.O. (1995). Bonding to enamel and dentine: a brief history and state of the art. *Quint. Int.* **26**, 95–110.

Eich, J.D., Guinnett, A.J. Pashley, D.H. & Robinson, S.J. (1997) Current concepts in adhesion to dentine. *Crit. Rev. Oral Biol. Med.* **8**, 306–35.

Jordan, R.E. (ed.) (1991) Eight articles on bonding to various substrates. *J. Esthet. Dent.* **3**, 117–155.

Barkmeier, W.W. (ed.) (1992) 22 articles on bonding to enamel and dentine. *Oper. Dent.*, Suppl. 5. *Proceedings of the International Symposium on Adhesive Dentistry*, 1–198.

ISO TR 11405 Dental Materials – Guidance on Testing of Adhesion to Tooth Structure.

Chapter 24

Glass Ionomer Restorative Materials (Polyalkenoates)

24.1 Introduction

Glass ionomer restorative materials have been available since the early 1970s and were derived from the silicate cements (Section 20.8) and poly-carboxylate cements (Chapter 30). Polycarboxylates were developed several years earlier and were the first dental cements for which an inherent adhesion to tooth substance could be demonstrated. They quickly gained popularity as luting cements but could not be used as restoratives because of high solubility, poor mechanical properties and unacceptable appearance caused by the residual opaque zinc oxide. It was soon discovered that when the zinc oxide of the polycarboxylate material was replaced with a reactive ion-leachable glass similar to that used previously in silicate cements a stronger, less soluble and more translucent cement could be produced.

24.2 Composition

These materials may be supplied as a powder and liquid or as a powder mixed with water. The composition is outlined in Table 24.1. For powder/liquid materials the powder consists of a sodium alumino-silicate glass of similar composition to that used in silicate materials. The ratio of alumina to silica in the glass is increased compared to that used in silicates. This increases the reactivity of the glass to a level where it reacts rapidly with polyacrylic acid, which is a weaker acid than the phosphoric acid used in silicate materials. As for the silicates, the glasses contain significant levels of fluoride which, although not directly involved in the setting reaction, may have an effect on the caries susceptibility of the surrounding tooth substance.

In the original glass ionomer material the liquid component was a 50% aqueous solution of poly-

Table 24.1 Composition of glass ionomer cements.

Powder/liquid materials

Powder	Sodium aluminosilicate glass with about 20% CaF and other minor additives
Liquid	Aqueous solution of acrylic acid/itaconic acid copolymer
	or
	Aqueous solution of maleic acid polymer and
	Tartaric acid in some products to control setting characteristics

Powder/water materials

Powder	Glass (as above) + vacuum-dried polyacid (acrylic, maleic or copolymers)
Liquid	Manufacturers supply a dropper bottle which the operator fills with water
	or
	The manufacturer supplies a dilute aqueous solution of tartaric acid

acrylic acid. Unfortunately, gelation of the polyacid occurred after only a few months, probably by intermolecular hydrogen bonding. Gelation can be reduced or eliminated by using copolymers instead of homopolymers. This creates sufficient steric hindrance to prevent hydrogen bonding.

Nowadays the liquid component may consist of an aqueous solution of acrylic acid or of a maleic acid/acrylic acid copolymer. Tartaric acid, which is used to control setting characteristics, is also included in the liquid component by many manufacturers. Other products are supplied as a powder/water preparation. The powder/water materials are of two types; both consist of a powder which contains vacuum dried polyacid, in addition to the glass powder. For some materials this is mixed with water and the manufacturers supply a dropper bottle to aid proportioning. With other products, the manufacturer supplies a dilute aqueous solution of tartaric acid. For products in which the polyacid forms part of the powder component, the manufacturers are able to revert to the use of homopolymers of acrylic or maleic acid as there is no problem of gelation in this solid form. Cements formed from these homopolymers tend to have improved physical characteristics when compared to those formed from acid copolymers.

Most glass ionomers for restorative use are now available in encapsulated form. This offers a great advantage – for these materials probably more than any others. The proportions are set and controlled by the manufacturer and mixing is a quick and clean process.

24.3 Setting reaction

The structure of polyacrylic acid is shown in Fig. 24.1a. It consists of repeating units derived from acrylic acid with reactive carboxylic acid groups at alternate carbon atoms along the polymer chain. Polymaleic acid has a similar structure except that there are acid groups at every carbon atom on the polymer chain. Hence, for a given chain length there are twice as many carboxylic acid groups in polymaleic acid compared with polyacrylic acid. The setting reaction involves the formation of a salt through reaction of the acid groups with cations released from the surface of the glass. The nature of the cross-linked polyalkenoate salt is illustrated in Fig. 24.1b.

On mixing the powder and liquid or powder and

(a) $- CH_2 - CH - CH_2 - CH - CH_2 - CH -$
$\qquad\qquad CO_2H \quad\ CO_2H \quad\ CO_2H$

(b)

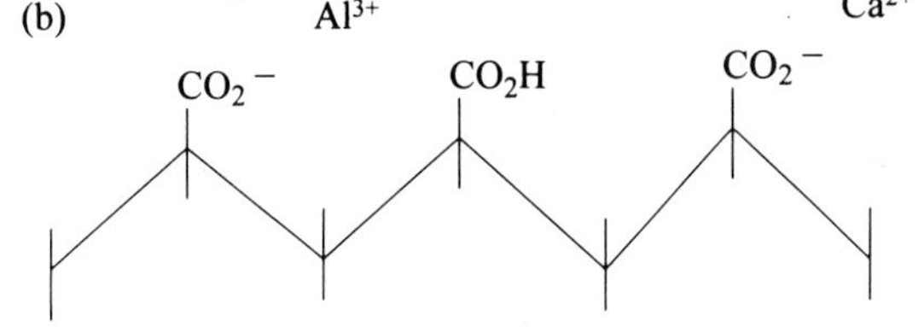

Fig. 24.1 Structural formula of (a) polyacrylic acid and (b) its cross-linking through calcium and aluminium ions.

water the acid slowly degrades the outer layers of the glass particles releasing Ca^{2+} and Al^{3+} ions. During the early stages of setting, Ca^{2+} is released more rapidly and is primarily responsible for reacting with the polyacid to form a reaction product akin to that shown in Fig. 24.1. Al^{3+} is released more slowly and becomes involved in setting at a later stage, often referred to as a secondary reaction stage. The set material consists of unreacted glass cores embedded in matrix of cross-linked polyacid. The stages of setting are illustrated in Fig. 24.2. The matrix region is composed of the salt reaction product shown in Fig. 24.1b. The second stage of the setting reaction involves the incorporation of significant quantities of aluminium in the matrix structure and results in a marked maturation of the physical properties of the material. Prior to this stage, the materials remain very weak and soluble. In order to ensure that the reaction proceeds to full maturity it is essential that the setting cement is protected from excessive moisture contamination since the presence of disproportionate quantities of water at this stage can interfere with salt formation.

The presence of tartaric acid plays a significant part in controlling the setting characteristics of the material. It helps to break down the surface layers of the glass particles, rapidly liberating aluminium ions with which it undergoes complex formation. Hence the aluminium ions are not immediately available for reaction with the polyacid so the working time of the cement is maintained. The initial onset of setting is further inhibited by the tartaric acid preventing unwinding and ionization of the polyacid chains. When the concentration of solubilized aluminium reaches a certain level the second stage of the setting reaction proceeds rapidly. The tartaric acid aids complex formation between the polyacid and the trivalent aluminium ions by overcoming steric hindrance problems which may occur when an aluminium ion attempts salt formation with three carboxylic acid groups. Hence many of the aluminium salt links consist of an aluminium ion bound to two carboxylate groups and one tartrate group. This mechanism is supported by the fact that there is very little unbound tartaric acid left in the set cement. The release of fluoride ions from the glass particles results in the matrix phase of the set material becoming a reservoir for fluoride. After setting the matrix is able to release this fluoride into the surrounding environment or to absorb fluoride from the surroundings when the ambient fluoride concentration is high (e.g. from a fluoride containing toothpaste). In addition to the potential therapeutic effects of the fluoride concentrated in the matrix

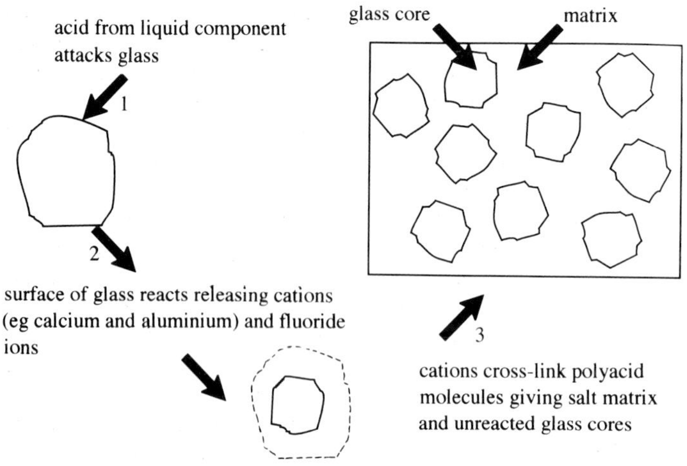

acid from liquid component
attacks glass

surface of glass reacts releasing cations
(eg calcium and aluminium) and fluoride
ions

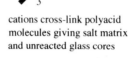

cations cross-link polyacid
molecules giving salt matrix
and unreacted glass cores

Fig. 24.2 Diagrammatic illustration of the setting of glass ionomer cement.

phase, its presence is also thought to contribute towards optimizing the setting characteristics by maintaining workability for a longer period followed by a relatively sharp increase in viscosity.

24.4 Properties

Some of the property requirements of glass ionomer cements are embodied in the ISO Standard for dental water-based cements (ISO 9917). These requirements are given in Table 24.2 along with those for the glass ionomer luting materials and cavity lining/base materials. Since glass ionomers and composites may be considered for similar applications – both being tooth coloured restorative materials – their properties are compared qualitatively in Table 25.1.

Like many dental cements the properties of glass ionomers are critically dependent upon the powder/liquid ratio. Unfortunately hand mixing at optimal powder/liquid ratios may result in a dry and apparently crumbly mix which dentists do not like. Hence

there is a tendency for dentists to add too much liquid to give a wetter consistency with a deleterious effect on the physical properties of the material. This problem is surmounted by the use of encapsulation and mechanical mixing.

The powder/liquid ratio should be high in order to optimize strength and solubility, but there should be sufficient free polyacid available to form a bond with tooth substance. The materials are often difficult to mix at the ratios recommended (typically around 3:1 by weight). The powder/water materials tend to be easier to handle than the powder/liquid products. Aqueous solutions of polyacids should not be stored in a refrigerator since this may initiate crystallization. The variability of material properties with powder/liquid ratio and the difficulties of mixing by hand suggest there are definite advantages to be gained by using the materials in encapsulated form. Here the proportions are fixed by the manufacturer and mixing takes only a few seconds in an electrically-powered mixer of the type available in most dental surgeries.

Table 24.2 Requirements of glass ionomer cements as outlined in ISO 9917.

Property	Restorative cement	Luting cement	Lining/base cement
Film thickness* (μm)	—	25 max	—
Setting time (min)			
minimum	2	2.5	2
maximum	6	8	6
Compressive strength (MPa)	130 (min)	70 (min)	70 (min)
Acid erosion (mm/h)	0.05 (max)	0.05 (max)	0.05 (max)

* No requirement for restorative or lining/base cements.

The setting reaction is rather protracted despite a fairly rapid initial hardening. The material must be protected from moisture contamination during the first hour, otherwise strength and solubility are adversely affected. Hence it is necessary to varnish the surface of the filling immediately after initial hardening. The varnishes used consist of a water resistant resin dissolved in a volatile solvent such as ether or ethylacetate. These varnishes can be expected to afford protection to the glass ionomer for a variable period of time, from a few seconds to an hour or more depending on how quickly they become dislodged. A more long-term protective effect can be achieved by using a resin-bonding agent or fissure sealant of the type described in Chapter 23.

One of the most important properties of these materials is their ability to adhere to both enamel and dentine, although the precise mechanism of bonding is still somewhat unclear. One theory is that polyacid molecules chelate with calcium at the tooth surface (Fig. 24.3). Support for this mechanism stems from the fact that the formation of the interfacial calcium polyalkenoate salt would involve a reaction similar to that thought to occur during the setting of the cement. Also, the significantly greater bond strength achieved with enamel than with dentine suggests that it is the calcium of tooth substance which is involved in bond formation. Another theory is that the outer layers of the apatite on the tooth surface become solubilized in the presence of acid. As more apatite dissolves and as the cement begins to set the pH begins to rise. This may cause reprecipitation of a complex mixture of calcium phosphate (from the apatite) and calcium salts of the polyacid onto the tooth surface. Thus the polyacid chains would be bound to a reprecipitated layer on the tooth surface. This mechanism could operate on enamel or dentine surfaces and could thus also be supported by bond strength data. It has been suggested that in the case of dentine there may also be some bonding between carboxylic acid groups of the cement and reactive groups within collagen, either by hydrogen bonding or by metallic ion bridging.

Various surface treatments have been used in an attempt to improve the strength and reliability of the bond between glass ionomer cements and dentine. One feature of dentine is the presence of a smear layer, as mentioned in Chapter 23. Many suggested surface treatments attempt to remove the smear layer or dissolve and reprecipitate it in order to give better binding to the underlying dentine. Citric acid solutions have been advocated for 'cavity cleansing' and their use will almost certainly lead to the disruption of the smear layer. The use of citric acid produces no improvement in bond strength however, probably due to the fact that the dentine surface is partially demineralized and starved of calcium required for bond formation. Treatment of the surface with a solution of polyacrylic acid has been found to be more effective in improving bond strengths. The mode of action is unclear but probably involves dissolution and reprecipitation of the smear layer. Another attempt to improve bond strengths to dentine involved artificially increasing the mineral content of the dentine surface by applying solutions from which calcium phosphate or calcium sulphate could crystallize to give a surface layer which is potentially more reactive towards polyacids.

There are limits to which the bond strength of glass ionomer cements to tooth substance can be improved. The tensile strength of the cement itself is only around 12 MPa and during tensile bond strength testing with enamel failure often occurs cohesively within the cement at a stress of around 5 MPa. This suggests that there is a zone of stress concentration within the cement which is set up as a result of bonding to the tooth. Hence it would appear that there is only limited scope for improving the bond strength of the cements to dentine (normally measured at around 1–3 MPa). Certainly there seems little scope for increasing the bond strength to values approaching that for resins to acid-etched enamel (16–20 MPa).

Most authorities consider glass ionomers to have acceptable biocompatibility despite their acidic nature. Attitudes towards the tolerance of acids by the dental pulp are changing rapidly as outlined in Chapter 23. However, the cements based on polyacids have traditionally been considered less harmful than those based on phosphoric acid for two reasons. First, the acids used are weaker acids than phosphoric acid. Second, the polyacid chains are large and immobile, their mobility being further restricted by their affinity for calcium ions in the tooth to which the material is applied. Pulpal studies indicate that glass ionomer cements cause a mild inflammatory

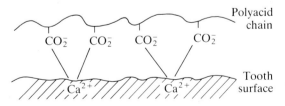

Fig. 24.3 Diagram illustrating one possible mechanism of bonding to tooth substance for glass ionomer cements.

response which is normally resolved within 30 days. The response is moderated according to the thickness of residual dentine. Only in very deep cavities having a thin residual layer of dentine is it considered necessary to use a cavity lining. In these cases, the lining of choice is normally one of the calcium hydroxide materials. The amount of calcium hydroxide material used is limited to that required to just cover any dentine which is considered close to the pulp. Covering large areas of the dentine with calcium hydroxide cement would negate any beneficial effect which could be gained by creating adhesion between the glass ionomer and dentine. These views will almost certainly be modified as a greater understanding of acid tolerance by the pulp is obtained.

The raw materials from which the glasses used in the products are derived sometimes contain small quantities of arsenic and lead. In appreciation of the potential harmful effects of such heavy metals the ISO Standard allows only 2 parts per million of acid soluble arsenic and 100 parts per million of acid soluble lead in the cements.

The thermal diffusivity value for glass ionomer cements is close to that for dentine. Hence the material has an adequate thermal insulating effect on the pulp and helps to protect it from thermal trauma. Although the setting reaction for the materials is exothermic it is considered that the temperature rise created for an average sized cavity (about 2–5°C) would not be great enough to cause serious damage. The value of the coefficient of thermal expansion for glass ionomer cements (13–16 ppm $°C^{-1}$) is quite a close match to the value recorded for tooth substance (8–11 ppm $°C^{-1}$). This, coupled with adhesion to enamel and dentine, helps to prevent invasion of the pulp by microleakage.

The matrix phase of a set glass ionomer cement contains significant amounts of fluoride ions which are fairly mobile since they are not involved in salt formation. The mobile fluoride ions readily diffuse to the surface of the cement where they may be washed away with saliva or undergo reactions with the surrounding tooth substance. Fluoride ions may replace hydroxy groups in the apatite structure and this change renders the apatite more resistant to acid attack. The presence of glass ionomer cements is likely therefore to reduce the chance of caries developing in the surrounding tooth substance. The cement can be considered as applying a long term topical fluoridation effect on the tooth substance with which it is in contact.

As stated earlier, not only can the matrix phase of the cement gradually release fluoride but it can also absorb fluoride from an aqueous medium which has a high fluoride concentration. Hence the level of fluoride in the cement can be 'topped up' as it absorbs ions released from toothpastes, mouthwashes, and drinking water. The amount of fluoride release required in order to give a beneficial therapeutic effect is not known – a fact which makes product optimization difficult. Also, in the UK, manufacturers rarely claim a therapeutic effect for glass-ionomer products, for to do so *may* result in the materials being classified as pharmaceutical products.

The glass ionomers are relatively brittle, having a flexural strength of only 15–20 MPa (cf >70 MPa for composites), and cannot be considered suitable as general-purpose filling materials for permanent teeth but more to answer a specific need for certain applications. The brittleness of the material, for example, would preclude the use of these products for restoring fractured incisal edges. Cavity designs for glass ionomer restorations should ideally avoid the production of thin sections of the material such as would occur in a filling with a knife-edge margin.

The tests required in the ISO Standard are unable to predict these problems as only compressive strength is measured (Table 24.2). Brittle materials often have relatively high values of compressive strength, but fail at much lower stress in tension or when subjected to a flexural stress. The difference between the compressive strength value for restorative cements (130 MPa minimum) and luting or lining/base cements (70 MPa minimum) is mostly due to the different powder/liquid ratios used. Whereas a ratio of about 3:1 by weight is normal for a restorative cement the ratio for luting and lining/base cements is closer to 1.5:1. This marked effect of powder/liquid ratio on mechanical properties highlights the need to achieve the ratio recommended by the manufacturer.

The glass ionomers have relatively poor abrasion resistance which results not only in a change of anatomical form but also in considerable surface roughening. Roughening may also be caused by polishing, leaving hard glass cores protruding from the softer matrix material.

Glass ionomers, like their close relatives the silicates, are susceptible to acid erosion. This is an inherent property in materials which are effectively inorganic salts formed by an acid–base reaction. Factors which affect the rate of erosion include the pH of the eroding medium (e.g. saliva, plaque or drinks) and the maturity of the cement at the time it contacts the acid. The worst possible conditions are when a freshly placed cement is bathed in a highly acidic fluid such as fruit juice. To reduce the risk of acid erosion it is essential that cements are protected with varnish or resin during setting. The situation is further improved if the material has a short setting time. Also, the cement should be used at the correct powder/liquid ratio, which is pre-set in the case of encapsulated materials.

In the ISO Standard (ISO 9917) the resistance to acid erosion is determined using the *jet test*. This involves preparing a sample of the cement in a mould with one surface of the cement exposed and then subjecting this surface of the cement to an impinging jet of aqueous lactic acid solution at a pH of 2.7. The standard requires that less than 0.05 mm of material be lost per hour (Table 24.2)

In terms of appearance, glass ionomers offer a reasonable match for the natural tooth, particularly to dentine, although most authorities agree that a better match is achieved with resin matrix composites. The translucency of the restorative cements is achieved through the presence of unreacted glass cores which are able to transmit light. Attempts to improve the properties of glass ionomers have involved changes to the composition of the glass in order to enhance reactivity with the acid component. These attempts are often frustrated by the fact that altering the reactivity of the glass may also result in an unacceptable change in the translucency. Nevertheless, the aesthetic nature of the materials, although not perfect, has improved significantly since the time when the materials were first introduced.

The conventional glass ionomer restorative cements lack radiopacity and cannot readily be detected using dental radiographic techniques. The diagnosis of caries around glass ionomer restorations can therefore prove difficult. The low radiopacity of the cements is due to the presence of metallic ions having relatively low atomic numbers and therefore having relatively few electrons capable of absorbing X-rays. The incorporation of metals of greater atomic number either in metallic form (e.g. silver) or oxide form (e.g. barium oxide) can be used to impart radiopacity but with a significant loss of translucency and colour match. This may not be acceptable for many restorative applications but may be perfectly acceptable for applications in which the appearance of the cement is of little consequence – e.g. cavity linings (Chapter 27) or core build up. There is one commercially available restorative material which exhibits some radiopacity.

24.5 Cermets

Cermets are essentially metal-reinforced, glass ionomer cements. The metal used in the commercially available material is silver, although many other metals such as tin, gold, titanium and palladium have been tried. The cermet powder is manufactured by mixing and then pelletizing under pressure a mixture of glass and metal powder. The pellets are fused at around 800°C, then ground to a fine powder. The powder particles consist of regions of metal firmly bonded to the glass. A closely related material consists of a blend of an aluminosilicate glass and an amalgam alloy powder containing silver and tin. In this product there is no attempt to bind the glass and alloy phases together. The setting reaction for the cermet material is identical to that for other glass ionomers. Because of the presence of metallic phases within the materials they tend to be grey in colour and are therefore unsuitable for use as aesthetic restorations. Attempts have been made to improve appearance using pigments although the opacity cannot be reduced. In one respect the poor appearance has been used to advantage since the manufacturers are able to use a more reactive glass (which would spoil the appearance of a conventional cement) in order to produce a faster setting material. The presence of silver also imparts a degree of radiopacity to cermet materials which is not present in conventional glass ionomers.

The cermets were developed in the hope that the dispersed phase of a relatively tough, ductile metal within the material may have a significant effect on some mechanical properties, particularly brittleness and abrasion resistance, whilst maintaining adhesion to enamel and dentine. The materials appear to have a greater value of compressive strength and fatigue limit than conventional glass ionomers. However, flexural strength and resistance to abrasive wear appear to be no better than values recorded for conventional glass ionomers. The rapid setting which occurs with these materials is probably responsible for their marked improvement in erosion resistance when compared with most other glass ionomers.

The cermets based on silver have been shown to have a much lower fluoride release rate than equivalent conventional glass ionomers. This is probably due to the fact that the acid–base setting reaction, which releases fluoride into the cement matrix, occurs quickly but less extensively in the cermets since part of the glass is replaced by metal.

24.6 Applications and clinical handling notes

The major applications of the glass ionomer filling materials reflect the advantage of their adhesive nature coupled with an inherent brittleness and a less than perfect aesthetic quality. They are widely used to restore loss of tooth structure from the roots of teeth either as a consequence of decay or the so-called cervical abrasion cavity. Both of these lesions tend to occur close to the gingival margins of teeth. Root caries tends to spread laterally across the root as well as centrally towards the pulp. Once it has been removed the resultant cavities tend to be broad and shallow. *Abrasion cavities* were once thought to be the product of over zealous tooth brushing, possibly in association with the use of an abrasive dentifrice. It is now recognized that both dietary factors and functional loading of teeth (causing the teeth to bend) can be co-factors in their aetiology. The morphology of such lesions is variable: some are relatively dish-shaped and shallow whilst others are more v-shaped and tend to be deeper. In both cases the tooth surface is likely to be caries free and highly burnished.

Cavities for glass ionomer cements should be of sufficient depth at their margins to give adequate bulk to the restorative material. A knife-edge finish is not suitable and hence both abrasion and carious cavities may need to be modified to give a butt joint margin of 0.75 mm depth or greater.

The use of glass ionomers for restoring class III cavities has been advocated. The early materials were far from ideal, being more opaque than either silicates or composites. Newer products are more satisfactory and are now sometimes used for this type of cavity.

Glass ionomer cements are gaining wide acceptance as filling materials for *deciduous teeth*, often being used in preference to amalgam in deciduous molars. They allow the trauma of cavity preparation to be reduced to a minimum and, although they are probably not durable enough to withstand forces of mastication in adults, they are probably adequate for the limited life of deciduous teeth.

Some new restorative techniques offer alternatives to traditional class I and class II cavities in posterior teeth in adults. Cavity preparation takes the form of a tunnel with its origin either from the occlusal surface a short distance away from the marginal ridge or from the buccal aspect. The tunnel leads into the area of carious dentine which is removed using rotary and hand instruments. An injectable glass ionomer cement is then inserted into the cavity with an appropriate matrix as required. The principal advantage of this approach is maintenance of the marginal ridge of the tooth. The clinical manipulation of glass ionomer cements should be designed to maximize their clinical acceptability whilst doing minimal damage to the set material. One of the key issues is to take care to maintain an appropriate level of hydration of the material's exposed surface.

Dentine surface treatment

Glass ionomer cements are frequently placed in non-undercut cavities, with reliance being placed upon their adhesive characteristics to ensure their retention. Dentine surfaces that are burnished (e.g. those from cervical wear lesions that have not been mechanically prepared) and both dentine and enamel surfaces that are contaminated with saliva are not receptive to bond formation. Even transient wetting with saliva during cavity preparation will inhibit good bond formation. These surfaces should be prepared to remove the precipitated salivary protein and/or the eburnated dentine surface. A variety of agents have been used for this purpose, including citric acid. However, the most effective agent seems to be 10–15% poly(acrylic) acid. This is applied to the tooth surface for 30 seconds then washed off and the tooth dried, but not dessicated, to achieve a receptive surface for bonding.

Matrix techniques

Generally, glass ionomer cements are used to restore proximal cavities on anterior teeth and defects on root surfaces, whether the product of wear or decay. The matrix technique for proximal cavities on anterior teeth is very similar to that for composites, using transparent flexible film made from either cellulose acetate or polyester. The matrix is inserted between the teeth adjacent to the prepared cavity usually before any dentine surface conditioning. Once the material has been placed in the cavity to slight excess, the matrix is drawn round the tooth root and held in place using firm digital pressure until the material sets.

The problems of adapting preformed, curved matrixes to teeth for cervical cavities have already been mentioned. An alternative that is available for these chemically-setting materials is an aluminium cervical matrix . These are malleable at room temperature and hence can be pressure formed around the root face of the tooth using hand instruments giving a *custom* matrix for each tooth. This is particularly useful where a cervical cavity extends into the junction between the roots of molar teeth. The cavity margin in this area will be concave towards the furcation. This form of malleable matrix offers the only possibility of achieving a reasonable contour of the restoration with a matrix rather than by post placement finishing. The matrix is adapted to the tooth surface at the completion of cavity preparation. It is then set to one side, and the dentine prepared for bonding and the material placed in the cavity to slight excess. The matrix is then replaced, taking care to ensure that the gingival portion of the matrix is lying on the outside of the tooth, not sitting on the cervical floor of the cavity (Fig. 24.4). These relatively rigid metal foils are very good for insertion into the gingival crevice to help to form the restoration in that area but care must be taken to ensure that the inferior portion of the matrix does not get caught on the gingival floor of the cavity. If this happens then a negative ledge will be formed, i.e. the tooth will be wider than the restoration. It can be helpful to control the position of the gingival tissues using an appropriate retraction cord or by *troughing* the gingival crevice using an electrosurgery unit to assist with this process.

The matrix should be left undisturbed until the material has set fully and can then be removed carefully using a sharp probe or an excavator. Matrix techniques for tunnel preparation require a thin metal strip to be passed between the teeth and then adapted to conform to the tooth using wedges.

Finishing and polishing

Glass ionomer cements are water-based and hence are highly susceptible to either desiccation or excessive moisture contamination during the early phase of their setting reaction. They achieve a *clinical* set part way through the chemical process of cement formation. Maturation continues for at least an hour and, with some materials, up to 24 hours.

The surface of the cement should be protected during that time period.

A variety of materials have been suggested for moisture protection – from cocoa butter through copal-ether and resin varnishes to unfilled methacrylate-based resins. This latter group is by far the most effective at delaying water flow into and out from the cement. The unfilled resin should be applied to the surface of the cement as soon as the matrix is removed. Light-activated resins are easiest to use for this purpose because of their command set after placement. Any finishing that is required will remove this protected layer; consequently early finishing should be confined to removal of gross excess alone (this can usually be avoided with careful matrix placement). If gross excess is present it should be removed either with a sharp-bladed hand instrument or, if necessary, a bur in a hand piece. It is best to use steel burs in slow hand pieces lubricated with petroleum jelly for this purpose. Water cooling should be avoided. As soon as the gross excess has been eliminated the finishing procedures should stop and a protective layer of resin or varnish should be re-applied to the surface of the material.

Once the material is fully mature any final finishing that is required can be undertaken. This is achieved using the same range of burs, strips, discs and abrasive points that are used for composites. However, care should be taken to avoid excessive heating of the cement if at all possible. All abrasives should be lubricated with petroleum jelly if water cooling is not being used.

Whilst GICs are not as susceptible to desiccation once setting is complete, it is sensible to coat a GIC

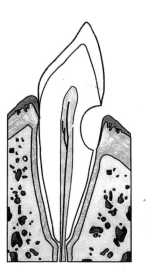
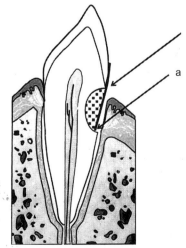

Fig. 24.4 Adaptation of a matrix for a cavity with subgingival margins can be complicated by negative ledge formation. The left-hand diagram illustrates a large cavity on the root face of a tooth, extending beneath the gingival margin. When a matrix is adapted to that cavity (b) it is important to ensure that it extends beyond the gingival extent of the cavity, otherwise a negative ledge will be formed (a).

restoration with a protective layer of resin-based varnish or unfilled bonding resin if restorations are likely to be subject to a desiccating environment for a protracted period, e.g. if a tooth containing a GIC restoration is isolated using rubber dam during a restorative procedure or endodontic care elsewhere in the mouth.

Moisture control during placement

There is a dichotomy between the use of the best moisture control techniques (isolation with rubber dam) and the risk of desiccation of the restoration if a rubber dam is used. It is usually adequate to isolate a tooth carefully using cotton rolls or *dry guards* during the placement of GIC restorations. Obviously, great care is required to avoid contamination of a prepared cavity with saliva prior to placing the cement as the salivary pellicle will interfere with bonding. Salivary pellicle can be removed by treating the dentine with poly(acrylic) acid for 15 seconds.

Use as fissure sealants

Another suggested use of glass ionomers is as *fissure sealants*. The material is mixed to a more fluid consistency to allow flow into the depths of the pits and fissures of posterior teeth. Early cements were found to be unsuitable as fissure sealants if the fissures were less than 100 μm wide. The large glass particles of the cement prevented adequate penetration of the fissure pattern and it was necessary to consider enlargement of the fissures with a bur. Luting cements (Chapter 30) having much smaller glass particles may be a more sensible choice of material for this application. Studies show that whilst the retention of glass ionomer fissure sealants generally does not compare favourably with the resin types (see Chapter 23), their caries inhibiting effect is significant. This has been attributed to the presence of fluoride within the cement and its ability to change the composition of the enamel with which it comes into contact.

GICs as an adhesive cavity lining (the sandwich technique)

GICs have a number of advantages as a cavity lining as they bond to dentine and release fluoride which may help to reduce recurrent decay. They can be used beneath either a composite resin or an amalgam.

The so called *sandwich technique* involves using a GIC as a dentine replacement and a composite to replace enamel (Fig. 24.5). The purpose designed lining materials set quickly and can be made receptive for the bonding of composite resin simply by washing the material surface if the material is freshly placed (excess water results in some of the GIC matrix being washed out from around the filler particles giving a microscopically rough surface to which the composite will attach in an analogous manner to etched enamel). This surface should be coated with either an unfilled resin or a DBA to optimize attachment. It is only necessary to etch a GIC with acid if the restoration has been in place for some time and has fully matured.

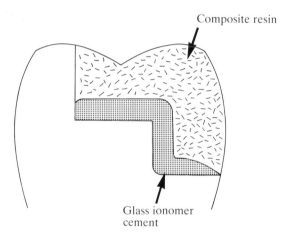

Composite resin

Glass ionomer cement

Fig. 24.5 Diagram illustrating the use of composite and glass ionomer cement for the restoration of a class II cavity – the sandwich technique. This combines the adhesive characteristics of glass ionomer cements with the better durability of composites.

The sandwich technique has a number of attractions, but it should be undertaken as a planned procedure rather than as a method to improve the appearance of an unsatisfactory GIC restoration. The principal reason for this is that most restorative-grade GICs are radiolucent; if these are cut back and a radiopaque composite placed over the top then the radiographic appearance is indistinguishable from recurrent decay beneath a restoration. This unfortunate coincidence could result in an otherwise perfectly satisfactory restoration being replaced. The purpose designed GIC base materials are radiopaque, alleviating this problem. Conversely these lining materials are not designed to survive exposed in the oral environment so should not be brought to the surface of the tooth even at a dentine interface.

ART

ART (the atraumatic restorative technique) is a method of caries management developed primarily for use in the Third World where skilled dental manpower and facilities are limited and the population need is high. The technique uses simple hand instruments (chisels and excavators) to break through the enamel and remove as much caries as possible. The cavity is isolated using cotton rolls. When excavation of caries is complete (or as complete as can be achieved) the residual cavity is restored using a modified GIC. These GICs are reinforced to give increased strength under functional loads and are radiopaque. Their aesthetic properties are poorer with the materials being optically opaque.

24.7 Suggested further reading

Knibbs P.J. (1988) Glass ionomer cement: 10 years of clinical use. *J. Oral Rehabil.* **15**, 103.

McLean, J.W. (1992) The clinical use of glass-ionomer cements. *Dent. Clin. North Am.* **36**, 693.

Walls, A.W.G. (1986) Glass polyalkenoate (glass-ionomer) cements: a review. *J Dent* **14**, 231.

Chapter 25

Resin-modified Glass Ionomers and Related Materials

25.1 Introduction

In the previous chapters we have considered two of the most important groups of tooth-coloured restorative materials – the composites and glass ionomers. Both products have advantages and disadvantages which are summarized in Table 25.1. The properties of these materials dictate that no single material from either group is suitable for all applications and that materials selection requires a decision on the part of the dentist which takes account of the limitations of the products. It was recognized that if it were possible to combine the characteristics of the two types of product it may be possible to produce a *hybrid* material which possesses the most advantageous properties of both materials whilst at the same time overcoming some of the disadvantages. Early attempts at producing hybrid products involved blending together components of commercially available glass ionomer and composite materials to produce a material which, though not viable as a clinically usable product, demonstrated

Table 25.1 Summary of the advantages and disadvantages of composites and glass ionomers.

Material	Advantages	Disadvantages
Composite	Strong Tough Insoluble Radiopaque Quick setting	No inherent adhesion Shrinkage No fluoride release
Glass ionomer	Inherent adhesion Little shrinkage Fluoride release Biocompatible	Brittle Soluble Not radiopaque Wear Water sensitive Slow setting

the possibility of combining two apparently dissimilar materials. Further research and development has led to a large new family of materials which are diverse in nature but which have a composition which lies somewhere on the continuum between resin–matrix type composites and acid–base reaction type cements. At the one extreme of the continuum they can be viewed as composite materials in which a modified resin and a reactive glass have been used. At the other extreme they can be viewed as acid–base cement matrix products with added resin.

25.2 Composition and classification

There has been considerable controversy over the terminology used to describe materials which fall into the categories lying between composites and glass ionomers. An ISO Standard (ISO 9917-2) for light-activated water-based cements describes the products as water-based and setting by multiple reactions which include an acid-base reaction and polymerization. An attempt has been made to further sub-divide products in these categories into *modified composites* and *resin-modified glass ionomers* (Table 25.2).

Modified composites. Some products are essentially resin–matrix composites in which the usual insert filler has been replaced by an ion-leachable aluminosilicate glass in order to encourage fluoride release. No acid–base reaction takes place during the setting of these materials. Setting is through free radical polymerization of methacrylate groups (often light-activated). In some materials the resin, in addition to the normal dimethacrylate components, also contains acidic (normally alkenoic) groups in order to generate the possibility of an acid–base reaction with the glass component. These products are often referred to as *acid-modified composites*. The term *compomer* has also been used to describe

Table 25.2 Summary of the nature of the available materials.

Material	Number of components	Require mixing	Active ingredients
Modified composites	1 or 2	2 components – yes 1 component – no (compomers)	Fluoroalumino silicate glass Methacrylate resin* (acid modified) Activators/initiators/stabilizers
Resin-modified glass ionomers	2 or 3	Yes	Fluoroaluminosilicate glass Methacrylate polyacid Hydroxyethylmethacrylate (HEMA) Water Activators/initiators/stabilizers

*Acid-modified products referred to as *acid-modified composites*.

these products. The primary setting reaction is still through polymerization of methacrylate groups in the resin component. The acid part of the modified resin is unable to enter into an acid–base reaction with the glass due to the absence of water from any of the material components. Indeed, the most widely used materials from this category are supplied pre-mixed in small single dose syringes. Since the modified resin and glass are pre-mixed and stored in the syringe before use, the exclusion of water is essential in order to prevent premature setting. This is normally achieved by packaging each small syringe in a waterproof foil container. Following setting through polymerization it is thought that some acid–base reaction can occur as the resin takes up water and the acid groups become ionized. This process may enable the surface of the glass particles to react in order to liberate fluoride.

Resin-modified glass ionomers. These products are considered by some authorities to be more truly based on a hybrid of the two parent groups of materials. In their simplest form they consist of a powder and liquid which require mixing prior to activation of polymerization (often by light activation). The most convenient of the restorative type resin-modified glass ionomers are provided in an encapsulated form in which the powder/liquid ratio is determined by the manufacturer and the mixing is carried out mechanically in only a few seconds. The powder consists primarily of an ion-leachable glass whilst the liquid contains four main ingredients:

(1) A methacrylate resin which enables setting to occur by polymerization.
(2) A polyacid which reacts with the ion-leachable glass to bring about setting by an acid–base mechanism.
(3) Hydroxyethylmethacrylate (HEMA), a hydro-

philic methacrylate which enables both the resin and acid components to co-exist in aqueous solution; the HEMA also takes part in the polymerization reaction.
(4) Water, which is an essential component required to allow ionization of the acid component so that the acid–base reaction can occur.

Other minor components include polymerization activators and stabilizers. Some products are simply formulated by blending together polyacids and dimethacrylates in aqueous solution. Most products, however, contain specially formulated resins in which both methacrylate and acid groups are present as active groups on a single polymer chain. This can be achieved, for example, as illustrated in Fig. 25.1, where some of the acid groups on the polyacrylic

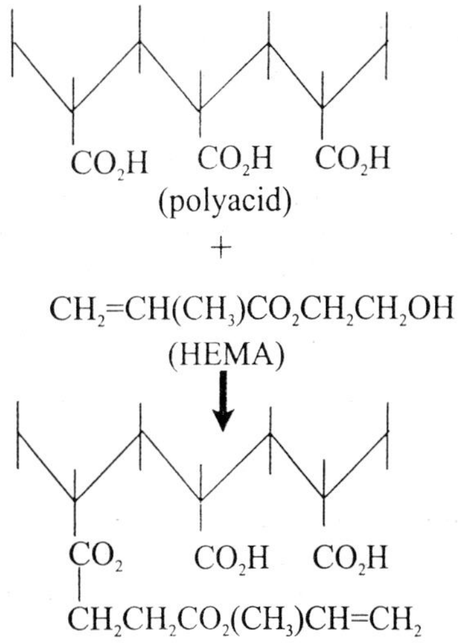

CO_2H CO_2H CO_2H
(polyacid)
+
$CH_2=CH(CH_3)CO_2CH_2CH_2OH$
(HEMA)

CO_2 CO_2H CO_2H
$CH_2CH_2CO_2(CH_3)CH=CH_2$

Fig. 25.1 Formation of a resin-modified polyacid chain by esterification of some acid groups with HEMA.

acid molecule are replaced with methacrylate groups by carrying out an esterfication with HEMA.

When the powder and liquid components of the cement are mixed together the acid–base reaction can begin immediately as the acid groups are able to react with the glass in the presence of water. Polymerization takes over as the primary setting reaction as soon as sufficient free radicals become available to initiate the reaction. For light-activated products this corresponds to the time at which light irradiation occurs. The light source used to activate polymerization is of the same type as that used for light activated composites (see Chapter 23). Polymerization involves the pendant methacrylate groups of the modified resin (as shown in Fig. 25.1) along with any free HEMA present in the liquid components. Most resin-modified glass ionomers contain activators which enable polymerization to occur both in the presence or absence of the activating radiation. Where the chemically activated polymerization plays an important part, the presence of three setting mechanisms may be claimed by the manufacturer:

(1) Acid-base setting;
(2) Light-activated polymerization;
(3) Chemically-activated polymerization.

The latter is sometimes described as a *dark cure*, but in essence it is similar to the chemically activated setting achieved with conventional two-component composites. In one product, mixing releases a previously microencapsulated persulphate/ascorbic acid redox catalyst system which activates polymerization in the absence of light.

The glass components of both modified composites and resin-modified glass ionomers have been modified in most materials in order to incorporate a heavy metal (e.g. strontium) which imparts radiopacity.

25.3 Setting characteristics

Although the resin-modified glass ionomers used for restorative applications are all light activated many do not possess the long working times associated with light-activated composites. There are three possible explanations for this behaviour. First, the acid–base reaction proceeds immediately after mixing and before exposure to activating light. Second, many materials contain chemical activators and initiators which enable a chemically-activated polymerization to proceed before exposure to activating light. Third, some materials are very sensitive to ambient visible light. Sensitivity to ambient light is tested as part of the ISO test for these materials (ISO 9917-2). The sensitive nature of the materials is identified by the fact that the material is required to remain homogenous for only 30 seconds when exposed to ambient light equivalent to that which would be found in the dental surgery.

In order to achieve acceptable results with these products it is best to carry out placement and shaping as soon as possible after mixing. Many encapsulated materials are provided with extrusion nozzles which allow the mixed material to be extruded directly from the capsule into the prepared cavity. The modified composite products have setting characterics similar to those for light-activated composites. In Chapter 22 the 'limited depth of cure' for light-activated composites was listed as one of the potential disadvantages of those materials. The resin-modified glass ionomers exhibit a similar behaviour except that unexposed material may set through an acid–base reaction or through a chemically-activated polymerization. Nevertheless, only the material properly activated by light will be optimally cured. The concept of 'depth of cure' can therefore be applied to these materials. The modified composites exhibit a similar behaviour to other composites. The setting reaction in all cases is highly exothermic and a temperature rise of 10°C above ambient can be readily produced in a medium sized cavity. An important feature of conventional glass ionomer products is their sensitivity to moisture contamination during and shortly after setting. Although the resin-modified glass ionomers contain water and set partly through an acid–base reaction, the presence of resin appears to protect the cement from the effects of contamination by moisture. Hence, protection with varnish or a resin is not advocated for most materials within this category. Another significant factor is that whereas finishing of conventional glass ionomers is best delayed for 24 hours to allow maturation of the cement, the light-activated resin-modified materials can be finished immediately after curing.

25.4 Dimensional change and dimensional stability

All categories of materials discussed in this chapter undergo a significant shrinkage on setting. The major component of the shrinkage is due to the polymerization of methacrylate groups in the resin component. Acid–base setting makes a minor contribution to the observed shrinkage. The magnitude of the shrinkage is similar to that observed for resin–matrix composites (Chapter 22) and the same arguments about shrinkage stress, cavity size and configuration factor apply.

The resin-modified glass ionomers undergo a rapid and marked expansion when placed in water. This more than compensates for the shrinkage and can result in the material protruding from the cavity and exerting a positive pressure against the cavity walls. This observation can be explained by a value of water absorption after 7 days of 100–250 μg mm^{-3} compared with a maximum of 40 μg mm^{-3} allowed for resin-based materials in ISO 4049. The large value of water absorption for the resin-modified materials is due to the use of the hydrophilic monomer, HEMA, as a primary constituent in these products. The clinical significance of the observed swelling is yet to be fully explained. Swelling does not occur to the same extent with modified composites as these products generally do not contain HEMA.

25.5 Mechanical properties

The flexural strength values for a range of resin-modified glass ionomers and modified composites are given in Table 25.3 along with the minimum values required in the ISO Standards. It is clear that whereas some of the weaker resin-modified glass ionomers are only marginally stronger than the conventional glass ionomer products (Chapter 24), some of the single component acid-modified composites have a strength value which clearly satisfies the requirement if ISO 4949 for resin-based materials. The latter products compare favourably with composites (Table 22.3). The values given in Table 25.3 support the hypothesis that the materials have a structure/property characteristic which would place them somewhere on a continuum which connects the purely acid–base reaction materials at one extreme and the purely resin–matrix products at the other. In general terms, incorporating increasing amounts of resin in a glass-ionomer system does seem to have the effect of strengthening and toughening these otherwise brittle materials. There is some evidence that the resin-modified glass ionomers become weaker after a period of water storage. This may be expected in light of the large water absorption values for these materials. The modified composites appear to be relatively unaffected by water storage.

25.6 Adhesive characteristics

Some of the products within the resin-modified glass ionomer groups give an inherent adhesion to enamel and dentine by a mechanism which is similar to that for conventional glass ionomers (Chapter 24). Free polyacid groups are thought to interact with the mineral of the tooth surface. When no conditioning or etching is used shear bond strengths of 4–10 MPa to both enamel and dentine are claimed for some products. Improvements in bond strength are obtained when the enamel and/or dentine are etched or conditioned and most manufacturers advocate the use of a conditioner such as aqueous polyacrylic acid in order to remove the dentine smear layer. Other manufacturers advocate conditioning and priming of dentine and enamel prior to placement of the restorative material. The primer may be a solution of the methacrylated polyacid (one of the major ingredients of the liquid component of the cement), which is able to partly demineralize the surface of the hard tissue and leave a surface which is more readily wetted by the restorative. The use of conditioning and priming can increase the shear bond strength into the range 8–24 MPa.

It is clear from the previous discussion that some

Table 25.3 Flexural strength (at 24 hours) of resin-modified glass ionomers and modified composites compared with the requirements of ISO 9917-2 and ISO 4949.

Material	Components	Mixing	Flexural strength (MPa)
Resin-modified glass ionomers	2	Yes	25–60
	3	Yes	65–80
Modified composites	2	Yes	35–40
	1*	No	100–120
Requirements of ISO 9917-2[†]	—	—	20 (minimum)
Requirements of ISO 4049[‡]	—	—	80 (minimum)

* Compomers.
[†] Light-activated water-based cements.
[‡] Resin-based filling materials.

materials must be treated in a similar way to composites in order to achieve an effective bond, i.e. special treatments of the enamel and dentine are required in order to produce effective bonding. To achieve adhesion with the modified composite products they must essentially be treated as composites and bonded using adhesive bonding agents similar to those described in Section 23.8. One system, for example, involves etching both enamel and dentine with 36% aqueous phosphoric acid solution followed by the application of a combined priming/bonding agent containing a phosphate type primer (PENTA). The same system is advocated as a bonding agent for composites (Table 23.3).

25.7 Fluoride release

Fluoride release has been considered a major advantage of the conventional glass ionomers. Various studies have demonstrated reduced levels of demineralization and caries around materials which are able to release fluoride ions *in vitro*. The pattern of fluoride release for conventional glass ionomers indicates a high initial release rate followed by a rapid reduction in the rate of release over time (Fig. 25.2). The relative importance of the 'initial burst' of greater levels of fluoride and the sustained release at a lower level over an extended period has not been fully explored. Furthermore the levels of fluoride release required to produce a therapeutic effect are not known and in the absence of such information it is often assumed that greater levels of release are better, whereas this may not be the case. One factor which may be significant is that fluoride release from

conventional glass ionomers is reversible and when these materials are bathed in an environment containing a high fluoride concentration (e.g. a topically applied fluoride gel) they are capable of taking up fluoride. Following such treatments the fluoride release rate of these cements can be significantly increased as they are able to slowly re-release the freshly absorbed fluoride. It is, therefore, said that conventional glass ionomers can act like a fluoride 'sink' which is capable of releasing fluoride but which can be 'topped up' at regular intervals.

Figure 25.2 shows daily (24 hours) fluoride release of small disc specimens of cements (10 mm diameter by 1.5 mm thick) into 5 ml of water as a function of time. The storage water is refreshed daily throughout the test. The results show that typically the resin-modified glass ionomers behave in a similar fashion to the conventional glass ionomers in terms of both the pattern of release and the daily amount of fluoride released. It is emphasized that results are for 'typical' materials and some considerable variation is seen between commercial materials. Key factors in the rate of fluoride release from resin-modified materials are the extent to which the acid–base reaction occurs during setting and the presence of HEMA, which results in the formation of a polymeric hydrogel through which water can diffuse quite rapidly. The fluoride release behaviour of the modified composite products is somewhat different to that of the other materials (Fig. 25.2). Hence, there is no initial burst, but there is a low and sustained level of fluoride release which typically, after about 40 days, becomes equivalent to that from a conventional glass ionomer. It has never been demonstrated that the modified composite products have any ability to act as a fluoride sink and so it is unlikely that their fluoride levels can be refreshed. The lower level of fluoride release from these products is a function of the limited extent to which any acid–base setting occurs combined with a lower rate of water diffusion through resins which do not contain the hydrophilic monomer HEMA.

25.8 Clinical handling notes

The handling characteristics and clinical techniques used for these materials are different to those for the conventional GICs, not least because they become hard, as a consequence of the visible-light-activated reaction, well before the acid–base reaction is complete.

Matrix techniques are similar to those used for composites with transparent cellulose acetate or polyester strips on proximal surfaces. Again, cervical

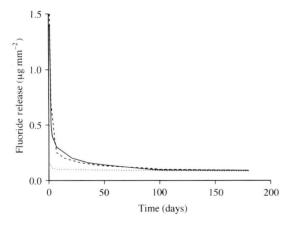

Fig. 25.2 Daily (24 hour) fluoride release over time for typical glass ionomers (solid-line), resin-modified glass ionomers (dashed line) and modified composites (compomer, dotted line).

cavities pose a problem because of the need for transparent matrix to permit light activation. One possibility is to use a small piece of kitchen film (*cling film*) as a physical separator that will allow contouring using hand instruments prior to light activation.

These materials are not as susceptible to desiccation as the chemically setting types and consequently surface finishing can be undertaken immediately after placement.

25.9 Suggested further reading

McCabe J.F. (1997) Resin-modified glass ionomers. *Biomaterials* (in press).

Sidhu, S.K. & Watson, T.F. (1995) Resin-modified glass ionomer materials. A status report for the American Journal of Dentistry. *Am. J. Dent.* **8**, 59.

Shaw, A.J., Carrick, T.E. & McCabe, J.F. (1997) Fluoride release from glass-ionomer and compomer restorative materials : 6 month data. *J. Dent.* (in press).

ISO 9917-2 (1998) Dental water-based cements Part 2 : light activated cements.

Chapter 26
Temporary Crown and Bridge Resins

26.1 Introduction

Temporary crown and bridge resins are used to provide immediate temporary coverage following tooth preparation for crowns or bridges.

The usual technique is to record an initial impression in an alginate material prior to tooth preparation. The major impression may be recorded then or subsequently using an elastomeric impression material. The mixed temporary crown or bridge resin is applied to the prepared areas by placing it into the desired area of the alginate impression which is reseated in the patient's mouth. After initial setting, the impression and the resin are removed and final hardening occurs outside the mouth. Temporary crowns can also be fabricated by placing the resins on to prepared teeth in clear plastic crown formers. In addition, the fit of prefabricated crowns can be improved by relining them with one of the temporary crown and bridge resins.

The temporary crowns and bridges are cemented into place with temporary cements, normally of a zinc oxide – eugenol composition.

26.2 Requirements

The product should ideally be non-injurious to oral tissues since it comes into direct contact with freshly cut dentine and the oral mucosa. During setting, it should not give an unduly large temperature rise whilst in contact with dentine, as this could damage the pulp. It should not undergo a large setting contraction which could make removal of the temporary crown or bridge difficult, particularly if the set material is rigid.

The material should also have convenient setting characteristics, including the following.

(1) Sufficient working time to allow mixing, placement into the impression and seating into the mouth.

(2) After seating in the mouth, rapid attainment of a 'rubbery' stage which facilitates its easy removal without distortion.

(3) Rapid hardening outside the mouth, enabling the trimmed crown or bridge to be cemented into place after a short time.

It should be strong and tough enough to resist fracture and wear in use and should, ideally, be tooth-coloured. Factors which affect durability and appearance are not of prime importance in view of the temporary nature of its use.

26.3 Available materials

Five types of material are available, as outlined in Table 26.1. The auto-cure acrylic material is essentially identical with that discussed on p. 169 as a restorative resin. A dual cure methacrylate material is now available. The liquid contains both chemical and light-sensitive initiators. The material undergoes a chemical setting reaction initially to achieve a partial set, the provisional restoration can be removed from its matrix (and the mouth) at this stage and final setting is achieved by visible light curing either in the mouth or at the chair-side. Care is required as the heat generated during this latter process is substantial.

The higher methacrylate resin is similar in many ways to the product sometimes used as a reline material for dentures and described on p. 108.

The composite material is different from those used as filling materials, which are not suitable for temporary crown and bridgework due to their unfavourable setting characteristics.

26.4 Properties

Setting characteristics: The composite materials have the advantage of exhibiting a distinct rubbery stage,

Table 26.1 Temporary crown and bridge resins.

Type	Dispensation method		Composition
Acrylic	Powder/liquid	Powder Liquid	Polymethylmethacrylate (PMMA) beads + peroxide Methacrylate monomer + activator
Acrylic	Single paste (light activated)		PMMA + monomer + light activators
Higher methacrylate	Powder/liquid	Powder Liquid	Polyethlmethacrylate beads + peroxide Isobutylmethacrylate + activator
Composite	Paste/paste (gun-mix)		Multi-functional methacrylate + fillers + initiators + activators
Composite	Single paste (light activated)		Multi-functional methacrylate + fillers + light activators

during which the temporary crown or bridge can be removed from the patient's mouth without distortion or damage.

This rubbery phase is achieved in the composite material by the use of a multifunctional acrylic monomer which produces a relatively high cross-link density early on in the setting reaction. Normal filling composites do not possess this characteristic and set rapidly to a hard rigid solid.

After removing the provisional crown during its rubbery stage, final setting can be accelerated by immersion in hot water for a few seconds.

The two types of acrylic material do pass through a rubbery stage, when removal is facilitated, but this stage is not as distinct as in the other two products. Automated mixing of provisional crown and bridge resins should enhance their properties by eliminating mixing porosity. The dual-cure composite material once again relies upon its chemical set to give the rubbery stage to facilitate removal of the provisional restoration. Final curing is achieved out of the mouth by visible-light activation.

None of the materials should be allowed to set completely *in situ* since they all undergo a significant setting contraction. This is greatest for the polymethylmethacrylate material where a volumetric shrinkage of about 5% occurs.

Each of the materials exhibits an exothermic reaction on setting, the temperature rise being greatest in the acrylic material. This may have important biological consequences, when a considerable bulk of resin is present, in constructing a large temporary crown or bridge on freshly cut vital dentine. One should ensure that the materials are removed from the patient's mouth well before their maximum temperature rise has occurred. This relies on being able to identify the commencement of the rubbery stage after which the maximum temperature is normally reached within a minute or two.

Biocompatibility: Certain components of some of the products are known to have an irritant effect when placed on freshly cut vital dentine. Methylmethacrylate monomer, for example, present in the acrylic material, falls into this category. When using this product it is necessary to either varnish the preparations or apply a surface layer of petroleum jelly as a protective measure. The isobutylmethacrylate monomer used in the higher methacrylate product is far less irritant than methylmethacrylate.

Mechanical properties: The mechanical properties of the materials become most significant when minimal tooth tissue removal or shoulderless crown preparations are used. There is a danger of fracture occurring in the thin areas at the tapered margin of such a temporary crown. This is most likely in the acrylic material which is weaker and more brittle than the other products.

Appearance: In terms of appearance the acrylic, higher methacrylate and composite materials are all available in a range of shades and a good match with tooth substance can be achieved.

Chapter 27
Requirements of Dental Cements for Lining, Base and Luting Applications

27.1 Introduction

Cements are widely used in dentistry for a variety of applications. Some products are used primarily for *cavity lining* whilst others are primarily used for *luting* applications. Other, more specialist products, are used for sealing root canals as part of a course of *endodontic treatment.*

Some cements are specifically formulated as filling materials. These products are discussed in Chapters 20, 24 and 25. Some of the materials described previously in those chapters are used for a variety of applications and some of the discussion related to their use as fillings will be relevant to other applications of the same or similar products.

27.2 Requirements of cavity lining materials

Certain filling materials are not suitable for placing directly into a freshly prepared cavity. In such circumstances, a layer of cavity lining material is placed in the occlusal floor of the cavity, and on the pulpal axial dentine wall for class II cavities, prior to placement of the filling. The requirements of the cavity lining material chosen for any specific application depend on the *depth of the cavity*, which determines the *thickness of residual dentine* between the base of the cavity and the dental pulp, and the *type of filling material* which is being used to restore the tooth.

The purpose of the cavity lining, or *cavity base*, is to act as a barrier between the filling material and the dentine which, by virtue of the dentinal tubules, has direct access to the sensitive pulp. Depending upon the specific circumstances, the lining may be expected to provide a *thermal, chemical* and *electrical* barrier as illustrated in Fig. 27.1. In addition, the cavity lining or base must have sufficient mechanical strength to resist disruption during the

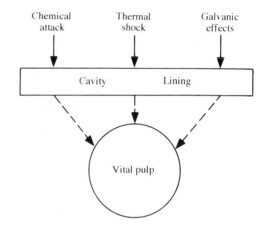

Fig. 27.1 Diagram illustrating the way in which a cavity lining protects the dental pulp.

placement of fillings and provide a firm, rigid base which will adequately support the filling above it.

Thermal barrier

The cavity lining or base is often expected to form a thermally insulating barrier in order to protect the pulp from sudden intolerable changes in temperature. The insulating properties of the cement are characterized by its value of thermal conductivity or thermal diffusivity (see Chapter 2).

A thermally insulating cavity lining is particularly required when a metallic filling, such as amalgam is used. Table 21.5 shows that the thermal diffusivity value for amalgam is about 40 times greater than that for dentine. In deep cavities, having only a thin residual layer of dentine, there is a danger of 'thermal shock' to the pulp when the patient takes hot or cold food. A layer of insulating cavity lining material of sufficient thickness helps to prevent this. Unfortunately this protective effect can be negated if a dentine pin is used to help to provide retention for a metallic restoration. The interface between the pin and the restoration cannot be insulated hence conduction of thermal change can occur rapidly into the tooth. In shallow cavities, where there is a relatively thick layer of residual dentine, it becomes less important to use a lining with thermal insulating properties. Indeed, for amalgam restorations in shallow cavities, the use of a thick layer of cavity lining may reduce the thickness of the overlying amalgam to such an extent that it becomes weakened and liable to fracture. Hence, in such shallow cavities, the base and walls of the cavity can be lined with a *varnish*.

The varnish consists of a solution of a natural or synthetic resin in a volatile solvent. It is painted into the cavity and the solvent evaporates to leave a very thin layer of resin which helps to seal the ends of the dentinal tubules. The varnishes do not provide adequate thermal protection in deep cavities since they form only a thin layer. The resin in the varnish will tend to swell in the presence of water; this may help to establish a marginal seal around an amalgam restoration immediately after its placement.

Another potential cause of thermal injury to the pulp is through the considerable amount of heat liberated by certain filling materials during setting. The acrylic resins, for example, can give a temperature rise of 10°C or more for a small cavity, whilst some light-activated composite materials can show a transient increase of 15°C for an average-sized cavity. Temperature rises of this magnitude may cause injury to the pulp and one function of the cavity lining is to form an insulating barrier against such stimuli.

One complicating factor is that many of the lining cements themselves set by an exothermic reaction.

Chemical barrier

Cavity lining materials may be required to form a protective barrier against potential chemical irritants present in some filling materials. Phosphoric acid in silicate materials, and acrylic monomers in some resin-based materials, are two such potential irritants. The situation may again be complicated if the cement itself contains irritants. Some cements may be suitable for use in shallow to medium depth cavities but totally unsuitable in deep cavities where they may be placed adjacent to the pulp.

Set against these conventional arguments is a gathering wealth of knowledge which suggests that conventional wisdom relating to the effects of some chemicals, particularly acids, on the pulp has been misguided. It is now accepted by most authorities that the dentine and pulp are able to survive contact with quite powerful acids (e.g. 37% phosphoric acid) providing that access to the pulp is effectively sealed at the end of the course of treatment. Hence, creating a chemical barrier is now seen in terms of generating an adhesive bond at the tooth/restorative material interface so that leakage at the margins can be reduced or eliminated.

Electrical barrier

When two dissimilar metals are placed adjacent to or opposing each other (e.g. amalgam/gold) it is possible to set up a galvanic cell which not only accelerates corrosion but can cause pain. The use of an electrically insulating lining material helps to prevent such activity. Unfortunately, most of the lining materials used are either water-based or contain polar organometallic compounds. They are not, therefore, ideal electrical insulators.

Varnishes consisting of less polar resins, such as polystyrene, may be used to provide some electrical resistance. These are sometimes painted onto the surface of metallic restorations giving temporary relief to the symptoms of 'galvanic pain'.

Strength and flow

The vast majority of cavity lining materials are supplied as two components which are mixed together, initiating a setting reaction. The setting characteristics should allow sufficient time for mixing and placing in the cavity followed by rapid setting in order that the filling material can be placed without too much delay.

The lining should remain intact during the placement of the filling material. The integrity of the lining depends on several factors.

(1) The degree of set achieved at the time the filling material is placed.
(2) The strength of the set material and its thickness.
(3) The type of cavity.
(4) The pressure exerted during the placement of the filling material.
(5) The degree of support from surrounding structures.
(6) The choice of correct operative techniques.

When an amalgam restoration is being placed it is important to ensure that the lining is fully set or there is every possibility that the material will undergo considerable flow due to the high pressures used. This is illustrated in Figs. 27.2 for a class I cavity and 27.3 for a class II cavity. It can be seen that in both cases the insulating layer of lining is lost and the amalgam comes into close contact with dentine. For the class II cavity, a further danger is the production of a thin section of amalgam as the lining flows upwards during the packing of the interproximal box (Fig. 27.3a) and is forced further upwards during the filling of the remainder of the cavity (Fig. 27.3b).

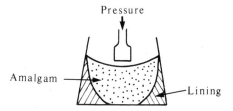

Fig. 27.2 Flow of an unset cement lining caused by the high pressure of condensation.

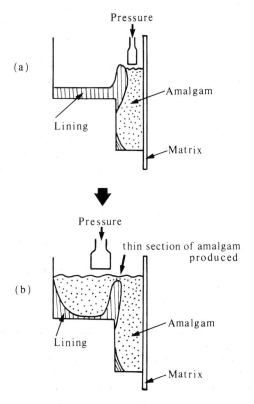

Fig. 27.3 Flow of an unset cement lining in a class II cavity caused by the high pressure of condensation. (a) Whilst filling the box. (b) Whilst filling the occlusal part of the cavity.

If the lining material has set at the time of amalgam condensation there is little chance of flow. The strength of the set material should be sufficient to resist fracture. For class I cavities there is little chance of fracturing a set lining, even though it may have relatively low strength, since it is supported on all sides by a rigid cocoon of tooth substance (Fig. 27.4). For class II cavities the situation is different, as illustrated in Fig. 27.5. The axial wall of lining is unsupported and attempts to condense amalgam directly onto this may cause fracture at the exposed corner. This technique not only destroys the integrity of the lining but may produce an incompletely filled cavity, having voids as shown.

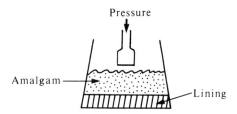

Fig. 27.4 There is little danger of fracturing a cement lining in a class I cavity since it is fully supported by dentine on all sides.

The correct technique is to condense amalgam into the interproximal box first, as shown in Fig. 27.6. This provides support for the lining of the axial wall which can then withstand direct forces.

The placement of other filling materials does not present problems as severe as those encountered with amalgam condensation since much smaller forces are used for adaptation. If the lining material is properly set, there is little chance of flow and fracture is also unlikely at lower pressures.

Radiopacity and compatibility

Cavity linings should, ideally, be radiopaque in order that the dentist can observe them on radiographs, thereby aiding the diagnosis of caries around the filling. A radiolucent lining material may hinder the early detection of such lesions.

Finally, the cavity lining material chosen for any particular application must be compatible with the filling material which is placed above it. The constituents of the lining should not have any effect on the setting characteristics or properties of the filling.

A technique to increase the retention of amalgam restorations using zinc phosphate cement has been

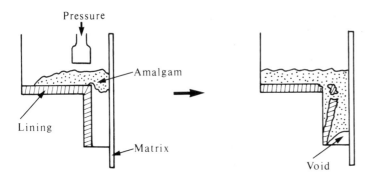

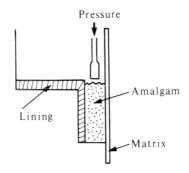

Fig. 27.6 The problem highlighted in Fig. 27.5 is overcome by condensing amalgam into the interproximal box first. This then provides support for the cement lining of the axial wall and the occlusal part of the cavity can be filled without causing fracture.

Fig. 27.5 When condensing amalgam into a class II cavity, the cement lining on the axial wall is most vulnerable to fracture.

described in which a thin lining is placed over the tooth and the amalgam packed immediately, whilst the lining is still fluid. This may result in some 'bonding' of the amalgam to the tooth. This approach has been 'rediscovered' with the advent of materials that can bond to the amalgam and tooth tissue. These materials are either glass-ionomer cements (Chapter 24) or chemically-active methacrylate-based luting agents (Chapter 23). Again, the amalgam is condensed against freshly mixed cement/resin with the deliberate intention of achieving a chemical union between the tooth and the amalgam to assist with the retention and in improving marginal seal.

27.3 Requirements of luting materials

Many dental appliances and restorations are constructed outside the patient's mouth and then fixed into place using a cement luting material. Examples include the fixing of porcelain and metal crowns, bridges, inlays and metal posts.

Many of the requirements of luting materials are

similar to those of cavity lining materials, for example, the material should, ideally, be non-irritant. This requirement is not as critical for luting as for cavity lining since the luting cement is normally applied to a thicker residual layer of dentine than would exist in a deep cavity.

The *setting characteristics* should allow sufficient time for mixing the material, applying to the restoration and/or tooth preparation and for seating the restoration in place in the mouth. The material should, ideally, be of low initial viscosity or be pseudoplastic, to allow flow of the cement lute so that proper seating can occur. If the viscosity of the cement is high at the time of insertion there is a danger of the restoration being incompletely seated. For crowns, a thick layer of cement may be produced at the margins as illustrated in Fig. 27.7. An indication of the ability of a cement to flow during seating is sometimes obtained by measurements of *film thickness*. A given volume of mixed cement is placed on a flat surface and at a predetermined time is compressed under a constant load. The thickness of the film of cement produced gives an indication of the flow during seating of a crown or other restoration.

Luting cements should, ideally, give thermal and electrical *insulation* since many of the restorations commonly cemented to teeth are based on alloys, for example gold crowns.

The *retention* of restorations depends on the correct design and accuracy of the restoration and on the strength of the cement. Figure 27.8 illustrates how the cement enters microscopic interstices on the rough tooth and restoration surface. On setting, the cement gives mechanical resistance to the displacement of the restoration, and must be strong enough to resist fracture when loads are applied to the restoration. Retention may be further improved if the luting cement adheres to the tooth surface and restoration.

The *solubility* of a luting cement should be low because cement margins are often exposed to oral fluids as illustrated in Fig. 27.7. Dissolution or ero-

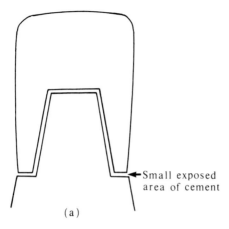

←Small exposed
area of cement

(a)

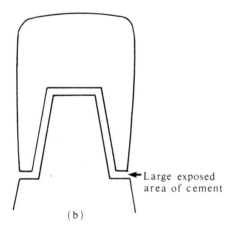

←Large exposed
area of cement

(b)

Fig. 27.7 The thickness of the cement lute may vary according to the viscosity of the cement at the time of seating the restoration. (a) Thin layer of cement. (b) Thicker layer of cement.

sion of the cement may lead to failure by loss of retention or by the initiation of caries in the tooth substance adjacent to the eroded lute.

27.4 Requirements of endodontic cements

Certain forms of treatment require removal of the pulp followed by preparation and disinfection of the root canal. The cleaned canal is then filled using a combination of an inert filler (most commonly gutta percha) and a cement as a sealant. The root canal system is a complex three-dimensional structure and the fluidity of both the filler and the sealant needs to be adequate to flow or to be pressed into such a complex structure. Alternative forms of treatment involve the sealing of the canal with cement sealer

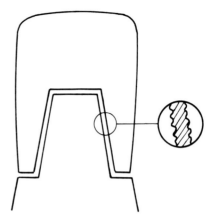

Fig. 27.8 Diagram illustrating how the cement lute gives mechanical retention of the restoration by entering small interstices in the tooth and restoration surface.

alone, but this is not a widely used or recommended procedure.

The requirements of the cement sealer are mainly concerned with its biocompatibility and its ability to resist dissolution and to form a good seal, both along the walls and at the apex of the canal. The material should also be radiopaque in order that the dentist can confirm the attainment of a satisfactory root filling radiographically.

Cements used for sealing root canals must have setting characteristics which enable them to be forced into the warm, moist environment of the root canal before setting. This would not be possible with some conventional cements which set almost instantaneously in the presence of moisture. Hence, specialist products have been developed for endodontic applications; these tend to have a very prolonged working time to allow the procedure to be completed (which may take 20–30 minutes for a multi-rooted tooth) and then for a check radiograph to be taken to ensure that the root filling is satisfactory. If it is not satisfactory then it can be removed immediately if the sealant has not set.

27.5 Requirements of orthodontic cements

Cements are used extensively in orthodontics for attaching bands and brackets. Materials used for this purpose have special requirements which are based on the fact that the brackets and bands must be held securely in place during the course of treatment but must be quite readily removed at the end of treatment without damaging the teeth. Furthermore, after removing the brackets and bands there should ideally be a minimal amount of residual cement attached to the teeth so that only a short time is required for 'clean up'. It would be an added advantage if the cement were able to exert a protective influence on the surrounding tooth substance during treatment as these areas are prone to plaque accumulations and decalcification of the enamel around brackets can be a problem.

The rheological properties of orthodontic cements are important. The mixed cement should have a viscosity which is low enough to enable positioning of the bracket and the creation of a low film thickness of cement. Likewise, it should be possible to make minor adjustments to the position of the bracket before cement setting occurs. Once positioning is complete there should be no drift in the position of the bracket and this will be most easily achieved if the cement has pseudoplastic characteristics or a significant yield stress (Bingham characteristics). Rapid setting (e.g. through light activation) will also help to ensure that the position of the bracket does not change.

In order to create an effective bond between bracket/band and tooth, the bond strength to enamel and to the material of the band or bracket (alloy, ceramic or plastic) must be adequate. The bonding surfaces of bands or brackets are often provided with mechanical undercuts (e.g. in the form of a mesh) or are treated with adhesion promoters (e.g. silane for ceramics), in order to give an adequate bond. Ideally, bond failure should not occur during treatment, but on completion of treatment debonding should occur readily. If debonding occurs at the cement/enamel interface leaving the enamel surface 'clean' a minimal clean up is required. One danger of trying to encourage debonding at the interface is that fracture can occasionally occur partly within the tooth. Fracture within the cement may require some clean up of the enamel but will help to ensure that fracture of the enamel does not occur. Many cements used for orthodontic bonding are of the resin type described in Chapter 23. Acid–base type cements and resin-modified cements are attracting more attention as it is recognized that some of these products are capable of matching the ideal characteristics more closely.

Chapter 28
Cements based on Phosphoric Acid

28.1 Introduction

One group of widely used cements is based on the vigorous reaction which occurs between certain basic oxides and phosphoric acid to form phosphate salts of low solubility. The three products considered in this section are the *zinc phosphate* cements, *silicophosphate* cements and *copper phosphate* cements. The *silicate* filling materials described in Chapter 20 are closely related, having a liquid component which is essentially an aqueous solution of phosphoric acid and a powder which is a glass derived from amphoteric or basic oxides, but these are considered separately due to their different applications.

28.2 Zinc phosphate cements

Composition: These materials are generally supplied as a powder and liquid which are mixed together by hand. Encapsulated products are available but are rarely used due to the extra cost involved. They do, however, give both a greater speed and consistency of mix which has the dual benefits of more reliable performance and an increased working time. This is of particular benefit when using these cements as luting agents.

The composition of powder and liquid in a typical cement are given in Table 28.1. The major reactive component of the powder is zinc oxide. Small quantities of other oxides such as magnesium oxide

may also be present. The liquid is essentially an aqueous solution of phosphoric acid buffered by adding small quantities of zinc oxide or aluminium oxide. These compounds form phosphates which stabilize the pH of the acid and reduce its reactivity.

Setting reaction: On mixing the powder and liquid together a vigorous reaction occurs, resulting in the formation of a relatively insoluble zinc phosphate as follows:

$$3ZnO + 2H_3PO_4 + H_2O \rightarrow Zn_3(PO_4)_2 \cdot 4H_2O$$

Only the surface layers of the zinc oxide particles react, leaving unconsumed cores bound together by the phosphate matrix.

The reaction is rapid and exothermic although its rate is tempered somewhat by the presence of buffers in the acid and a special process of deactivation of the zinc oxide powder involving heating and sintering with other, less reactive, oxides.

Manipulative variables: The powder/liquid ratio depends on the application. For cavity lining a putty-like consistency having a powder/liquid ratio of about 3.5 : 1 is used. For luting, a more fluid mix, with lower powder/liquid ratio, is employed to ensure flow of the cement during seating of the restoration. It is not normal practice to measure the proportions of powder or liquid but rather to assess the suitability of the mix 'by experience'. When proportioning, it is important to remember that lowering the powder/

Table 28.1 Composition of zinc phosphate cements.

Powder	Zinc oxide	Approximately 90% as main active ingredient
	Other metallic oxides	Approximately 10%
Liquid	Aqueous solution of phosphoric acid	50–60% concentration
	$AlPO_4$ $Zn_3(PO_4)_2$	Up to 10% as buffers

liquid ratio produces a weaker, more soluble and more irritant material.

The powder is best incorporated into the liquid in small increments until the desired consistency is reached. This method has the effect of delaying the set slightly and creating more working time, since the concentrations of zinc phosphate produced during the early stages of setting are not sufficient to cause a noticeable increase in viscosity. When all the powder has been incorporated mixing should be quickly discontinued, since continuing to mix after zinc phosphate has started to form can significantly weaken the cement. Mixing is easier if carried out on a cooled glass mixing slab. Care must be taken, however, not to cool the mixing slab below the dew point, since water may condense from the atmosphere into the mix of cement below this temperature. Excess water affects both the setting characteristics and the physical properties of the set material. Proportioning and mixing are greatly simplified by using pre-encapsulated materials. Some products are supplied pre-encapsulated in syringes which enable the mixed material to be syringed into place following mechanical mixing for 5 or 10 seconds.

For hand-mixed powder/liquid systems it is necessary to take precautions over the handling of the liquid. The cap should be removed from the bottle only long enough to dispense sufficient liquid for one mix, and then replaced immediately. If the liquid is left open to the atmosphere for extended periods, water will either be lost or gained depending upon the ambient humidity. Such changes in the water content of the liquid may alter the setting characteristics and physical properties of the material. In a hot, dry atmosphere crystallization of phosphates may be observed on the sides of the bottle as water evaporates. If this occurs the remaining liquid is useless and should be discarded. Only a small change in the water content of the liquid is required to produce a large and unacceptable change in the properties of the cement.

When using the materials for luting, the working time is optimized by adding the cement to the fitting surface of the restoration, which is initially at room temperature, and not to the tooth preparations which are at mouth temperature (37°C). If the cement is added to the tooth preparations first, there is every chance that its viscosity will have increased considerably before the restoration can be seated. In extreme cases the cement may even be completely set. This demonstrates the marked effect of temperature on the rate of reaction for these products. Cast or all-porcelain restorations are usually designed to have a reasonable space between the casting and the preparation for the cement lute (approximately 30–40 μm). This space is generated for castings by painting the surface of the working die with a varnish or *die spacer* which dries in a single coat to give a reliable film thickness. Multiple coats are often required to achieve the desired spacing. The platinum foil achieves the same purpose for porcelain jacket crowns. For those crowns that are made on a refractory die the dental stone model of the prepared tooth is coated in die space before the preparation is replicated. The luting agent should be loaded into/onto the restoration in sufficient quantity to fill this 'defect', but not in gross excess otherwise there may be problems seating the restoration.

Properties: Some of the important properties of zinc phosphate cements, as required in the ISO Standard (ISO 9917), are outlined in Table 28.2.

Providing the materials are manipulated correctly, the phosphate cements have sufficient working time to allow placement of a cavity lining or cement lute before the viscosity has increased markedly. The ISO Standard (ISO 9917) carries no requirement for working time. However, there is a minimum setting time of 2.5 minutes for luting cements and 2 minutes for lining cements which is designed to ensure that there is sufficient working time. The evaluation is

Table 28.2 Requirements of cements as specified in ISO 9917.

Cement	Maximum film thickness* (μm)	Minimum compressive strength (MPa)	Maximum acid erosion (mm/hour)
Zinc phosphate	25	70	1.0
Polycarboxylate	25	70	2.0
Glass ionomer	25	70–130[†]	0.05
Silicophosphate	—	170	0.05

* Requirement for luting cements only.
[†] Lower limit for luting and lining, higher limit for restorations.

made by determining the resistance to penetration of 1 mm diameter probe under a load of 400 g. The material is considered set when it can fully support the loaded probe. At the lower powder/liquid ratio used for luting, the material is sufficiently fluid to allow seating of the restoration and formation of a thin film of lute.

Film thickness, which is an important property for luting cements, is not only controlled by powder/liquid ratio but also by particle size of the zinc oxide powder. Large grains of powder tend to form a thick layer of cement and prevent proper seating of a crown. In order to achieve adequate seating it is important that cements with fine grain zinc oxide powders are used. Such powders have relatively high exposed surface areas and react rapidly with phosphoric acid. Adequate working time is achieved by manufacturers reducing the reactivity of the acid with buffers. Proper material selection and manipulation should result in a cement film thickness of less than 25 µm as required by the ISO Standard. This is determined in the standard by the application of a force of 150 N across two circular glass plates (area 200 mm^2) with a sample of mixed cement sandwiched between them. Another factor which can seriously affect the seating of crowns is an incorrect convergence angle of the axial walls of the prepared tooth. This should ideally be 10° (5° taper on each side); any angle which is considerably smaller than this will make proper seating of the crown difficult due to no fault of the cement.

Initial hardening of the material normally occurs within 4–7 minutes, although the strength continues to increase for some time after that. The ISO Standard requires a maximum setting time of 6 minutes for lining cements and 8 minutes for luting cements. The compressive strength ultimately reaches a value of about 80 MPa for luting cement and 140 MPa for lining material, reflecting the differing powder/liquid ratios used. As seen in Table 28.2, the ISO Standard requirement for compressive strength (at 24 hours) is only 70 MPa and the difference between this and some typical values given above reflects the variation in properties which can be seen when comparing different brands. For lining materials used beneath amalgam restorations, the mechanical properties at between 3 and 6 minutes after placing are important, since this is the time at which amalgam is normally condensed. This time has been reduced over the years by the increased use of mechanically mixed amalgams requiring only a few seconds trituration. At about 5 minutes after placement a typical zinc phosphate lining cement has a compressive strength of only 30 MPa. This value is comparable with the stress used by some practitioners during amalgam condensation with lathe-cut alloys. Obviously the packing pressures required for spherical particle alloys are lower. Fracture of lining is unlikely since it is almost totally constrained in both class I and class II cavities providing a correct technique is used (see Figs 27.5 and 27.6). The materials have generally achieved a sufficient degree of set at 5 minutes to resist flow during amalgam condensation.

The mechanical properties of the cement play a part in determining the retentive properties of a cement luting agent. Phosphate cements are not adhesive to tooth substance or to restorative materials. The cement flows into the myriad of fine undercuts naturally occurring on the fitting surface of the restoration and on the cut tooth surface. The importance of an element of surface roughness on these two surfaces which are to be joined is clear. Polished surfaces are not easily joined by cement luting agents. Tags of set cement, along with a correct design of taper to the preparation, prevent displacement of the restoration. It is important therefore that the tags should resist fracture in function. Experience suggests that phosphate cements are sufficiently strong to resist such fracture. As mentioned earlier, the strength increases with increasing powder/liquid ratio up to a maximum, then reaches a plateau before falling again if insufficient acid is present to bind all the zinc oxide particles together. Maximum strength can only be achieved therefore at high powder/liquid ratios but these cannot be used for luting cements because of the adverse effect on film thickness. As a general rule it follows that the cement should be as thick as practicable for the particular work being carried out.

The set material has a small, though significant, solubility in water and cement lute margins may erode slowly in the mouth by a combination of dissolution and abrasion. The cement lute is, potentially, the weak link of any indirect restoration since it normally joins two resistant materials, for example, gold and enamel or dentine, or porcelain and dentine. Erosion, leading to loss of the cement lute and failure of the restoration, is not, however, a problem particularly associated with zinc phosphate cement. Loss of restorations is more likely to occur due to a poorly retentive design of the preparation. An important consequence of cement lute erosion is that the crevice formed is a potential site for caries development. One problem with evaluating cement erosion and solubility is that it is notoriously difficult to reproduce in laboratory experiments. The simplest of tests for solubility involve suspending discs of cement in water for 24 hours, at which time the weight loss of the cement is recorded. In such a test a phosphate cement would be expected to give a solubility of about 0.1% whereas in a similar test a solubility of around 0.3% would be normal for a silicate cement. It is known, however, that in the clinical situation the relative rankings of solubility for the two cements is reversed. A better indication of solubility and erosion is achieved by testing the materials in acidic media (e.g. pH 2.7 lactate buffer) in the presence of mildly abrasive conditions. The method currently used in the ISO Standard employs the use of impinging jets of buffered lactic acid which can both dissolve material at the surface and at the same time wash away the solubilized material to expose a fresh surface. The maximum values of material loss (Table 28.2) allowed in the standard are determined using this method. It can be seen that whereas the erosion rate is expected to be smaller than that for a polycarboxylate cement it is significantly greater than that for a glass-ionomer cement.

Zinc phosphate cements may have an irritant effect on the dental pulp, particularly when used as cavity lining materials. The pH value of the cement at the time of application to the tooth is between 2 and 4 depending on the particular brand and the powder/liquid ratio. The degree of irritation depends on the depth of the cavity and the thickness of residual dentine. It is necessary to remember that attitudes towards the acid tolerance of the dentine and pulp are changing (Chapters 23, 24 and 27), although many experts still feel that zinc phosphate cements are unsuitable for use as linings in deep cavities unless a sublining of a less irritant material such as calcium hydroxide or zinc oxide/eugenol cement is used (see Fig. 29.3). The powders of zinc phosphate cements often contain small quantities of a fluoride salt. This is thought to leach out from within the set cement and to afford some protection to the surrounding tooth substance. The quantity of fluoride leached is generally much less than that leached from silicate or glass-ionomer cements.

The phosphate materials have adequate thermal insulating properties when used under metallic restorations. The value of thermal conductivity is approximately 1.17 $Wm^{-1}{}^{\circ}C^{-1}$ compared with 0.63 $Wm^{-1}{}^{\circ}C^{-1}$ for dentine and 23 $Wm^{-1}{}^{\circ}C^{-1}$ for dental amalgam. The value of thermal diffusivity does not differ markedly from that of tooth substance. They are not able to form an effective chemical barrier, however, due to their inherent acidity.

The set material is opaque due to a high concentration of unreacted zinc oxide. This may detract from the aesthetic appeal of a porcelain crown having a zinc phosphate lute, particularly if the cement lute margin is visible. Consequently crown margins should be placed within the gingival crevice if they are going to be visible in order to hide any exposed cement lute.

Zinc phosphate cements are widely used for all types of lute applications, and as cavity linings under amalgam fillings.

28.3 Silicophosphate cements

Silicophosphate cements are, essentially, hybrids of zinc phosphate and silicate materials. They are supplied as a powder and liquid. The liquid is an aqueous solution of phosphoric acid, containing buffers, whilst the powder is, essentially, a mixture of zinc oxide and aluminosilicate glass. The setting reaction produces a matrix of zinc and aluminium phosphates enclosing unreacted cores of zinc oxide and glass particles.

As seen in Table 28.2, the silicophosphate cements are stronger and less soluble than the phosphate cements. Their properties are more akin to those of the silicates (Chapter 20). The aluminosilicate glass particles also contain a significant amount of fluoride. The leaching of fluoride ions imparts a significant anticariogenic influence on the surrounding tooth substance.

These materials are used, primarily, as temporary filling materials.

28.4 Copper cements

These materials are closely related to the zinc phosphate cements. They are supplied as a powder and liquid. The liquid is an aqueous solution of phosphoric acid whilst the powder is a mixture of zinc oxide and black copper oxide. The setting reaction is similar to that for zinc phosphate materials.

The two properties which distinguish these products from simple zinc phosphate materials are their black appearance and their bactericidal effects, produced by the presence of copper.

The materials are not widely used nowadays, although they can be used as filling materials in deciduous teeth where it has not been possible to remove all caries. Their durability is not good but they are capable of preserving such teeth until they exfoliate. Another application is the cementation of orthodontic appliances, although they have been largely superseded by other materials for the latter application. Finally they can be used for the cementation of cast silver cap splints that are used occasionally during the management of facial fractures.

28.5 Suggested further reading

Going, R.E. & Mitchem, J.C. (1975) Cements for permanent luting: a summarizing review. *J. Am. Dent. Assoc.* **91**, 107.

Øilo, G. (1991) Luting cements: a review and comparison. *Int. Dent. J.* **41**, 81.

Chapter 29

Cements based on Organometallic Chelate Compounds

29.1 Introduction

Many cements used in dentistry can be characterized by setting reactions which involve the formation of chelate compounds between zinc ions and *ortho*-disubstituted aromatic compounds. Three types of aromatic compound are commonly used, delineating the three groups of materials.

(1) Zinc oxide/eugenol cements.
(2) *Ortho*-ethoxybenzoic acid (EBA) cements.
(3) Calcium hydroxide cements, in which the aromatic ligands are silicylates.

29.2 Zinc oxide/eugenol cements

Composition and setting: These products may be supplied as a powder and liquid or as two pastes. The composition of a typical powder/liquid material is given in Table 29.1. The small quantity of zinc acetate in the powder acts as an accelerator by helping to create an ionic medium in which the setting reaction can occur. Some commercial products contain hydrogenated rosin or polystyrene and are known as *resin-reinforced* zinc oxide/eugenol cements. The relative proportions of powder and liquid are not normally measured accurately,

although some manufacturers provide a scoop which gives a known volume of powder to which a given number of drops of liquid are added. Thin mixes, having a low powder/liquid ratio, should be avoided since they produce inferior properties – lower strength and higher solubility. The past/paste materials are similar to the impression pastes described on p. 130. These have the advantage of easier proportioning and mixing.

The setting reaction involves chelation of two eugenol molecules (see Fig. 17.2) with one zinc ion to form zinc eugenolate (see Fig. 17.3). This reaction proceeds very slowly in the absence of moisture. When the mixed material contacts water, however, setting is often completed within a few seconds.

Properties: The setting characteristics of the zinc oxide/eugenol cements are, to some extent, ideal. They offer a combination of adequate working time, during which very little increase in viscosity occurs, coupled with rapid setting after placing into the cavity. The latter is caused by residual moisture in the cavity and the higher temperature of the mouth compared to room temperature. The effect of cavity moisture is noteworthy, particularly since efforts are generally made to dry the cavity before placement of a lining. Only very small amounts of water are required to cause the accelerating effect.

The ultimate compressive strength values for the zinc oxide/eugenol cements are somewhat lower than those recorded for zinc phosphate materials, typically 20 MPa for unreinforced materials and 40 MPa for reinforced materials. The nature of the setting reaction is such, however, that the materials develop their strength rapidly and the reinforced materials in particular are unlikely to flow or fracture during amalgam condensation, providing correct technique is used.

Zinc oxide/eugenol cements may be used as linings

Table 29.1 Composition of zinc oxide/eugenol cements.

	Component	Function
Powder	Zinc oxide	Primary reactive ingredient
	Zinc acetate (1–5%)	Accelerator
Liquid	Eugenol	Primary reactive ingredient
	Olive oil (5–15%)	To control viscosity

in deep cavities without causing harm to the pulp. Unconsumed eugenol is able to leach from the set material and although this substance has been shown to be irritant under certain conditions, it appears to have an obtundant effect on the pulp. The free eugenol is also bacteriocidal which helps to minimize the effects of bacterial ingress and the production of exotoxins causing pulpal damage as a consequence of microleakage.

The ease with which eugenol can gain egress from the material is responsible for its relatively high solubility. Leached eugenol is replaced by water which, under certain conditions, can cause hydrolysis of the zinc eugenolate and disintegration of the cement structure. The materials are, therefore, not suitable for luting applications except on a temporary basis.

Free eugenol may also have an effect on resin-based filling materials, interfering with the polymerization process and sometimes causing discoloration. Clinically this can also result in softening of the surface of the composite. In addition there can be problems with resin-based adhesive luting systems that are being used increasingly, if a provisional restoration is luted using a zinc oxide eugenol temporary cement.

The materials form an effective thermal barrier under metallic restorations having a value of thermal diffusivity similar to that for dentine.

The main uses of these cements are for linings under amalgam restorations, either used alone or as a sublining overlaid with a zinc phosphate material. They are also used as temporary luting cements and as temporary filling materials.

Root-canal pastes: These pastes, used alone or in combination with gutta-percha or a silver point, are often modifications of zinc oxide/eugenol cavity lining materials. They contain additives, such as barium sulphate or bismuth trioxide which render the materials radiopaque, and small quantities of water-absorbing compounds which effectively increase the working times of the materials under moist conditions. Some materials contain therapeutic agents such as anti-inflammatory drugs and disinfectants. *Para*-formaldehyde has been used as a disinfectant in some products, the utilization of which has been criticized because of the highly irritant effect which this substance can have on periapical tissues if the root filling inadvertently goes beyond the apex.

Reinforced zinc oxide–eugenol cements are being used increasingly to provide the retrograde seal during surgical endodontics. Traditionally amalgam has been used in this role, but concerns have been expressed about the advisability of implanting a toxic material containing free mercury within the tissues.

29.3 *Ortho*-ethoxybenzoic acid (EBA) cements

Composition: These cements are generally supplied as a powder and liquid. The composition of a typical material is given in Table 29.2. The ratio of *o*-ethoxybenzoic acid to eugenol in the liquid may vary from one product to another but is usually about 2 : 1. The structural formula of *o*-ethoxybenzoic acid is given in Fig. 29.1. Comparison with Fig. 17.2 shows the similarity between the structure of *o*-ethoxybenzoic acid and eugenol. Both compounds are able to form chelate compounds with zinc ions.

Table 29.2 Composition of an *ortho*-ethoxybenzoic acid (EBA) cement.

	Component	Function
Powder	Zinc oxide (approximately 60%)	Primary reactive ingredient
	Quartz (approximately 35%) Hydrogenated rosin (approximately 5%)	Reinforcing agents
Liquid	0-Ethoxybenzoic acid Eugenol	Reactive ingredients

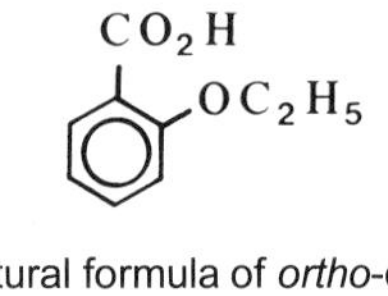

Fig. 29.1   Structural formula of *ortho*-ethoxybenzoic acid.

The structural formula for zinc eugenolate is shown in Fig. 17.3. The structure of zinc *o*-ethoxybenzoate is very similar.

Properties and applications: The setting characteristics are similar to those of the zinc oxide/eugenol materials and are similarly affected by moisture. It is possible to achieve a higher powder/liquid ratio with these products since much of the powder consists of inert, reinforcing filler.

The set material is significantly stronger than even the reinforced zinc oxide/eugenol products due to the high powder/liquid ratio and the presence of fillers. A typical commercial product has an ultimate compressive strength of around 85 MPa. In addition, the lower level of residual eugenol, coupled with a greater resistance to hydrolysis of the zinc *o*-ethoxybenzoate, produces a cement with lower solubility than that observed for zinc oxide/eugenol products. Thermal characteristics are similar to those of the zinc oxide/eugenol materials.

The materials form a suitable cavity lining for amalgam condensation due to their adequate strength and resistance to flow, although they are primarily used as luting cements.

29.4 Calcium hydroxide cements

Composition: Some calcium hydroxide preparations consist simply of a suspension of calcium hydroxide in water. This is applied to the base of the cavity and dries out to give a layer of calcium hydroxide. These materials are both difficult to manipulate and form a very friable cavity lining which is easily fractured. A solution of methyl cellulose in water or of a synthetic polymer in a volatile organic solvent can be used instead of water. These additives produce a more cohesive cement but the compressive strength remains very low at about 8 MPa. This is well below the value of strength required to withstand amalgam condensation and when this filling material is to be used the calcium hydroxide preparation must be overlaid with a layer of a stronger cement. Most calcium hydroxide products in current use are supplied in the form of two components, normally pastes, which set following mixing to form a more substantial cavity lining. The composition of a typical commercial product is given in Table 29.3.

The structural formula of butylene glycol disalicylate, a glycol salicylate commonly used in one of the pastes, is given in Fig. 29.2. This is a difunctional

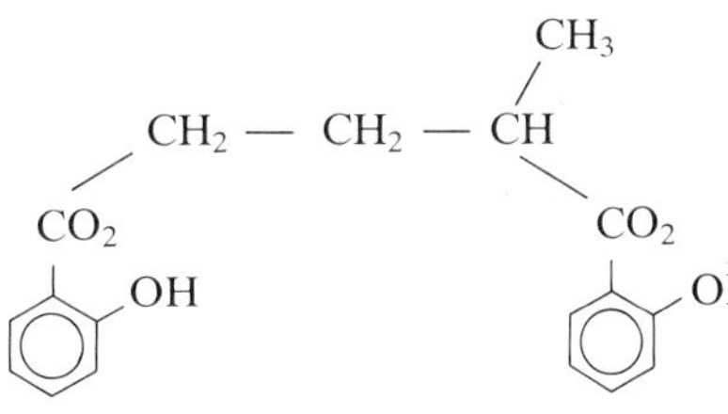

Fig. 29.2 Structural formula of butylene glycol disalicylate.

chelating agent having two aromatic groups with reactive groups in *ortho* positions. On mixing this with a paste containing zinc oxide and calcium hydroxide, chelate compounds with structures similar to that shown in Fig. 17.3 are formed. It is thought that zinc ions are primarily responsible for chelation, with calcium being largely unreacted.

The sulphonamide compound used in the zinc oxide/calcium hydroxide paste is present merely as a carrier and is not thought to have any therapeutic effect.

Some cements contain paraffinic oils instead of sulphonamides. These cements are more hydrophobic and release their calcium hydroxide more slowly. This may have an adverse effect on the antibacterial properties of the cement.

Light-activated calcium hydroxide cements are available. They carry brand names which suggest that they are chemically similar to the two-paste products. They are, however, based on a totally different setting reaction involving light-activated polymerization of a modified methacrylate monomer of the type used in resin based filling materials (see Chapter 22). A typical material contains dimethacrylate (e.g. Bis GMA) hydroxyethylmethacrylate (HEMA), polymerization activators and calcium hydroxide. The purpose of the HEMA is to produce a relatively hydrophilic polymer which can absorb water and release calcium hydroxide to create an alkaline environment.

Properties: The mixed materials have very low viscosity and setting can be relatively slow for some products. Moisture has a dramatic effect on the rate of setting however, and the materials set within a few seconds of being placed in the cavity, even when the cavity has been 'dried'. Setting of the light-activated materials is more under the control of the operator and residual moisture in the cavity does not have the same influence on setting time. An exposure to activating light for only a few seconds is required to activate polymerization of the thin layer of cement.

Table 29.3 Composition of a typical calcium hydroxide cement.

	Component	Function
Paste 1	Calcium hydroxide (50%)	Primary reactive
	Zinc oxide (10%)	ingredients
	Zinc stearate (0.5%)	Accelerator
	Ethyl toluene sulphonamide (39.5%)	Oil compound, acts as carrier
Paste 2	Glycol salicylate (40%)	Primary reactive ingredient
	Titanium dioxide	Inert fillers,
	Calcium sulphate	pigments and
	Calcium tungstate	radiopacifiers

One characteristic of these cements which has been largely ignored is the relatively high temperature rise produced on setting. This results from the heating effect of the light source and the exothermic setting reaction.

The set material is relatively weak compared to other cements, having a compressive strength of about 20 MPa. This strength is gained rapidly, however, and under the constrained conditions of a cavity the material is able to resist flow and fracture during amalgam condensation, providing correct technique is used. The light-activated materials in which the set material has a cross-linked resin matrix are less brittle than the two paste products.

The consistency of the materials makes them difficult to apply to cavities in thick section. In deep cavities, therefore, a commonly used technique is to apply a thin sublining of a calcium hydroxide cement and then to build up the base of the cavity with a zinc phosphate material prior to amalgam condensation, as illustrated in Fig. 29.3.

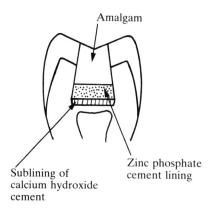

Amalgam

Sublining of calcium hydroxide cement

Zinc phosphate cement lining

Fig. 29.3 Diagram showing the use of a calcium hydroxide cement as a sublining beneath a zinc phosphate cement.

The set materials have a relatively high solubility in aqueous media. Calcium hydroxide is readily leached out, generating an alkaline environment in the area surrounding the cement. This is thought to be responsible for the proven antibacterial properties of these materials. This characteristic is utilized in very deep carious lesions, sometimes involving exposure of the pulp, or occasionally in cases of traumatic exposure of the pulp during cavity preparation. The calcium hydroxide cement is used as a *pulp capping* agent in such situations. It is sufficiently biocompatible to be placed adjacent to the pulp and capable of destroying any remaining bacteria. The material is also able to initiate calcification and for-

mation of a secondary dentine layer at the base of the cavity. This calcification process is a product of irritation of the pulp tissues by the cement, possibly mediated by the activation of TGFβ, a cellular growth factor. Calcium from the cement does not become bound into the mineralized tissues of the calcific barrier/secondary dentine. In pulp capping procedures the calcium hydroxide material is generally overlaid with a strong cement base material such as zinc phosphate cement before completing the restoration of the tooth with amalgam.

The resin-based calcium hydroxide materials are far less soluble than the conventional products. This is advantageous providing that the rate of calcium hydroxide release remains great enough to maintain the antibacterial and dentine regeneration properties of the material. One problem with the resin-based materials is that the unreacted methacrylate groups can become attached to a freshly placed composite resin restoration. The composite shrinks during its setting reaction and this can pull the calcium hydroxide material away from the tooth, leaving a void.

Calcium hydroxide cements are routinely used as lining materials beneath silicate and resin-based filling materials. Unlike the eugenol-containing cements they have no adverse effect on these filling materials and form an effective chemical barrier against acids and monomers.

The need for a lining material beneath a composite is controversial. As stated previously, some authorities would suggest that with modern dentine adhesives there is no need for a lining as the cavity margins are sealed by the adhesive, making microleakage unlikely. Obviously any lining that is placed will act as a barrier between the bonding agent and the dentine, reducing the potential area available for bonding. Indeed, it has been suggested that even exposed pulps can simply be etched and then coated with a resin adhesive to give a primary seal.

The converse of this argument is that pulp perfusion studies (a technique whereby fluid is pumped into the pulp chamber at physiological pressures during *in vitro* microleakage studies to mimic the effects of dentinal tubule fluid flow) have failed to demonstrate complete sealing of the dentine tubules, even under ideal laboratory conditions (i.e. despite bonding composite to a cut dentine surface there is continued egress of fluid from the pulp measured by monitoring fluid flow into the pulp chamber). This suggests that some of the tubules remain patent and hence the potential for microleakage remains.

At the time of writing the consensus view is

- That exposed pulps should be capped with a proprietary calcium hydroxide material before attempting to bond composite to the adjacent dentine.
- That where the dentine at the base of the cavity is superficial (judged to be some distance from the pulp) then a lining is *not* required beneath an adhesive restoration.
- That where a cavity is very deep and the dentine at the base of the cavity is judged to be 'close to the pulp', then it may be prudent to place a lining over that area alone.

This final point gives problems clinically as it can only be based on a dentist's subjective assessment of the depth of the cavity. This judgement is based on experience. Unfortunately the only way of validating the assessment would be to cut through the dentine until the pulp was exposed, which would be ethically unacceptable.

Calcium hydroxide preparations, similar to those used for cavity lining and pulp capping but containing retarders, are now available as root-canal sealing pastes. The retarders are required to extend the working times of the materials whilst they are being manipulated in the warm, humid environment of the root canal. The advantage of the calcium hydroxide products over some of the alternative pastes is that they have effective antibacterial properties without being irritant to apical tissues.

Non-setting calcium hydroxide pastes are also widely used during root-canal therapy either as a dressing for the canal between visits or as a temporary root filling when managing problems with teeth in very young patients. Teeth erupt into the mouth before the end of the root is fully formed. If such a tooth with an 'open apex' requires a root filling it is very difficult to achieve an adequate apical seal due to the canal morphology. However, if non-setting calcium hydroxide is packed into the canal then often apical development will continue providing there is no infection. The mechanism for this is probably similar to that outlined above for dentine bridge formation. Once this process is complete (apexification) then a conventional condensed gutta percha root filling can be placed.

The high solubility and low strength of the calcium hydroxide cements render them unsuitable for luting purposes.

29.5 Suggested further reading

Fisher, F.J. (1977) The effect of three proprietary lining materials on micro-organisms in carious dentine. *Br. Dent. J.* **143**, 231.

Milosevic, A. (1991) Calcium hydroxide in restorative dentistry. *J. Dent.* **19**, 3.

Chapter 30

Polycarboxylates, Glass Ionomers and Resin-modified Glass Ionomers for Luting and Lining

30.1 Introduction

Before reading this chapter, the attention of the reader is drawn to Chapters 24 and 25. Here, the glass ionomers and resin-modified glass ionomers used for restorative purposes are discussed in some detail. Much of the information given in these previous chapters is relevant to our discussion of luting and lining cements.

Two types of cement based on polyacids are in common use for both luting and cavity lining applications. The first products to be developed were the *polycarboxylate* cements which rely on the reaction between zinc oxide and a polyacid. The second group of products are described as *glass ionomer* or *polyalkenoate* cements. The setting reaction takes place between a polyacid molecule and cations released from an ion-leachable glass.

A new family of cements has been developed by producing cements which have a nature which lies somewhere between that of the purely salt matrix glass ionomers and that of the purely resin matrix composite systems. These newer cements may be viewed as hybrids of the two parent groups from which they are derived.

30.2 Polycarboxylate cements

These materials may be supplied as a powder and liquid or as a powder which is mixed with water. For powder/liquid materials, the powder is finely ground zinc oxide which sometimes contains minor quantities of other oxides such as magnesium oxide. The liquid is an aqueous solution of polyacrylic acid of about 40% concentration. In the powder/water materials the powder contains zinc oxide and freeze-dried polyacrylic acid. On mixing the powder with water, the polyacrylic acid dissolves and starts to react with zinc oxide. The setting reaction is similar to that reported in Chapter 24 for glass ionomers. Zinc oxide behaves as a basic oxide and undergoes an acid–base reaction with acid groups in the polyacid to form a reaction product which consists of cores of unreacted zinc oxide bound together by a

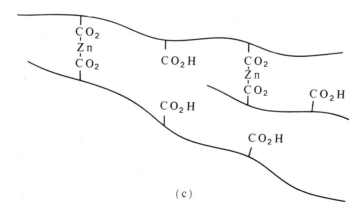

(c)

Fig. 30.1 Simplified structural formula of polyacrylic acid chains cross-linked with zinc ions.

salt matrix in which polyacrylic acid chains are cross-linked through divalent zinc ions (Fig. 30.1). Many recently developed products contain fluoride salts which may exert an anticariogenic effect on surrounding tooth substance.

The cements have sufficiently early strength to resist amalgam condensation and, allowing for product variations, have an ultimate compressive strength of about 80 MPa, a similar value to that recorded for the EBA materials.

The polycarboxylate materials are acidic, though not as irritant as phosphate cements, for two reasons. Polyacrylic acid is a weaker acid than phosphoric acid and the polyacid chains are too large and lack the mobility required to penetrate dentinal tubules. Despite the more biocompatible nature of these materials they are not widely used as linings in very deep cavities unless a sublining of a calcium hydroxide or zinc oxide/eugenol material is used. One reason for this is that they are difficult to handle well in a clinical setting. They tend to be rubbery during their setting reaction and they also adhere to stainless steel instruments, making their placement complex.

Laboratory tests show that the solubility values of polycarboxylate cements are greater than those for the zinc phosphate, silicophosphate and glass ionomer materials (Table 28.1). Despite this apparent disadvantage, the materials are widely used for luting without appearing to display an unduly high failure rate.

The materials form an adhesive bond with enamel and dentine but only a weak bond with gold and no perceptible bond with porcelain. Hence, the adhesive nature of the materials when used for the luting of gold or porcelain crowns is only utilized to a limited degree and cannot be considered an overwhelming advantage for such applications. They will, however, bond to non-precious metal alloys that are being used increasingly for porcelain fused-to-metal crowns. The materials form a strong bond with stainless steel which makes them useful for attaching orthodontic bands. Care must be taken when using steel instruments for mixing and placing. Excess material should be removed from such instruments before it sets, otherwise a tenacious bond will form.

As for most other cements, strength and solubility are optimized by achieving a high powder/liquid ratio. For polycarboxylate materials however, two restricting factors should be remembered. First, some free polyacid is required to form an adhesive bond and this will not be possible if a very dry mix is used. Secondly, a relatively low viscosity is required to allow seating of restorations during luting.

The set materials are opaque due to a high concentration of unreacted zinc oxided cores. This may detract from the appearance of porcelain crowns, particularly if the cement lute margin is visible.

The materials are primarily used as luting cements for attaching crowns, bridges and inlays or as cavity base materials. The adhesive properties of the materials are occasionally utilized for the attachment of *orthodontic bands*, since the material forms a strong bond with stainless steel as well as with enamel and dentine.

30.3 Glass ionomer cements

The use of glass-ionomer cements as adhesive restorative materials is discussed in Chapter 24. The cavity lining and luting cements are of broadly similar composition to that given in Table 24.1. One difference is that the luting and cavity lining cements contain glass of smaller particle size to allow the formation of a thinner film thickness during luting. Powder/liquid and powder/water materials are both available and widely used.

The set materials are stronger than the polycarboxylate products having a compressive strength value of about 130 MPa, although there may be wide variations from one product to another. The materials can withstand amalgam condensation and are occasionally used as cavity linings for amalgam restorations. Their biological properties are akin to those of the polycarboxylate cements which are covered in the previous section. Although they are considered relatively bland they are rarely used as linings in very deep cavities. The glass ionomer cements are now widely advocated as lining materials beneath posterior composite filling materials. They are claimed to give more rigid support than the calcium hydroxide cements. Their success in this situation has been further enhanced by the introduction of radiopaque glass ionomer cements containing either barium salts or metallic silver as the radiopacifying agents. Materials containing silver are grey in colour and may detract from the appearance of the composite restoration, although this is not very noticeable in molar and premolar teeth. Specialized techniques in which glass ionomers are used to form an adhesive 'sandwich' between dentine and restorative resins are described in Chapter 24.

The glass ionomer cements are less soluble than the polycarboxylates, and most of the other cement products, when measured under ideal laboratory conditions. The solubility can be adversely affected by early moisture contamination, however, as discussed in Chapter 24 for the glass ionomer filling materials. It is essential that cement lute margins are covered with a layer of a protective varnish immediately after seating the restoration. This can often be a difficult procedure, particularly if the margins lie subgingivally. Although the glass ionomers are theoretically capable of producing an insoluble cement lute this ideal may not be as easy to achieve in practice. There have been reports of pulpal damage associated with the use of some glass ionomer cement luting agents, particularly those based on poly(acrylic/maleic) acid as opposed to poly(-acrylic) acid alone. It is thought that the acrylic/maleic copolymers maintain a low pH for a relatively long time after mixing. Associated with the solubility of the cements is a slow and maintained release of fluoride which may help to protect adjacent tooth substance from attack by the acids of plaque.

The materials display the same adhesive properties as the polycarboxylates and are more translucent due to the presence of unreacted cores of glass rather than zinc oxide. The extra translucency is considered an advantage for luting porcelain crowns, although further improvements in appearance are required if the cement is to be truly able to match porcelain.

Glass ionomer cements are now widely used in orthodontics for the attachment of bands. The adhesive seal between the cement and tooth enamel, coupled with fluoride release, helps to maintain the banded teeth in good condition throughout a course of treatment. Several trials have been performed to evaluate the use of glass ionomers for bonding orthodontic brackets. It is felt that they could theoretically provide the ideal characteristics of a cement for this purpose, i.e. adequate bonding to ensure that debonding does not occur during treatment, coupled with easy debonding and rapid clean up of the teeth after treatment, combined with the benefits of fluoride release. In practice, however, the cements have not proved suitable for bonding brackets due to the unacceptable rate of debonding during treatment.

30.4 Resin-modified glass ionomers and compomers

In Chapter 25 the potential benefits of incorporating a significant resin component in a glass ionomer are explained. A new family of restorative materials has grown out of these findings. For each restorative material the manufacturers invariably produce a similar material for lining and/or luting purposes. Just as for those products described previously in Chapter 25, the materials available have a composition which lies on a continuum between the 'true' glass ionomers and the resin–matrix composites. Hence, some are adequately described as resin-modified glass ionomers whilst the term acid-modified composite better describes other products.

Whereas most restorative cements have a light-activated polymerization setting reaction as an important part of the setting procedure, the lining and luting cements may be chemically activated. In this case the material is likely to be provided as a powder and liquid containing the necessary monomers and polymerization initiators/activators. Setting begins when the components are mixed. The main advantages of resin-containing materials compared with conventional acid–base cements is that they are less soluble and less brittle. Many of the other potential benefits are outlined in Chapter 25. One disadvantage of their use relates to their bond to enamel and dentine. This is thought to be mediated through the acid–base setting reaction, which is relatively slow. Unfortunately the materials can be made hard by light activation before the bond has fully formed. If left undisturbed the bond would continue to form, but if a composite is placed over the base material it will bond well to the resin component of the cement and its contraction towards the curing light will place the bond interface between the cement and dentine under high stress before this bond has formed fully. This could result in disruption of this interface.

30.5 Suggested further reading

Millett, D.T. & McCabe, J.F. (1996) Orthodontic bonding with glass ionomer cement – a review. *Eur. J. Orth.* **18**, 385

Øilo, G. (1991) Luting cement: a review and comparison. *Int. Dent. J.* **41**, 8.

Index